ALSO BY NICK BERTOZZI

Lewis & Clark (2011)

The Salon (2007)

AS ILLUSTRATOR

Houdini: The Handcuff King (2007), with Jason Lutes

Stuffed! (2009), with Glenn Eichler

Jerusalem: A Family Portrait (2013), with Boaz Yakin

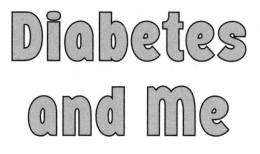

Diabetes and Me

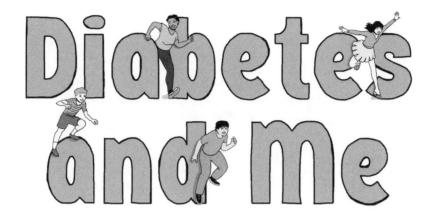

Diabetes and Me

AN ESSENTIAL GUIDE
FOR KIDS AND PARENTS

TEXT BY
KIM CHALONER

ILLUSTRATED BY
NICK BERTOZZI

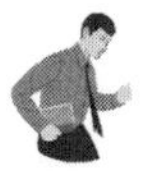

A Novel Graphic from Hill and Wang
A division of Farrar, Straus and Giroux
New York

Hill and Wang
A division of Farrar, Straus and Giroux
18 West 18th Street, New York 10011

Printed in the United States of America
Published simultaneously in hardcover and paperback
First edition, 2013

Library of Congress Cataloging-in-Publication Data
Chaloner, Kim, 1970–
Diabetes and me : an essential guide for kids and parents / written by Kim Chaloner & illustrated by Nick Bertozzi. — First edition.
pages cm
Includes bibliographical references.
ISBN 978-0-8090-2819-1 (hardcover) — ISBN 978-0-8090-3871-8 (pbk.) — ISBN 978-1-4668-4848-1 (ebook)
1. Diabetes in children—Juvenile literature. I. Bertozzi, Nick. II. Title.

RJ420.D5 C42 2013
618.92'4624—dc23

2012036543

Designed by Nick Bertozzi

Hill and Wang books may be purchased for educational, business, or promotional use. For information on bulk purchases, please contact the Macmillan Corporate and Premium Sales Department at 1-800-221-7945, extension 5442, or write to specialmarkets@macmillan.com.

www.fsgbooks.com
www.twitter.com/fsgbooks · www.facebook.com/fsgbooks

1 3 5 7 9 10 8 6 4 2

The information in this book is not intended to replace the advice of the reader's own physician or other medical professional. You should consult a medical professional in matters relating to health, diet, and nutrition, especially if you have existing medical conditions, and before starting, stopping, or changing the dose of any medication you are taking or adopting any nutritional changes based on information contained in this book. Individual readers are solely responsible for their own health care decisions. The author and the publisher do not accept responsibility for any adverse effects individuals may claim to experience, whether directly or indirectly, from the information contained in this book.

The fact that an organization or website is mentioned in this book as a potential source of information does not mean that the author or the publisher endorse any of the information they may provide or recommendations they may make. The stories in this book are composite fictional accounts based on the experiences of many individuals. Similarities to any real person or persons are coincidental and unintentional.

For Christian Blake Chaloner

CONTENTS

PREFACE

When I was diagnosed with Type 1 diabetes at the age of 16, I was already familiar with blood testing, endocrinologists, and preparing for low blood sugar reactions because my younger brother had been diagnosed when he was 7. Back then, I had a little window into diabetes: the whole family went through a typical education program, back when urine testing and refined pork insulin were still a regular part of treatment, and families practiced giving injections by piercing hapless oranges with syringes filled with water. My brother spent many hours learning how to care for his diabetes as well, time he would rather have spent drawing Spider-Man and playing baseball. Little did I know that I would be in his shoes just eight years later. Once diagnosed, I realized that injecting a few oranges with water in order to better understand my brother's routine was only the tip of the iceberg.

Now diabetes is just one part of the mosaic of my life. I am a science teacher, the mother of two daughters, an author, an environmentalist, a school dean, and an avid traveler. I am able to do things today that I never thought would be possible when I was first diagnosed. The landscape for diabetics has changed dramatically since my brother was 7. New technologies and more precise forms of treatment are making this disease more manageable and, in some surprising ways, actually fun to learn how to handle.

Yet with all of this in mind, diabetes is a disease that asks a lot of you, every day. Learning to successfully manage blood sugar is no cakewalk. I'm happy to be a healthy member of the diabetes community, but like other diabetics, I sometimes feel like managing this disease is a full-time job. Without the support of friends and family, it would be impossible. I will be forever grateful for the empathy and kindness my brother showed me. As we grew up together, he continued to teach me, through his attention, care, and advice, that an involved family is an important part of living with diabetes.

When friends suggested that my husband and I write and illustrate a graphic guide to diabetes for newly diagnosed kids, I thought about how much my brother and I would have preferred to approach the mountain of information we both had to learn in a format that made the task less intimidating. I hope that this guide offers kids (as well as the adults in their lives) an entry point to a disease that connects so many of us, and that it sparks conversations as well.

Our intent is to help diabetics and families of diabetics learn how to create healthy routines, explore new and delicious food choices, establish regular exercise as a part of their lives, and develop resilience when it comes to the ups and downs all diabetics encounter. I also hope that the guide encourages further research into diabetes causes and cures.

—Kim Chaloner

Diabetes and Me

PART ONE: WHAT IS DIABETES?

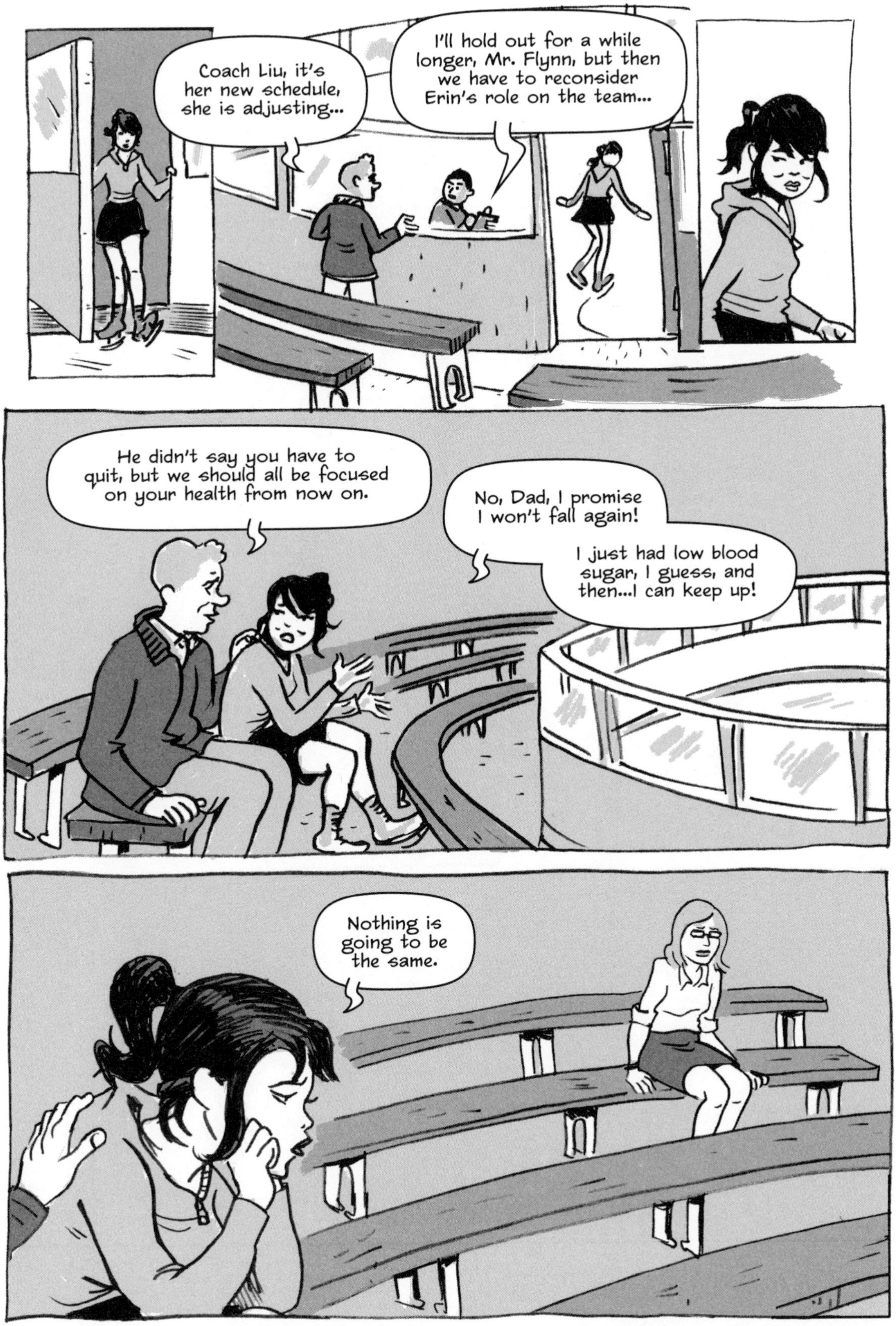
Coach Liu, it's her new schedule, she is adjusting...
I'll hold out for a while longer, Mr. Flynn, but then we have to reconsider Erin's role on the team...
He didn't say you have to quit, but we should all be focused on your health from now on.
No, Dad, I promise I won't fall again!
I just had low blood sugar, I guess, and then...I can keep up!
Nothing is going to be the same.

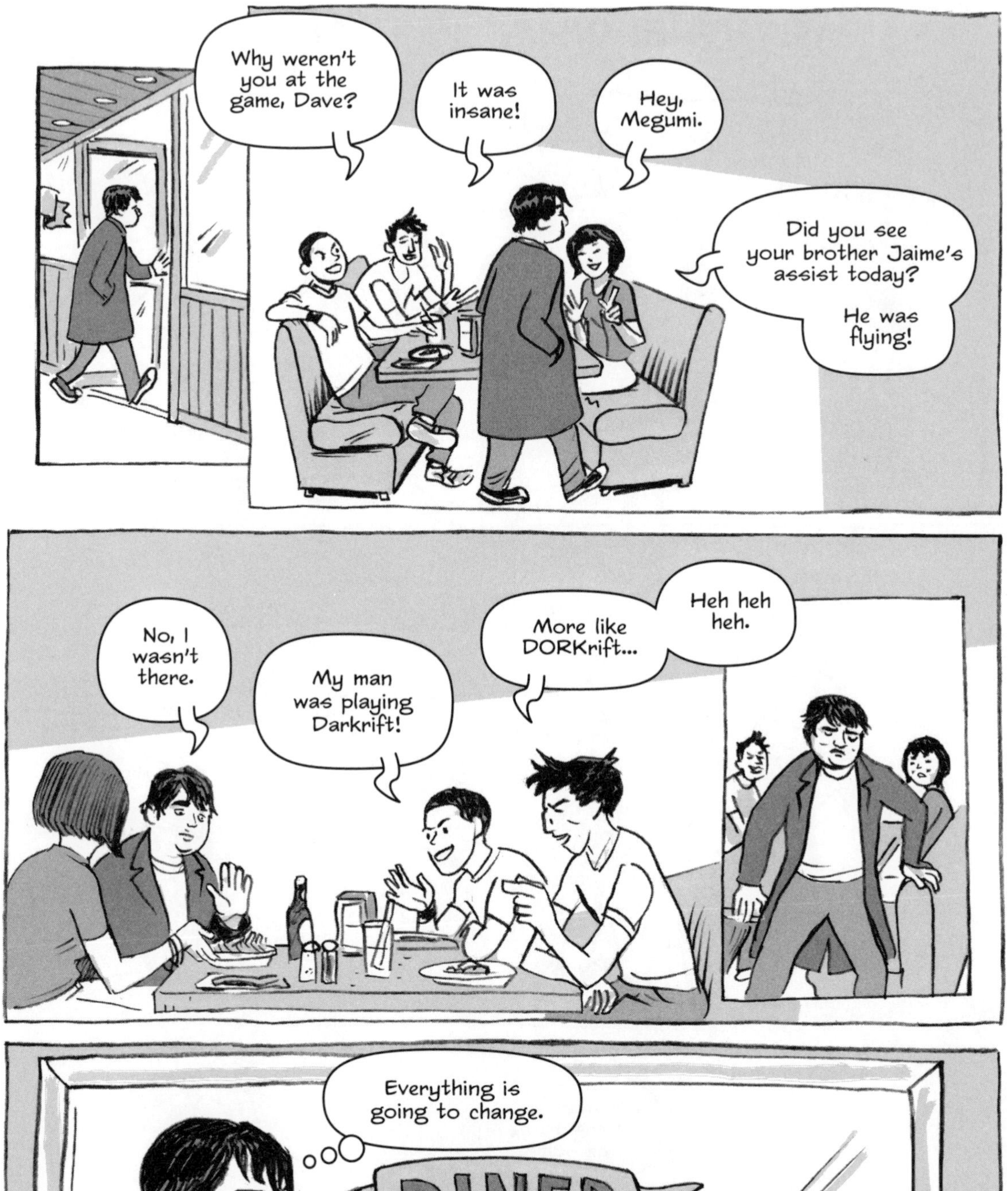
Why weren't you at the game, Dave?
It was insane!
Hey, Megumi.
Did you see your brother Jaime's assist today?
He was flying!
No, I wasn't there.
My man was playing Darkrift!
More like DORKrift...
Heh heh heh.
Everything is going to change.
DINER

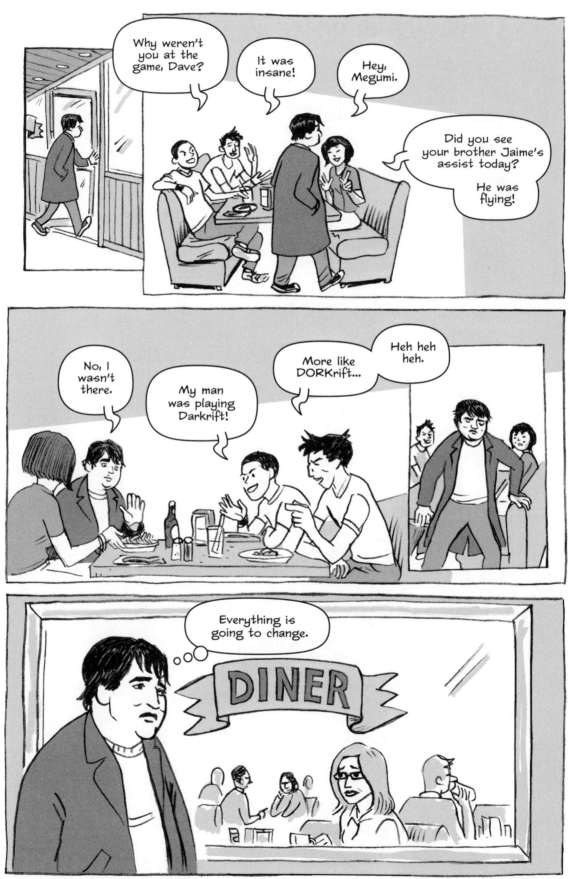

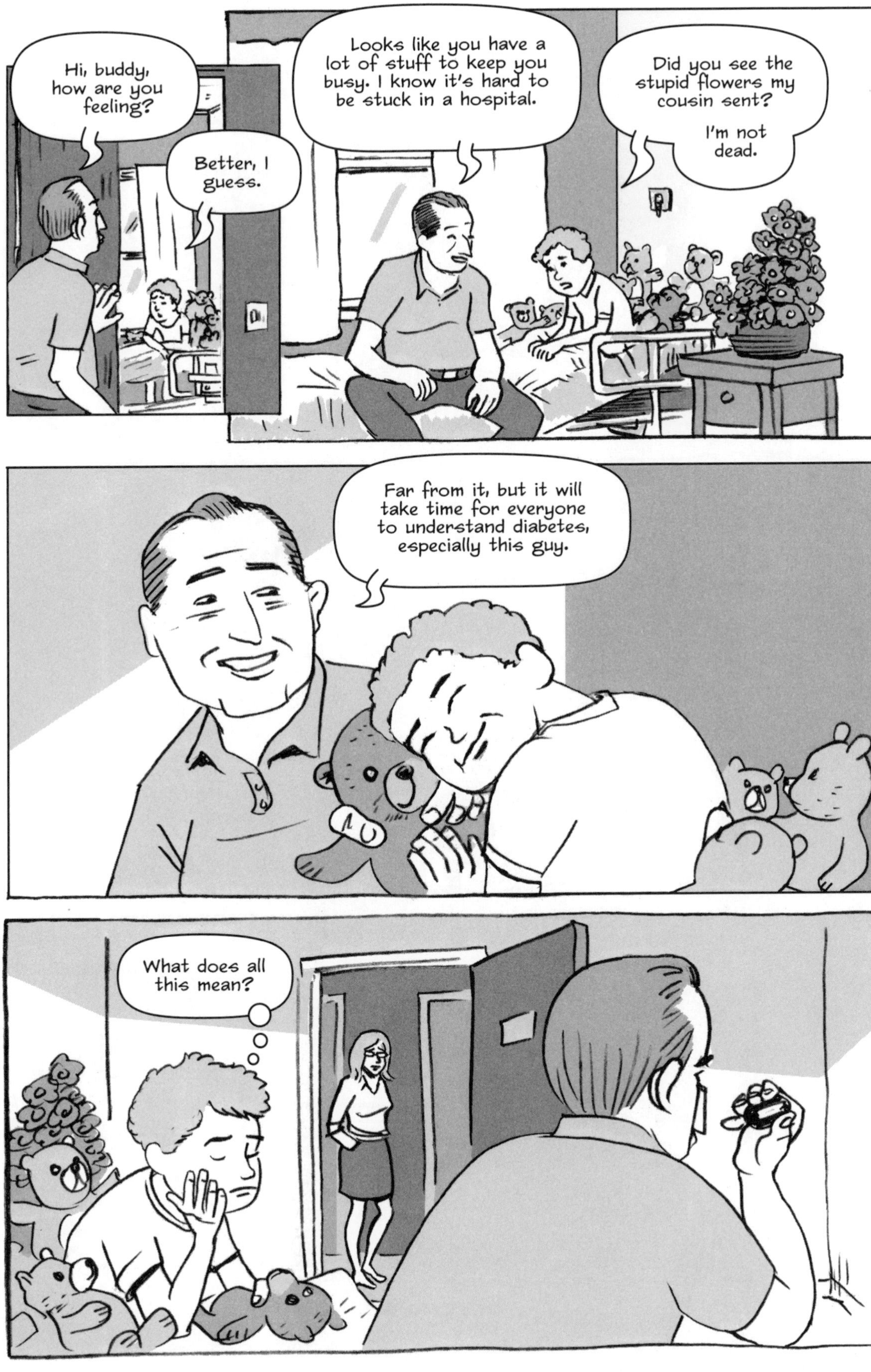
Hi, buddy, how are you feeling?
Better, I guess.
Looks like you have a lot of stuff to keep you busy. I know it's hard to be stuck in a hospital.
Did you see the stupid flowers my cousin sent?
I'm not dead.
Far from it, but it will take time for everyone to understand diabetes, especially this guy.
What does all this mean?

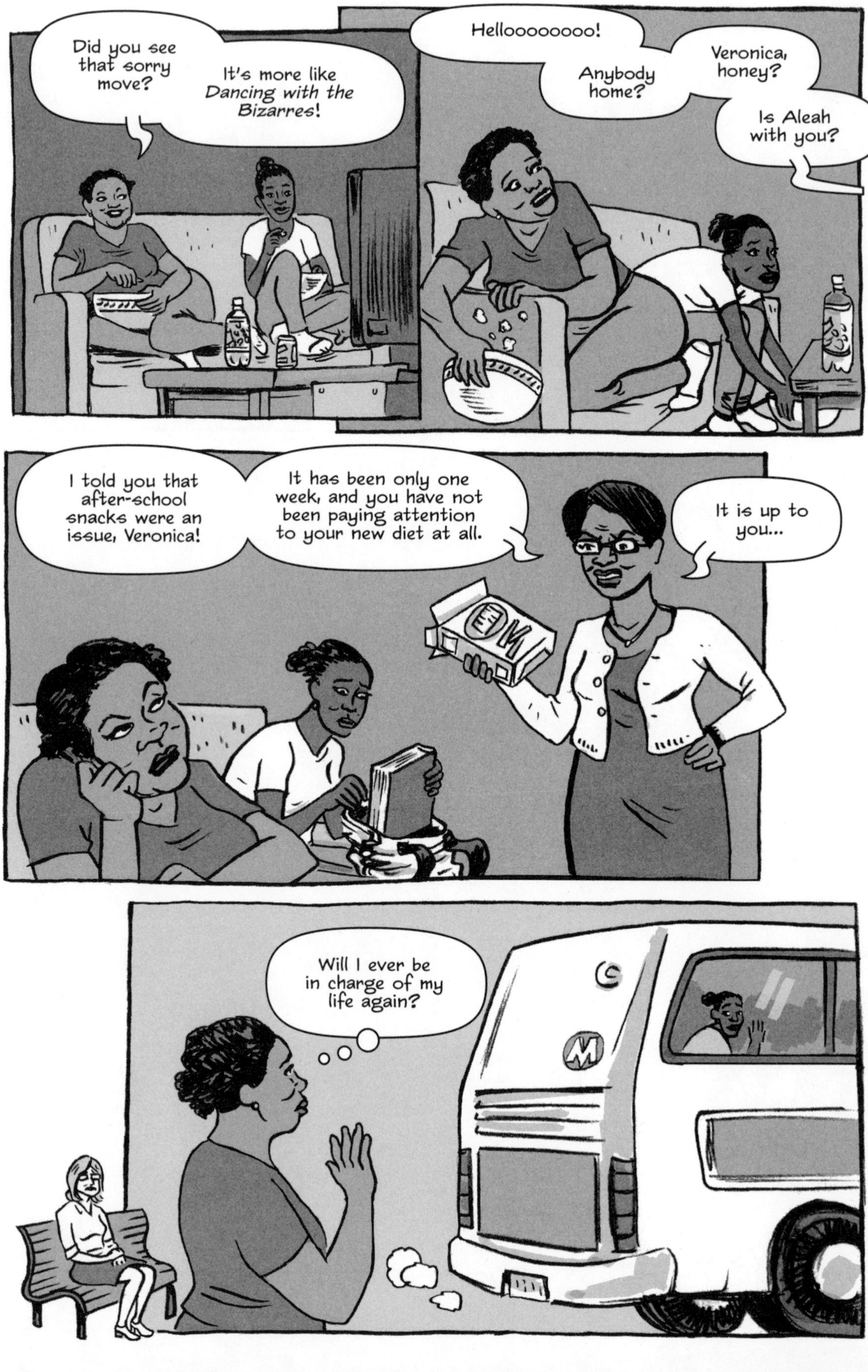
Did you see that sorry move?
It's more like *Dancing with the Bizarres*!
Helloooooooo!
Anybody home?
Veronica, honey?
Is Aleah with you?
I told you that after-school snacks were an issue, Veronica!
It has been only one week, and you have not been paying attention to your new diet at all.
It is up to you...
Will I ever be in charge of my life again?

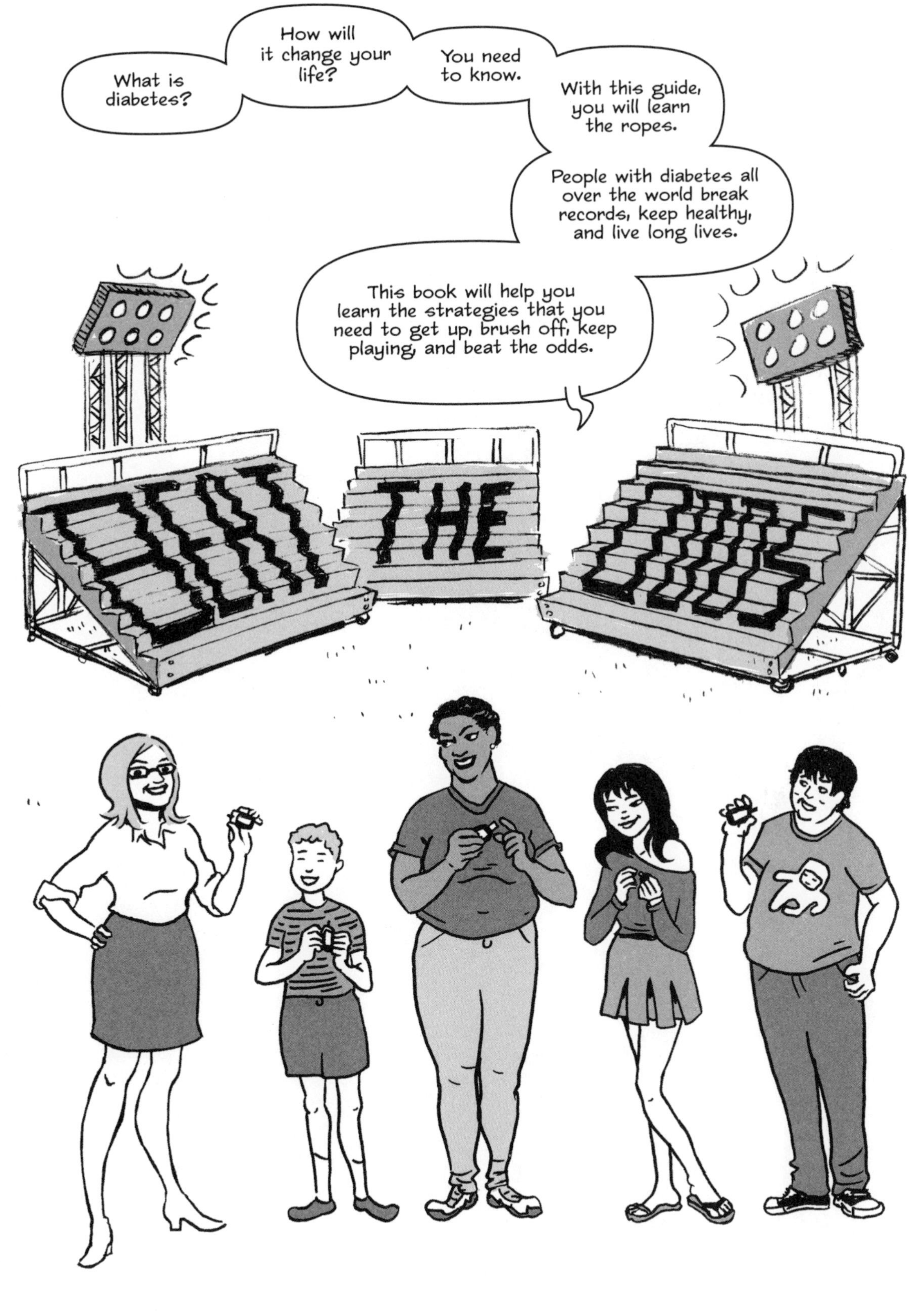
What is diabetes?
How will it change your life?
You need to know.
With this guide, you will learn the ropes.
People with diabetes all over the world break records, keep healthy, and live long lives.
This book will help you learn the strategies that you need to get up, brush off, keep playing, and beat the odds.
THE

WARM UP!

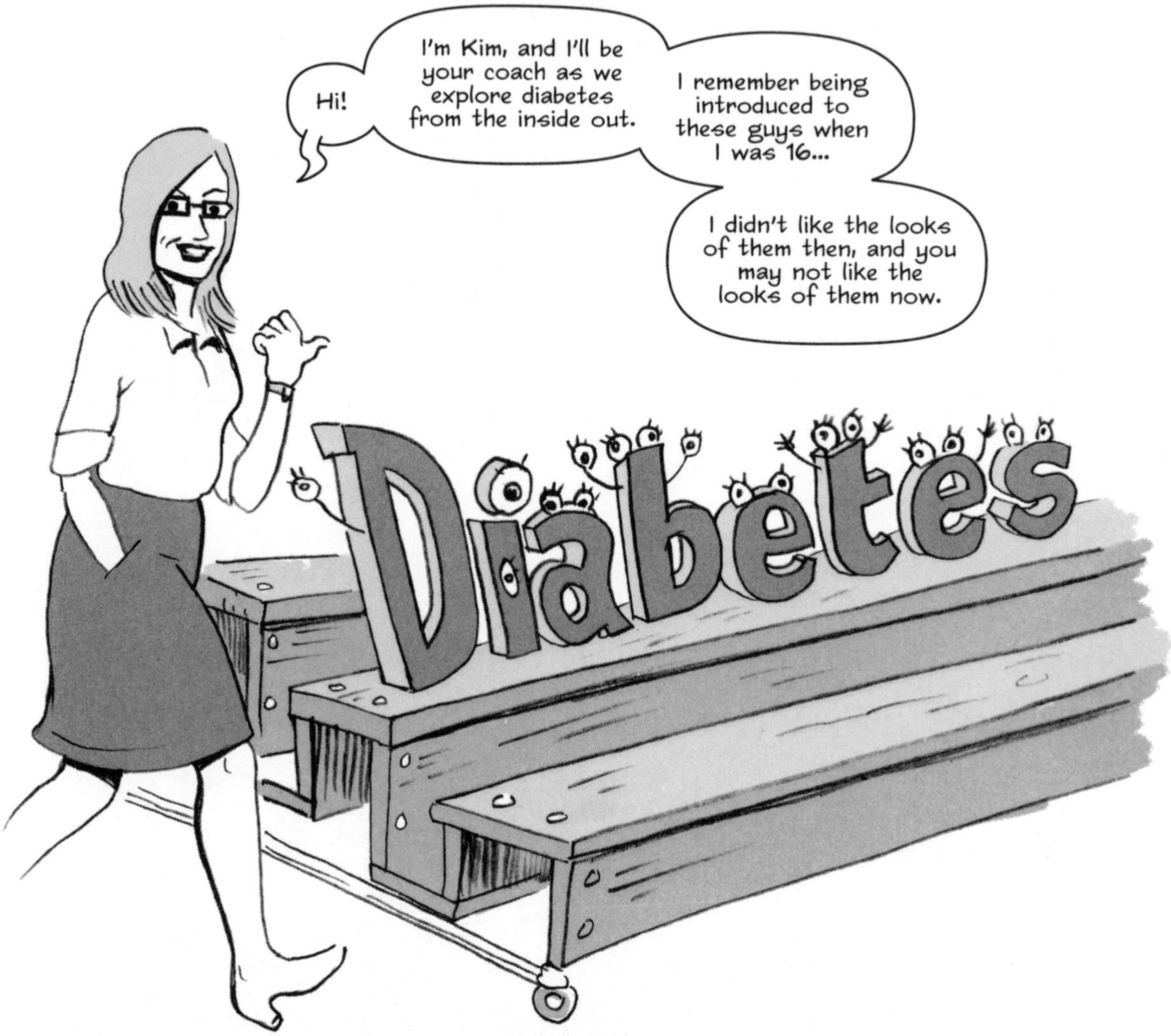
Hi!
I'm Kim, and I'll be your coach as we explore diabetes from the inside out.
I remember being introduced to these guys when I was 16...
I didn't like the looks of them then, and you may not like the looks of them now.
Diabetes

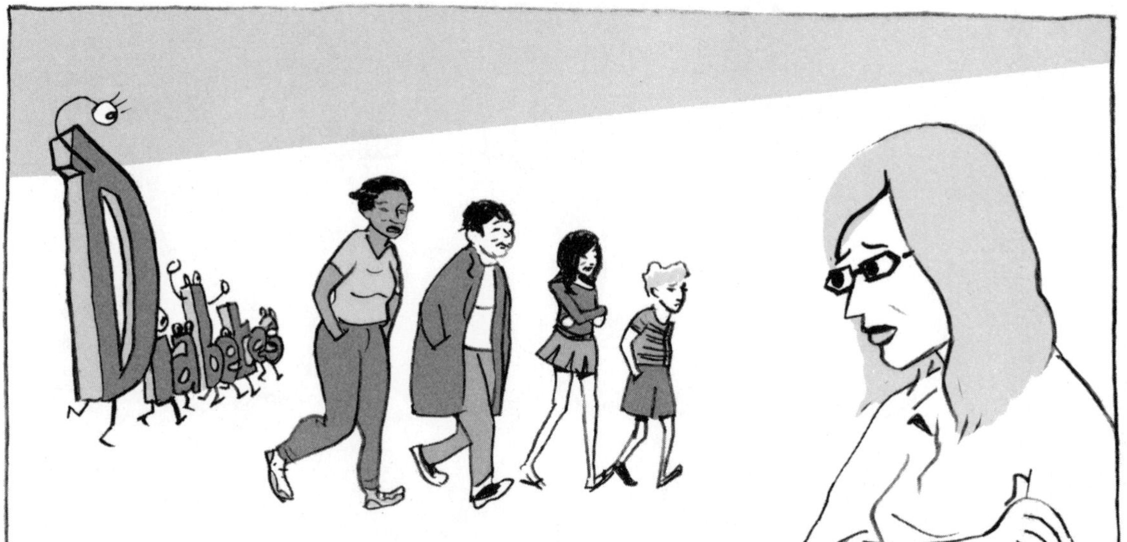
Diabetes

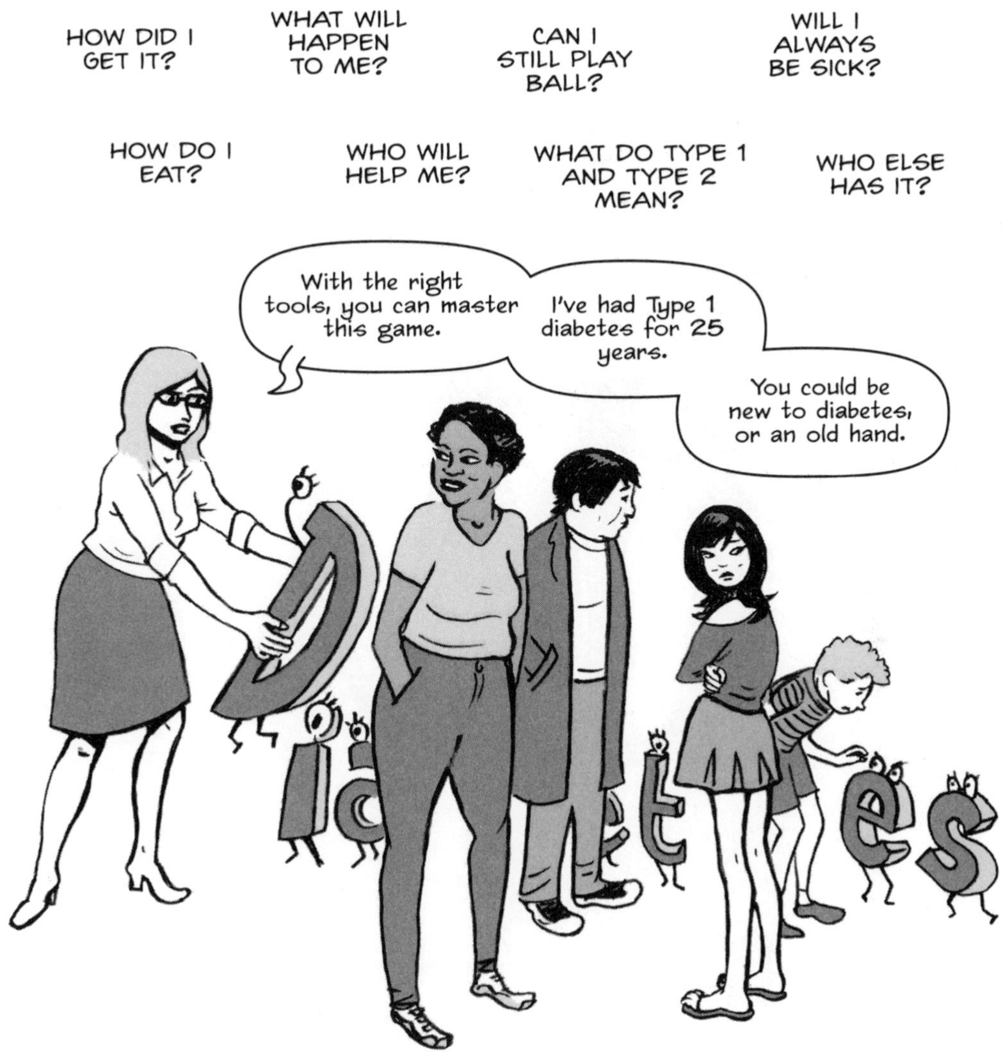
HOW DID I GET IT?
WHAT WILL HAPPEN TO ME?
CAN I STILL PLAY BALL?
WILL I ALWAYS BE SICK?
HOW DO I EAT?
WHO WILL HELP ME?
WHAT DO TYPE 1 AND TYPE 2 MEAN?
WHO ELSE HAS IT?
With the right tools, you can master this game.
I've had Type 1 diabetes for 25 years.
You could be new to diabetes, or an old hand.

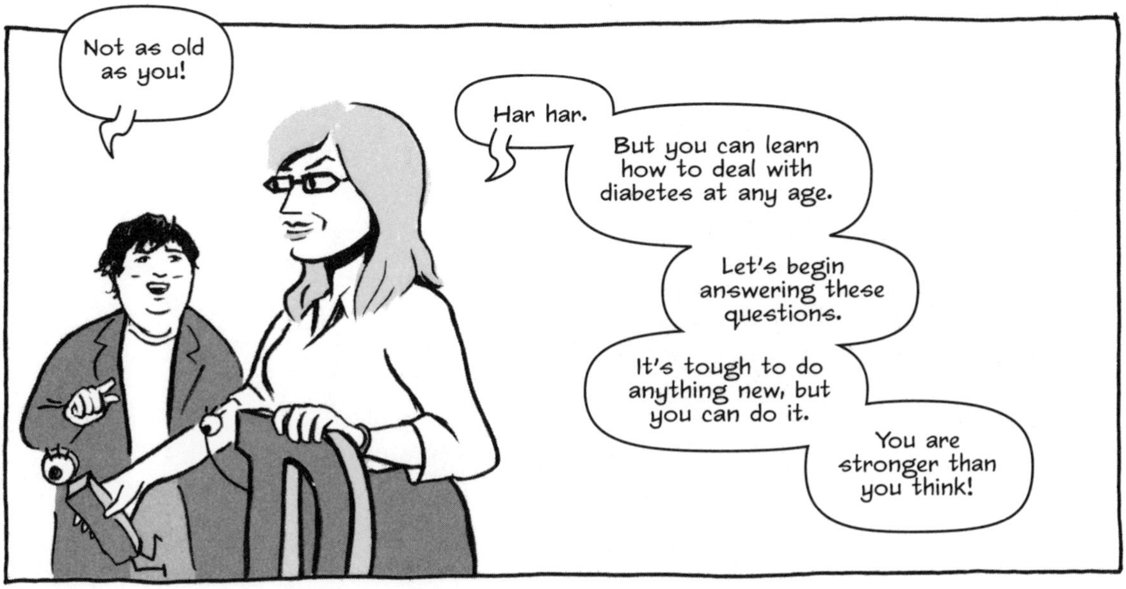
Not as old as you!
Har har.
But you can learn how to deal with diabetes at any age.
Let's begin answering these questions.
It's tough to do anything new, but you can do it.
You are stronger than you think!

I'm Veronica, 16 years old...
I found out I have Type 2 diabetes.
Will I be able to handle this disease?

I'm Marco. I'm 8.
My parents just found out I have Type 1.
My dog's name is Fifa.
Get it?
FIFA!*
I haven't told him I have diabetes yet.
Will I ever be able to play for FIFA?

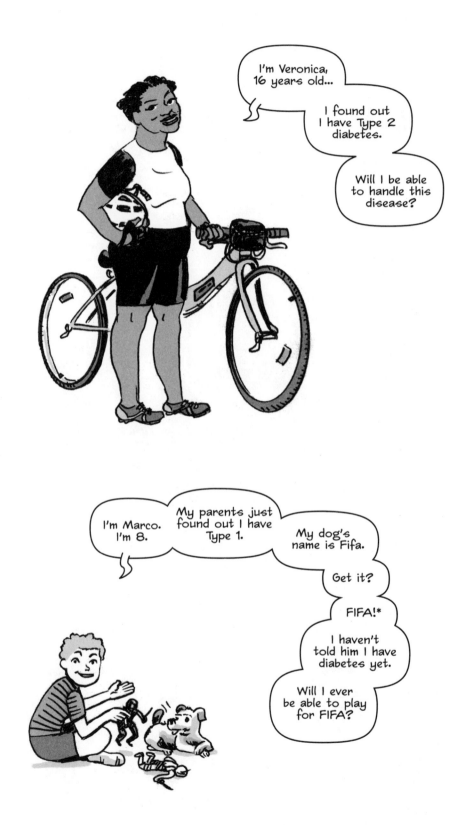

*FIFA: Fédération Internationale de Football Association.

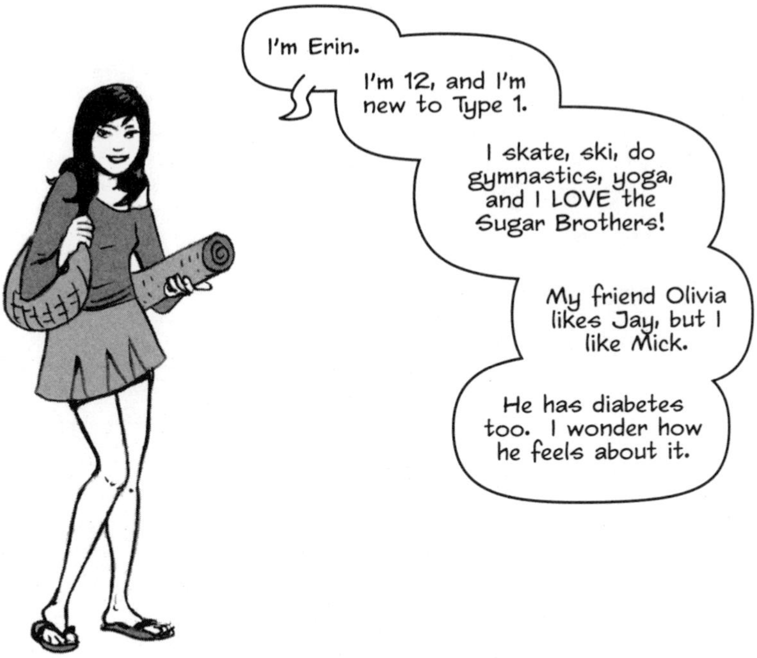
I'm Erin.
I'm 12, and I'm new to Type 1.
I skate, ski, do gymnastics, yoga, and I LOVE the Sugar Brothers!
My friend Olivia likes Jay, but I like Mick.
He has diabetes too. I wonder how he feels about it.

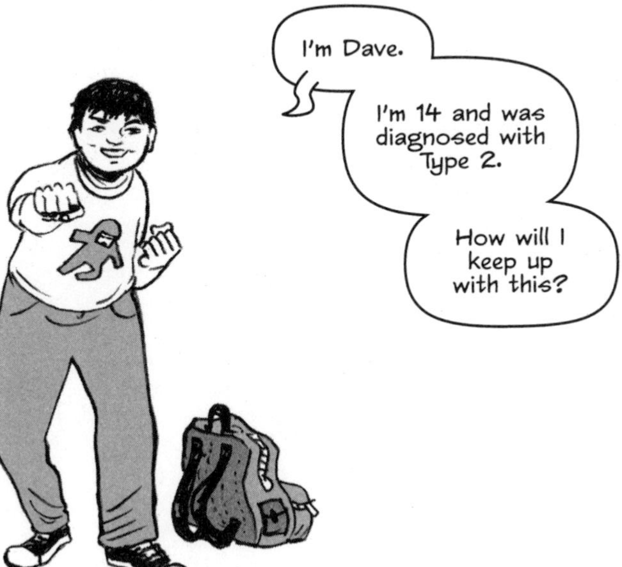
I'm Dave.
I'm 14 and was diagnosed with Type 2.
How will I keep up with this?

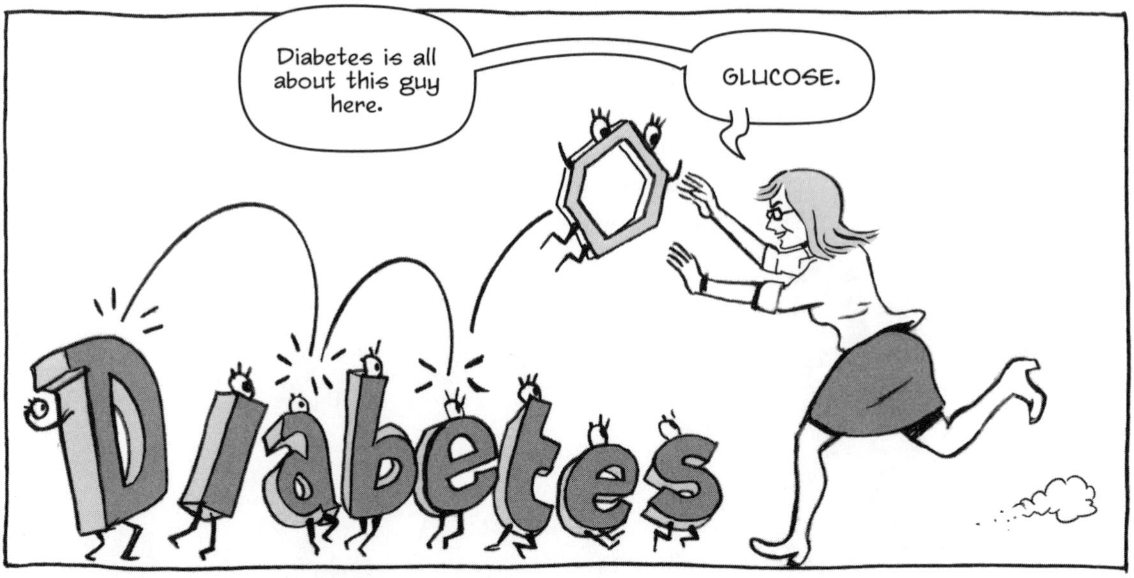
Diabetes is all about this guy here.
GLUCOSE.
Diabetes

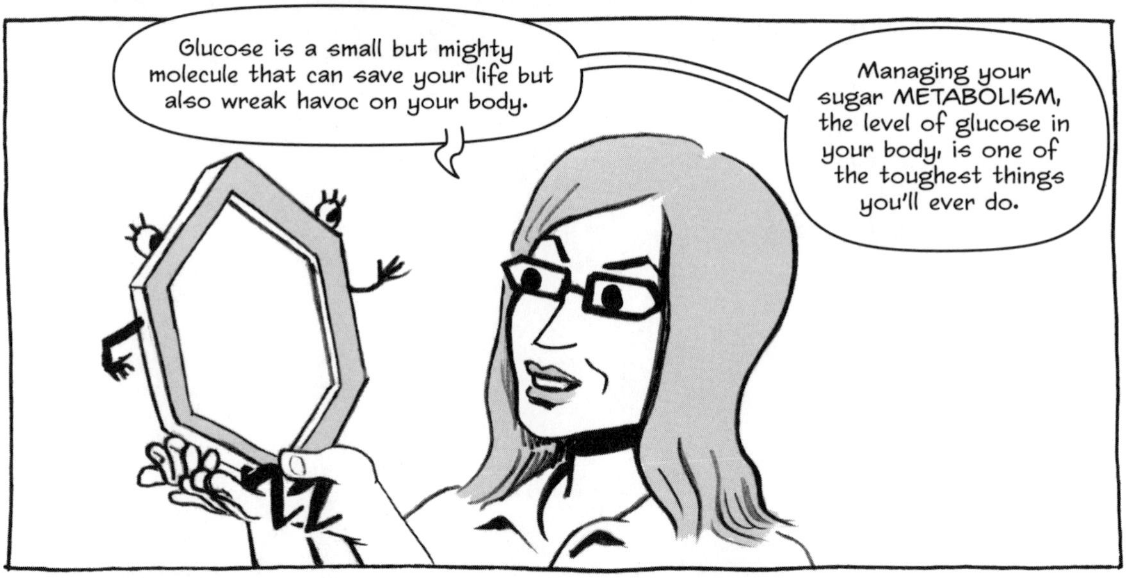
Glucose is a small but mighty molecule that can save your life but also wreak havoc on your body.
Managing your sugar METABOLISM, the level of glucose in your body, is one of the toughest things you'll ever do.

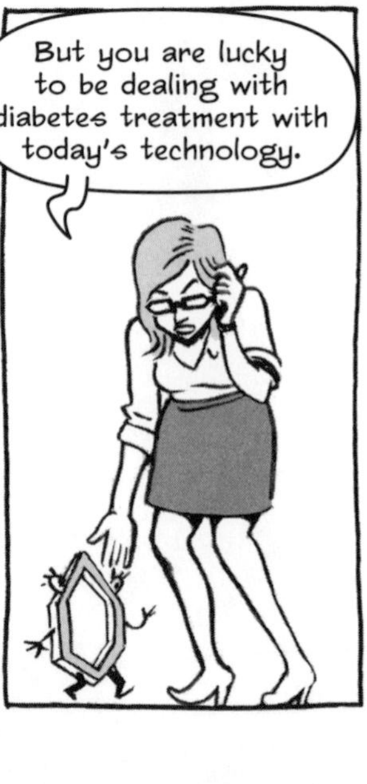
But you are lucky to be dealing with diabetes treatment with today's technology.

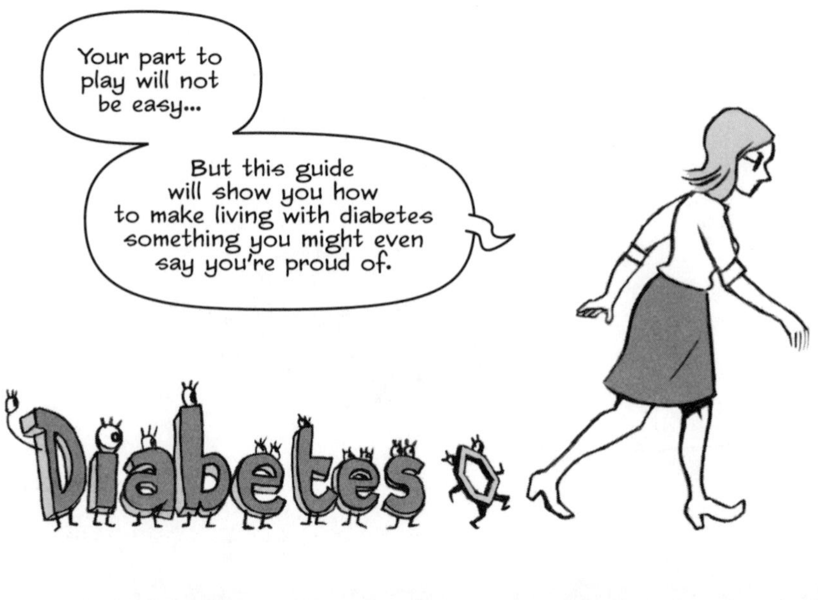
Your part to play will not be easy...
But this guide will show you how to make living with diabetes something you might even say you're proud of.
Diabetes

WHAT IS DIABETES?

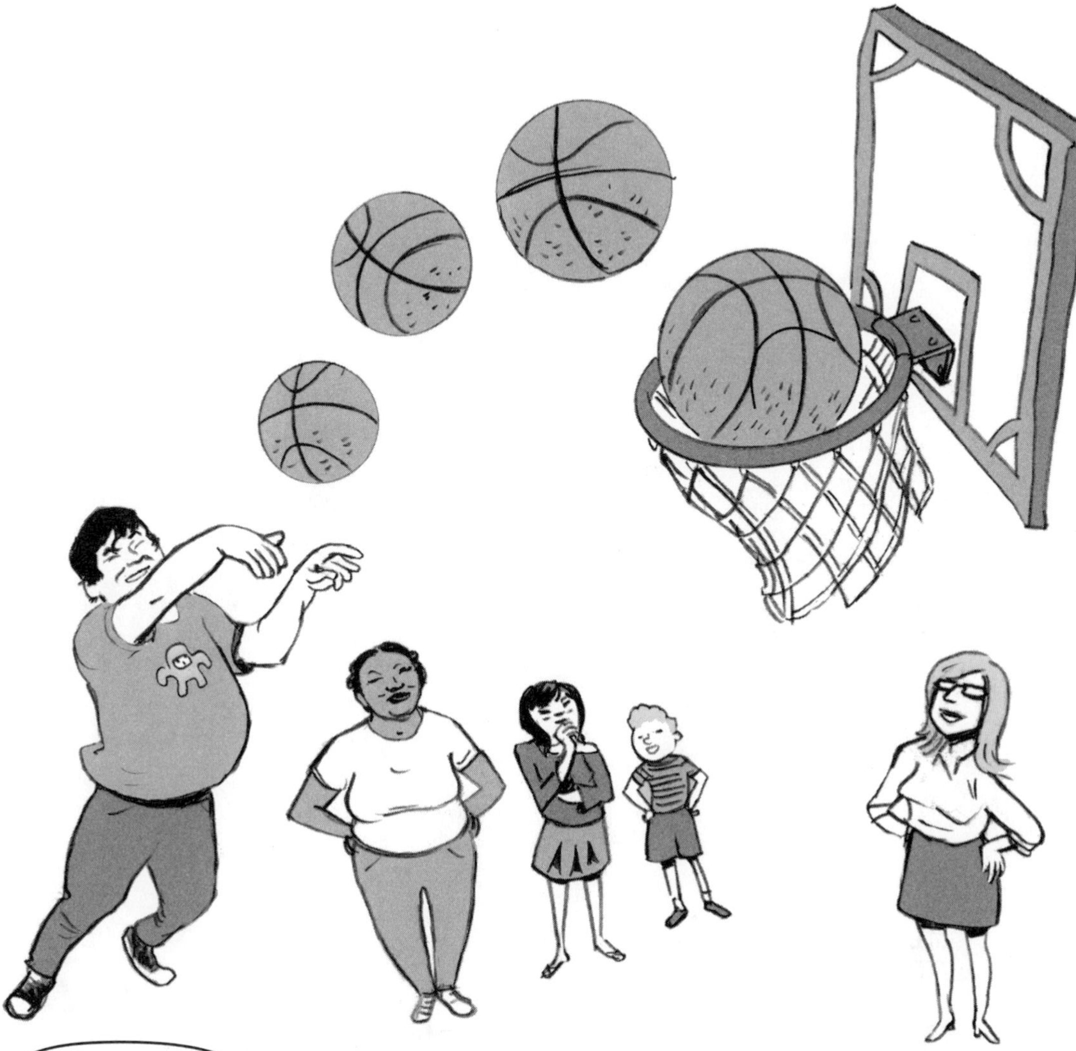

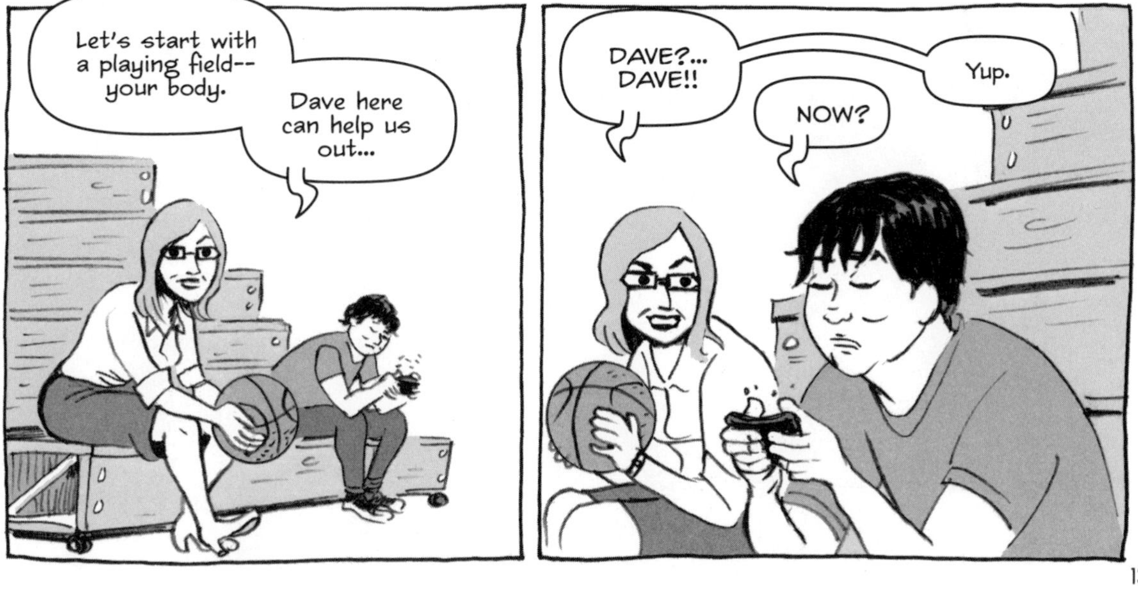
Let's start with a playing field-- your body.
Dave here can help us out...
DAVE?... DAVE!!
Yup.
NOW?

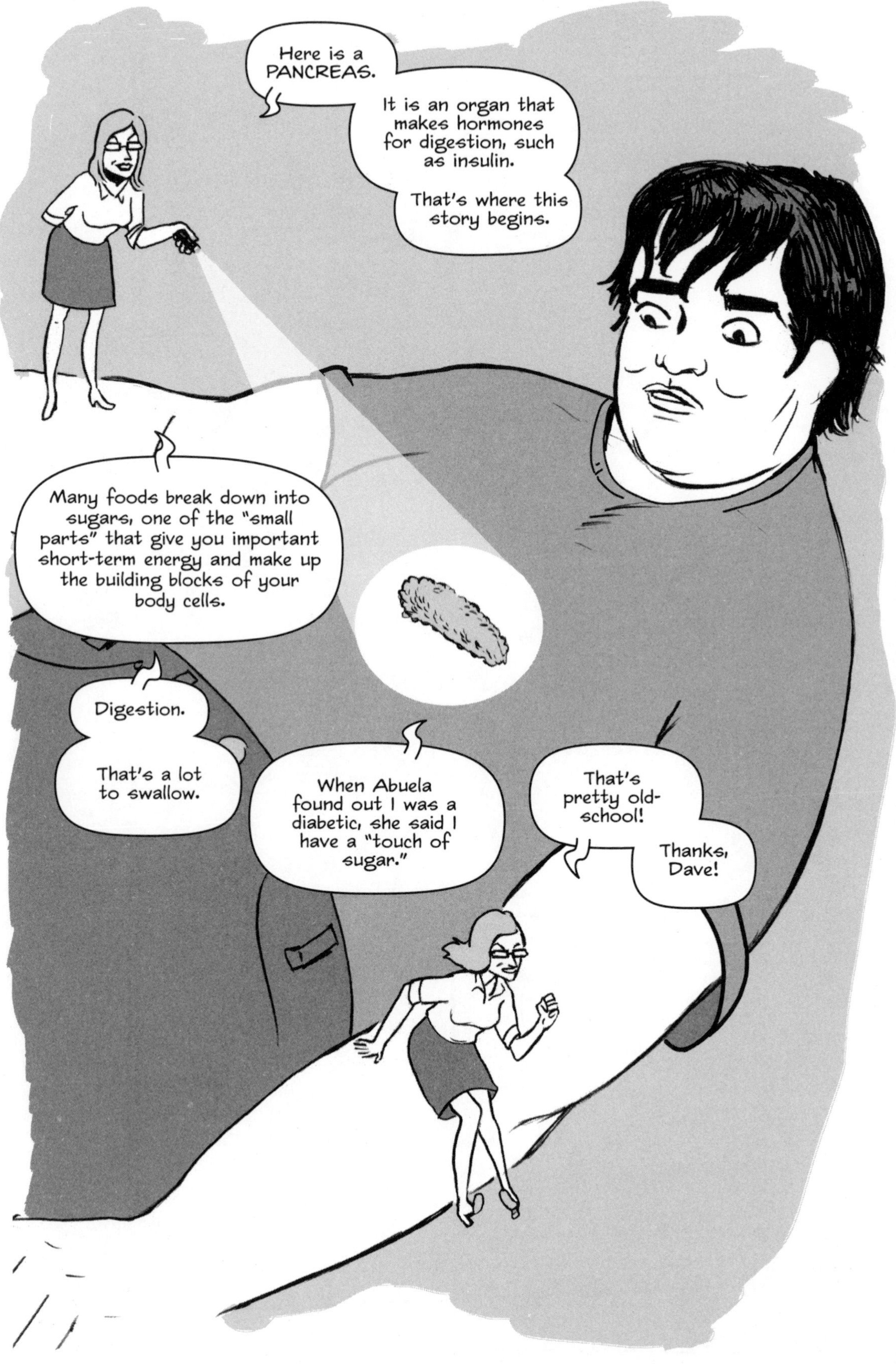
Here is a PANCREAS.
It is an organ that makes hormones for digestion, such as insulin.
That's where this story begins.
Many foods break down into sugars, one of the "small parts" that give you important short-term energy and make up the building blocks of your body cells.
Digestion.
That's a lot to swallow.
When Abuela found out I was a diabetic, she said I have a "touch of sugar."
That's pretty old-school!
Thanks, Dave!

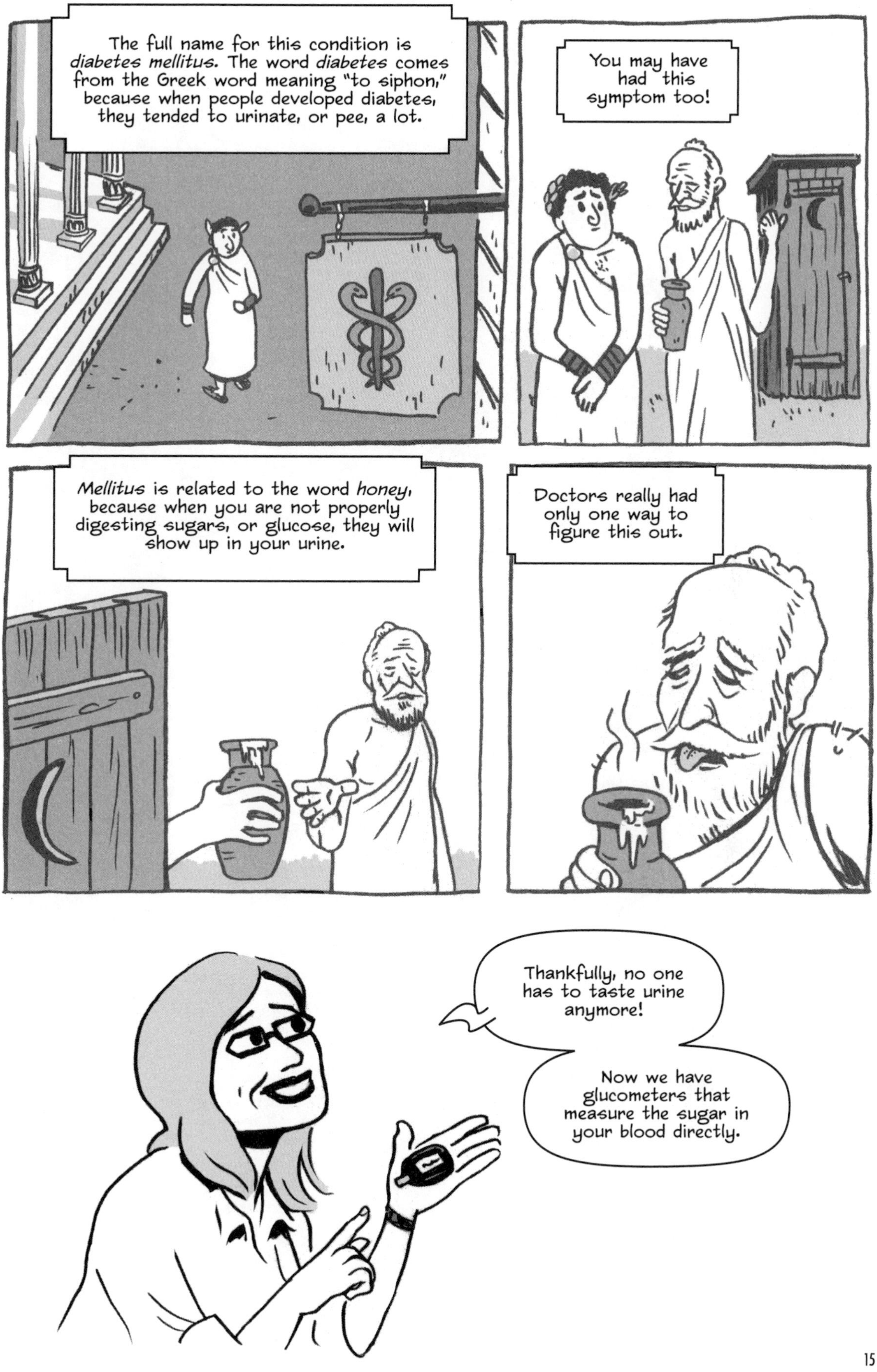
The full name for this condition is diabetes mellitus. The word diabetes comes from the Greek word meaning "to siphon," because when people developed diabetes, they tended to urinate, or pee, a lot.
You may have had this symptom too!
Mellitus is related to the word honey, because when you are not properly digesting sugars, or glucose, they will show up in your urine.
Doctors really had only one way to figure this out.
Thankfully, no one has to taste urine anymore!
Now we have glucometers that measure the sugar in your blood directly.

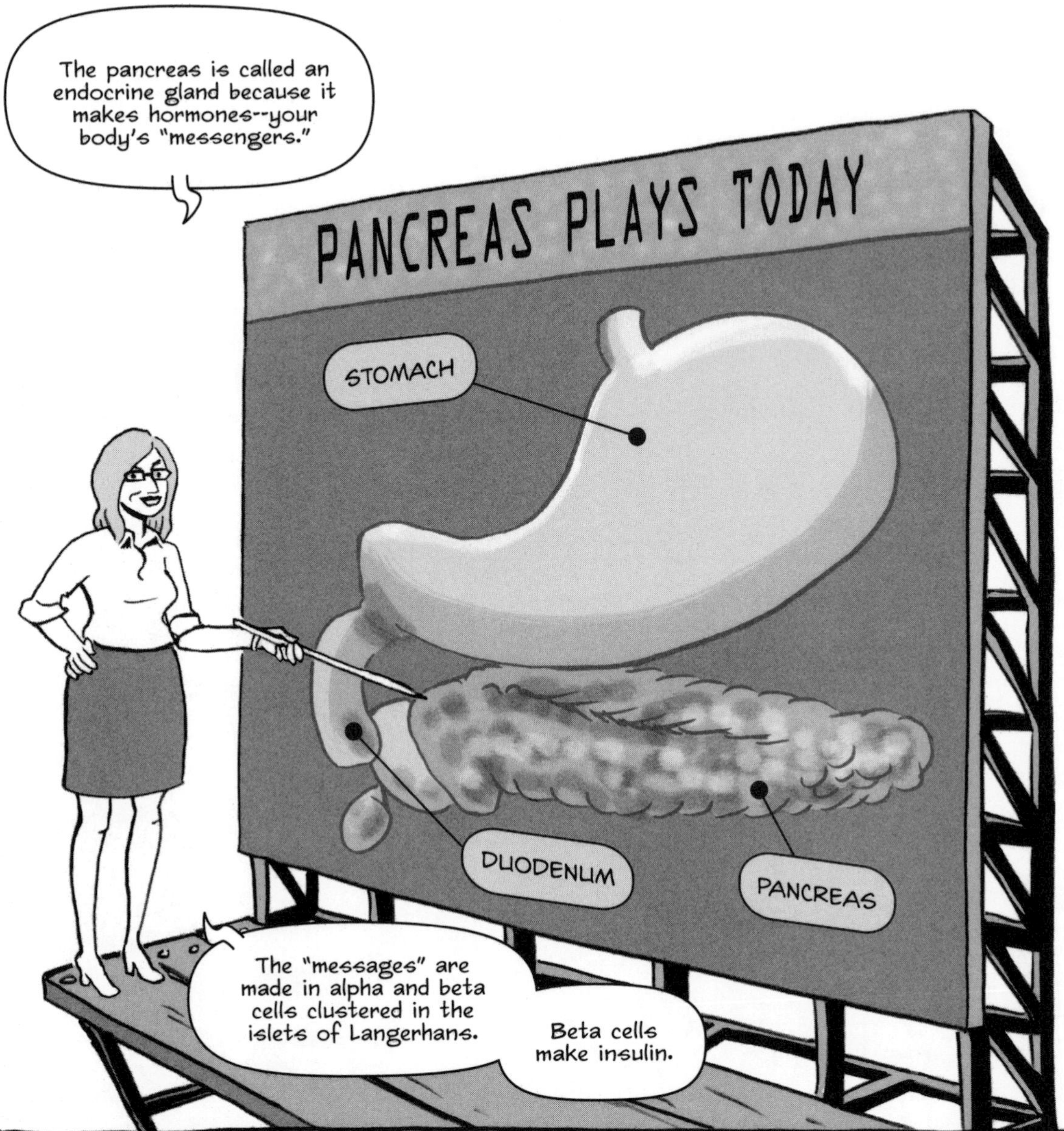
The pancreas is called an endocrine gland because it makes hormones--your body's "messengers."
PANCREAS PLAYS TODAY
STOMACH
DUODENUM
PANCREAS
The "messages" are made in alpha and beta cells clustered in the islets of Langerhans.
Beta cells make insulin.

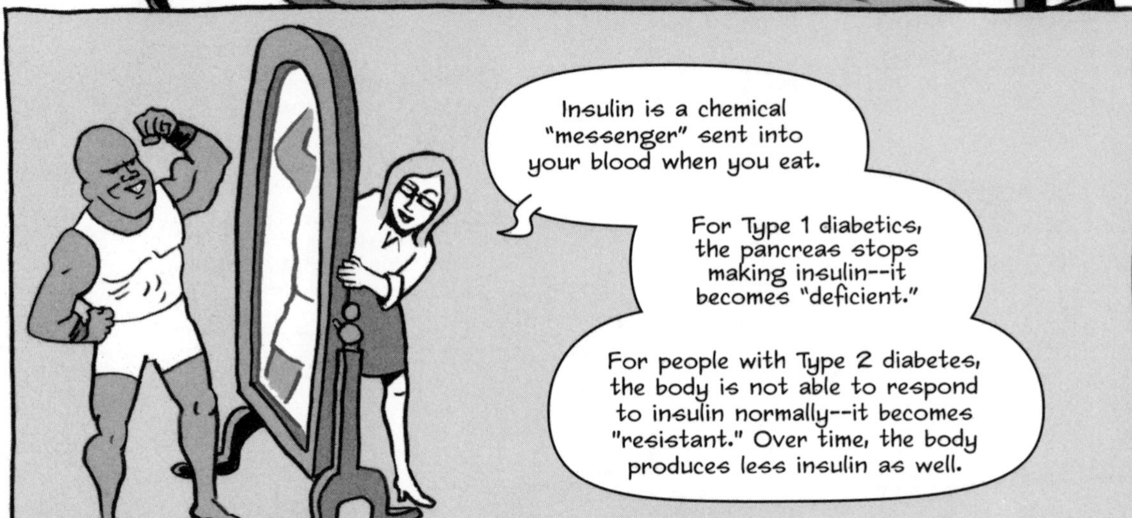
Insulin is a chemical "messenger" sent into your blood when you eat.
For Type 1 diabetics, the pancreas stops making insulin--it becomes "deficient."
For people with Type 2 diabetes, the body is not able to respond to insulin normally--it becomes "resistant." Over time, the body produces less insulin as well.

WHO HAS DIABETES?

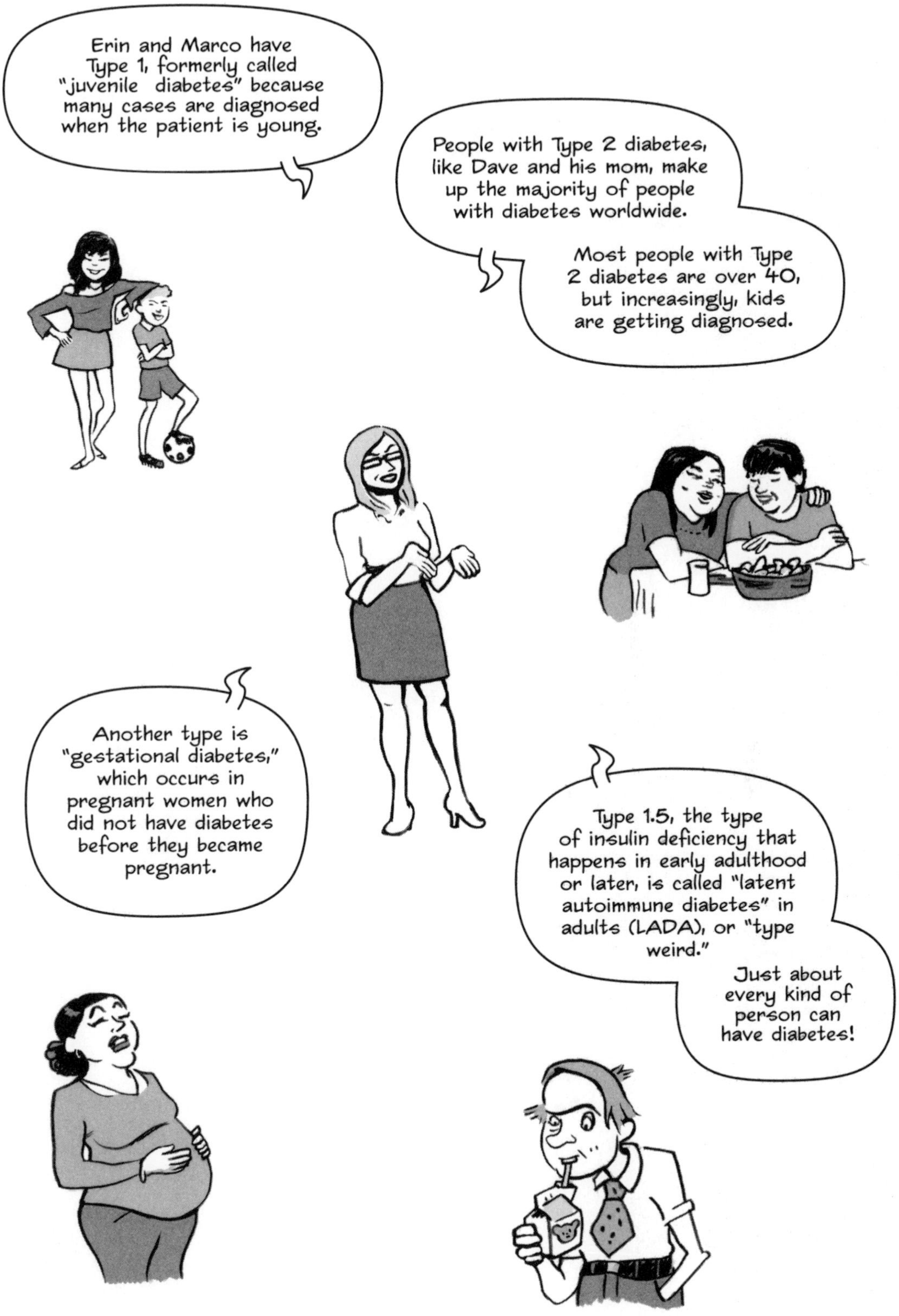
Erin and Marco have Type 1, formerly called "juvenile diabetes" because many cases are diagnosed when the patient is young.
People with Type 2 diabetes, like Dave and his mom, make up the majority of people with diabetes worldwide.
Most people with Type 2 diabetes are over 40, but increasingly, kids are getting diagnosed.
Another type is "gestational diabetes," which occurs in pregnant women who did not have diabetes before they became pregnant.
Type 1.5, the type of insulin deficiency that happens in early adulthood or later, is called "latent autoimmune diabetes" in adults (LADA), or "type weird."
Just about every kind of person can have diabetes!

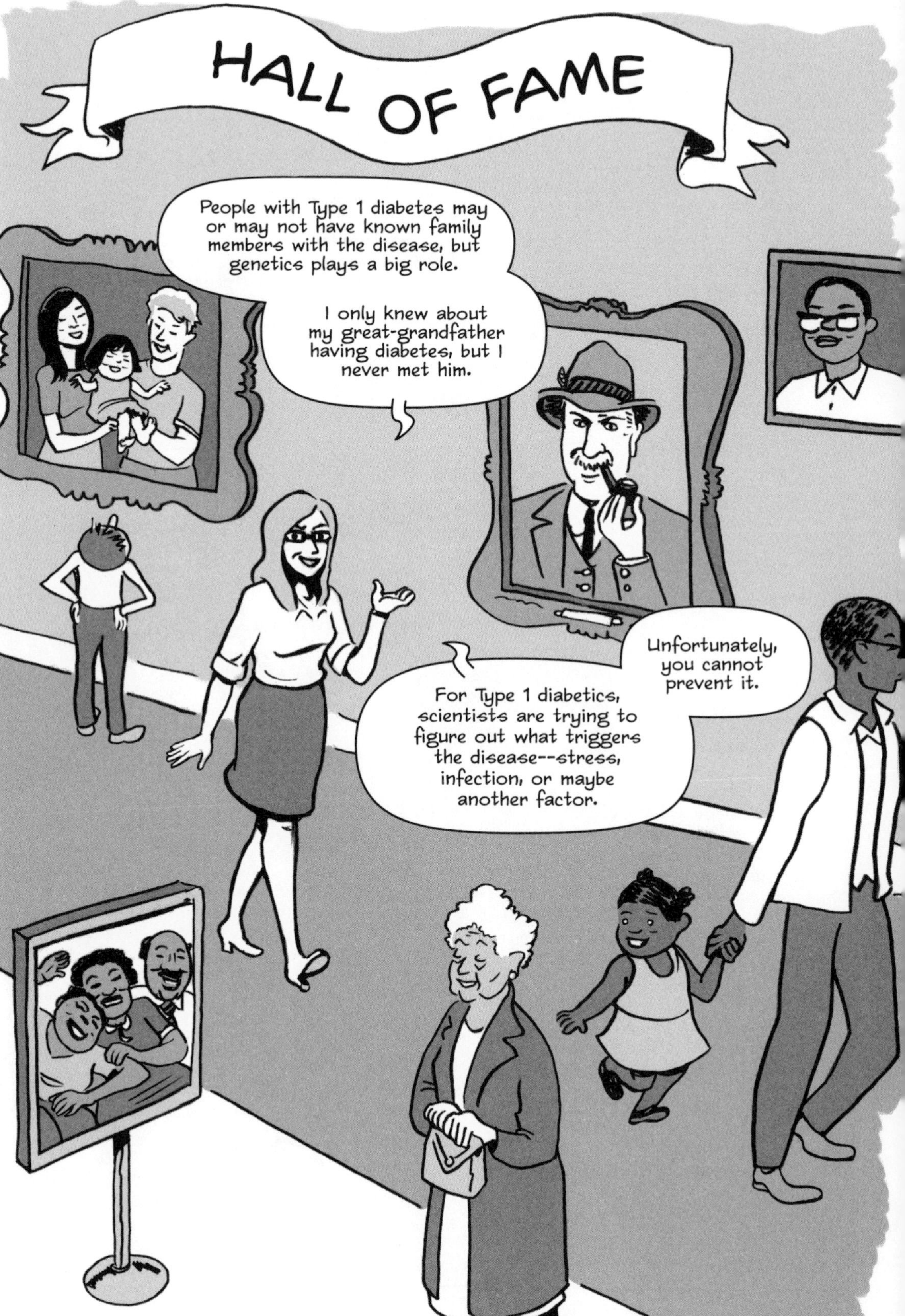
HALL OF FAME
People with Type 1 diabetes may or may not have known family members with the disease, but genetics plays a big role.
I only knew about my great-grandfather having diabetes, but I never met him.
For Type 1 diabetics, scientists are trying to figure out what triggers the disease--stress, infection, or maybe another factor.
Unfortunately, you cannot prevent it.

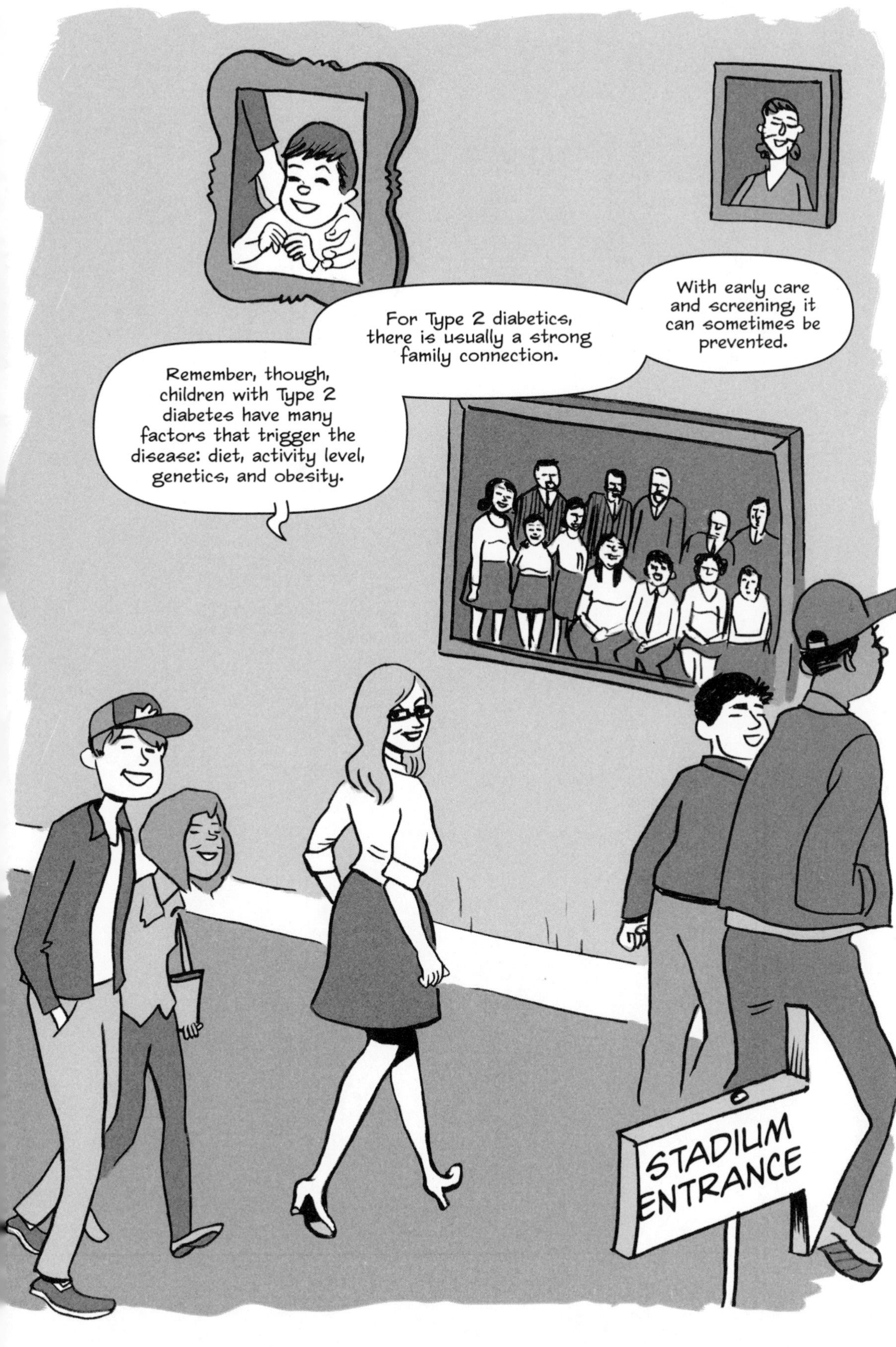
Remember, though, children with Type 2 diabetes have many factors that trigger the disease: diet, activity level, genetics, and obesity.
For Type 2 diabetics, there is usually a strong family connection.
With early care and screening, it can sometimes be prevented.
STADIUM ENTRANCE

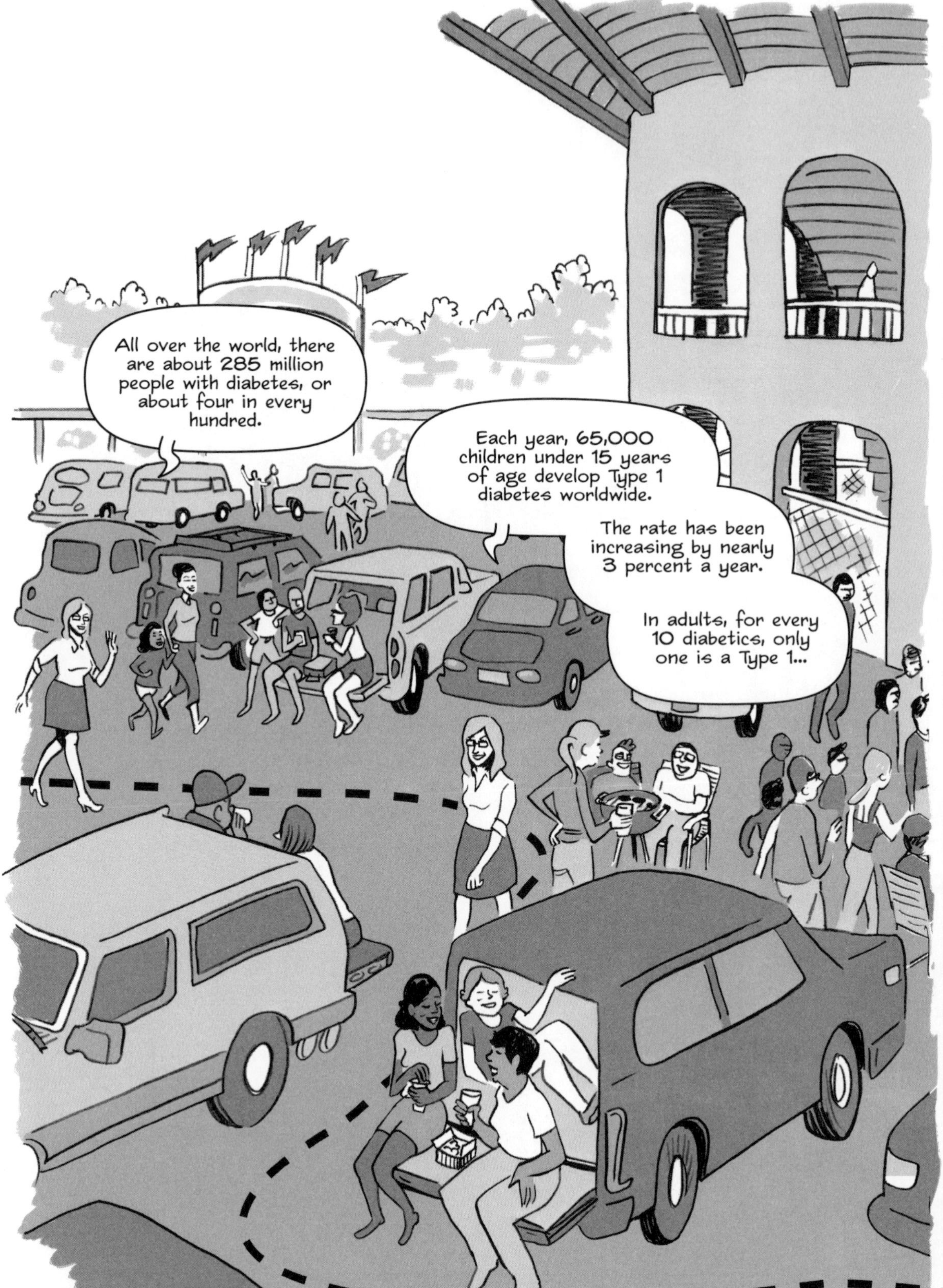
All over the world, there are about 285 million people with diabetes, or about four in every hundred.
Each year, 65,000 children under 15 years of age develop Type 1 diabetes worldwide.
The rate has been increasing by nearly 3 percent a year.
In adults, for every 10 diabetics, only one is a Type 1...

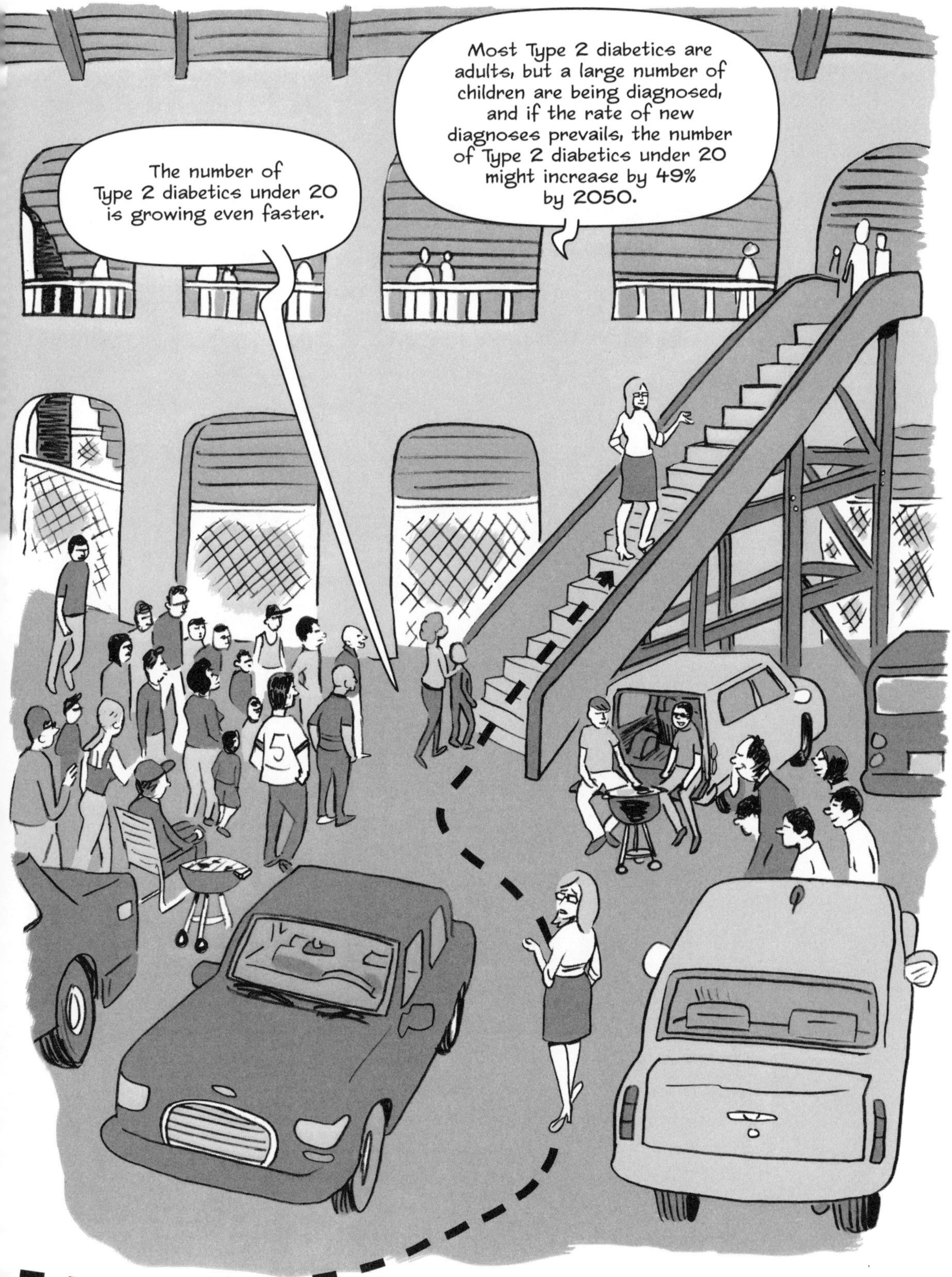
The number of
Type 2 diabetics under 20
is growing even faster.
Most Type 2 diabetics are
adults, but a large number of
children are being diagnosed,
and if the rate of new
diagnoses prevails, the number
of Type 2 diabetics under 20
might increase by 49%
by 2050.
5

People with Type 1 diabetes:
- are not necessarily overweight or inactive
- can be diagnosed from infancy to their late teens
- sometimes have a family member with the disease, but not always

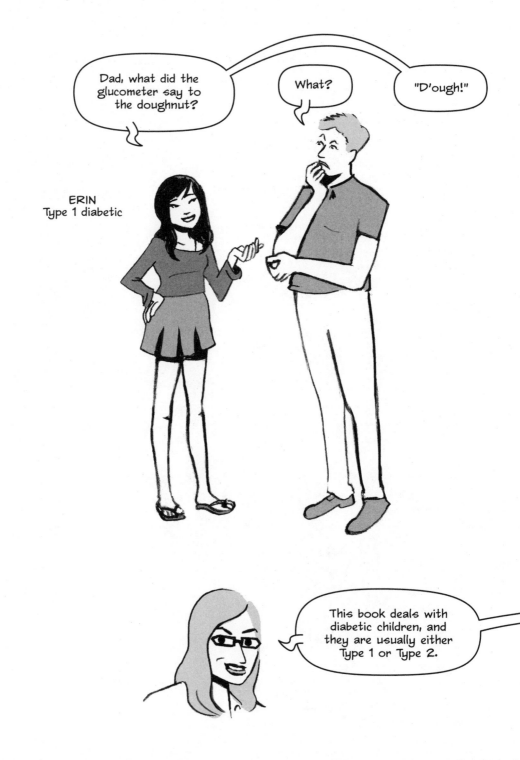

Dad, what did the glucometer say to the doughnut?

What?

"D'ough!"

ERIN
Type 1 diabetic

This book deals with diabetic children, and they are usually either Type 1 or Type 2.

People with Type 2 diabetes:

- are often overweight (but some Type 2 children are not overweight)
- are often inactive
- often have a family history of diabetes

VERONICA
Type 2 diabetic
ALEAH
Prediabetic
Aleah pre-took my fries at lunch.
Next I'll pre-kick your butt in calculus.
No chance.

Prediabetes means that a person's blood sugar levels are higher than normal, but not high enough to be diagnosed as Type 2 diabetes.

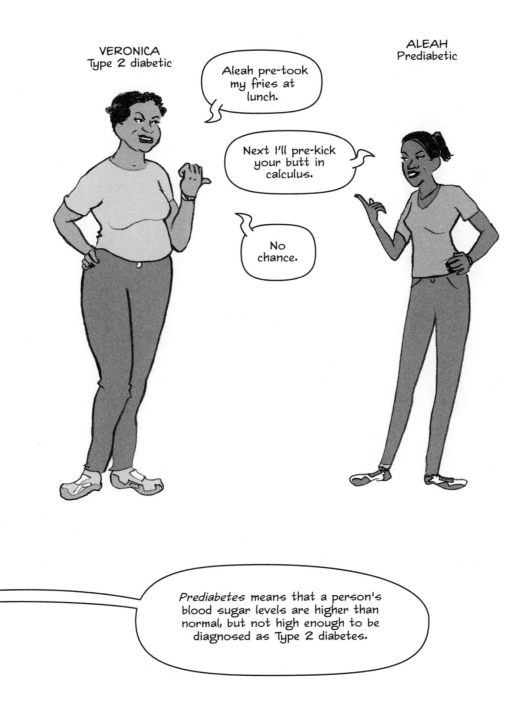

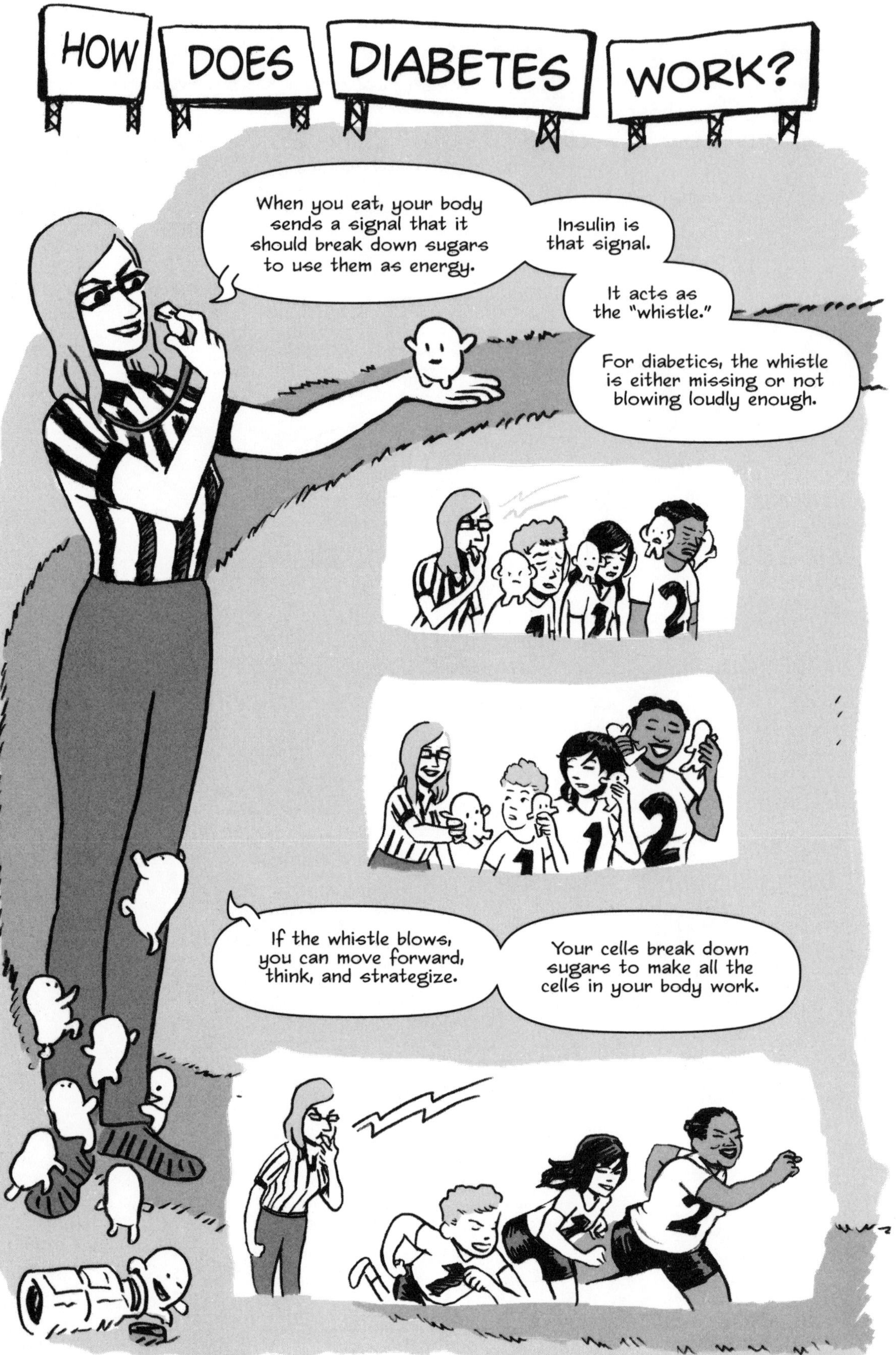
HOW DOES DIABETES WORK?
When you eat, your body sends a signal that it should break down sugars to use them as energy.
Insulin is that signal.
It acts as the "whistle."
For diabetics, the whistle is either missing or not blowing loudly enough.
1
2
1
2
If the whistle blows, you can move forward, think, and strategize.
Your cells break down sugars to make all the cells in your body work.
2

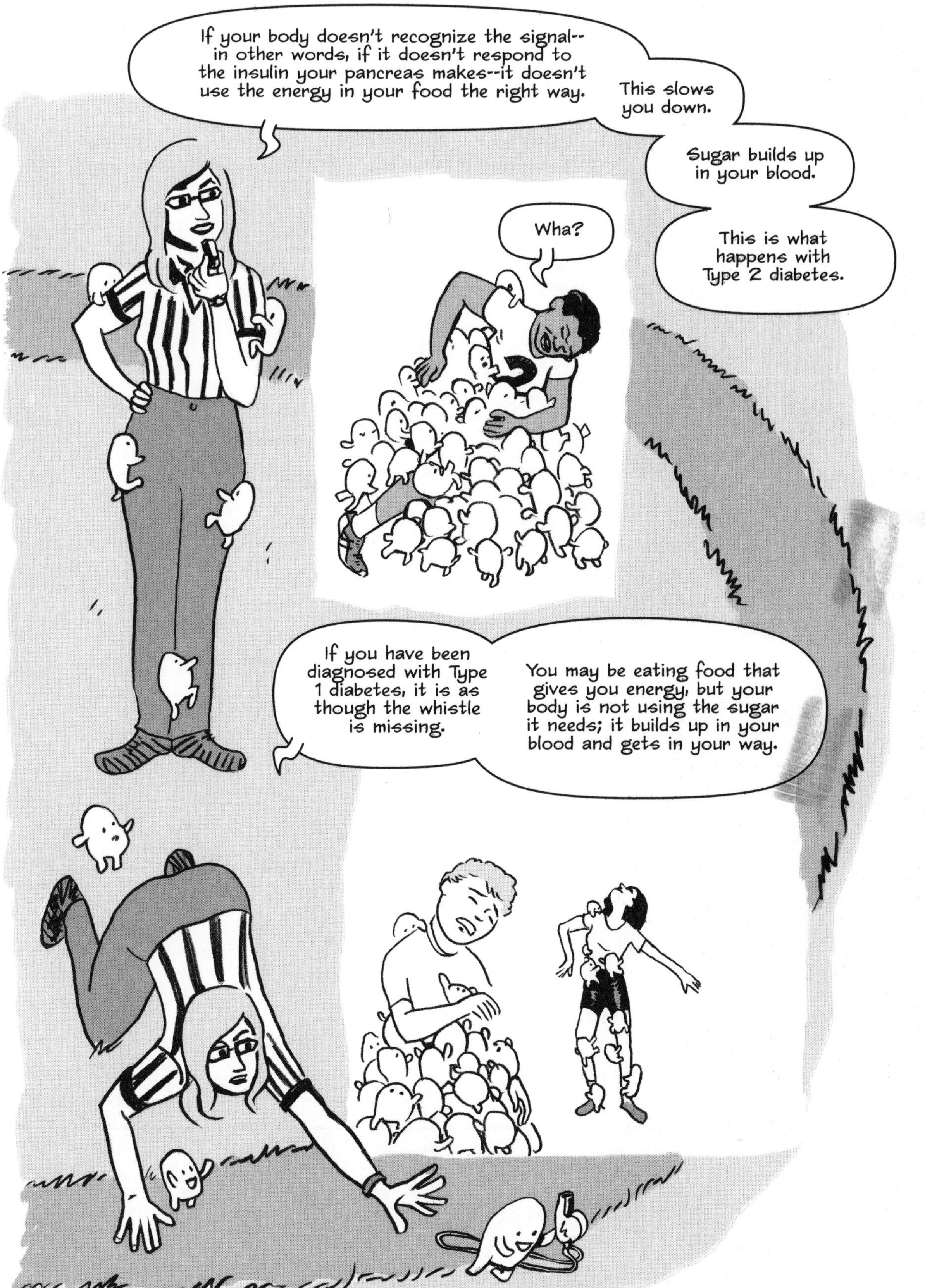
If your body doesn't recognize the signal--in other words, if it doesn't respond to the insulin your pancreas makes--it doesn't use the energy in your food the right way.
This slows you down.
Sugar builds up in your blood.
This is what happens with Type 2 diabetes.
Wha?
If you have been diagnosed with Type 1 diabetes, it is as though the whistle is missing.
You may be eating food that gives you energy, but your body is not using the sugar it needs; it builds up in your blood and gets in your way.

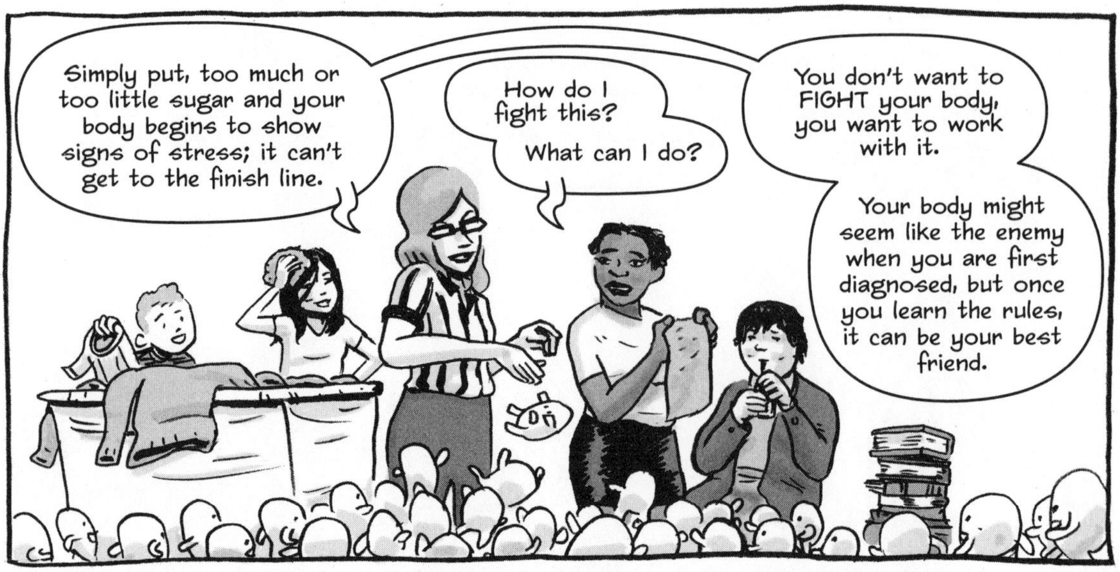
Simply put, too much or too little sugar and your body begins to show signs of stress; it can't get to the finish line.
How do I fight this?
What can I do?
You don't want to FIGHT your body, you want to work with it.
Your body might seem like the enemy when you are first diagnosed, but once you learn the rules, it can be your best friend.

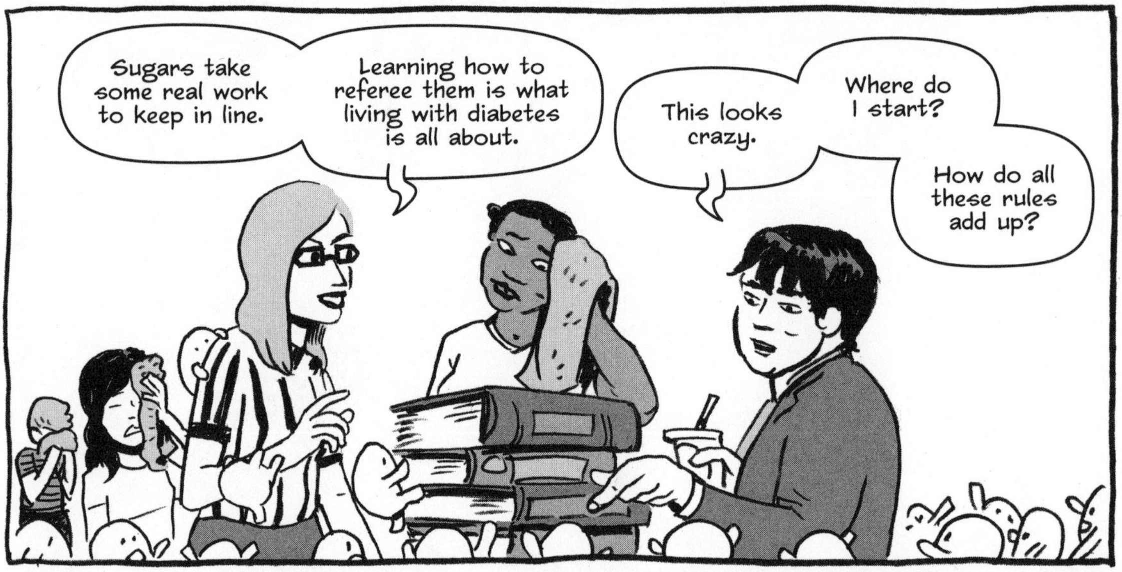
Sugars take some real work to keep in line.
Learning how to referee them is what living with diabetes is all about.
This looks crazy.
Where do I start?
How do all these rules add up?

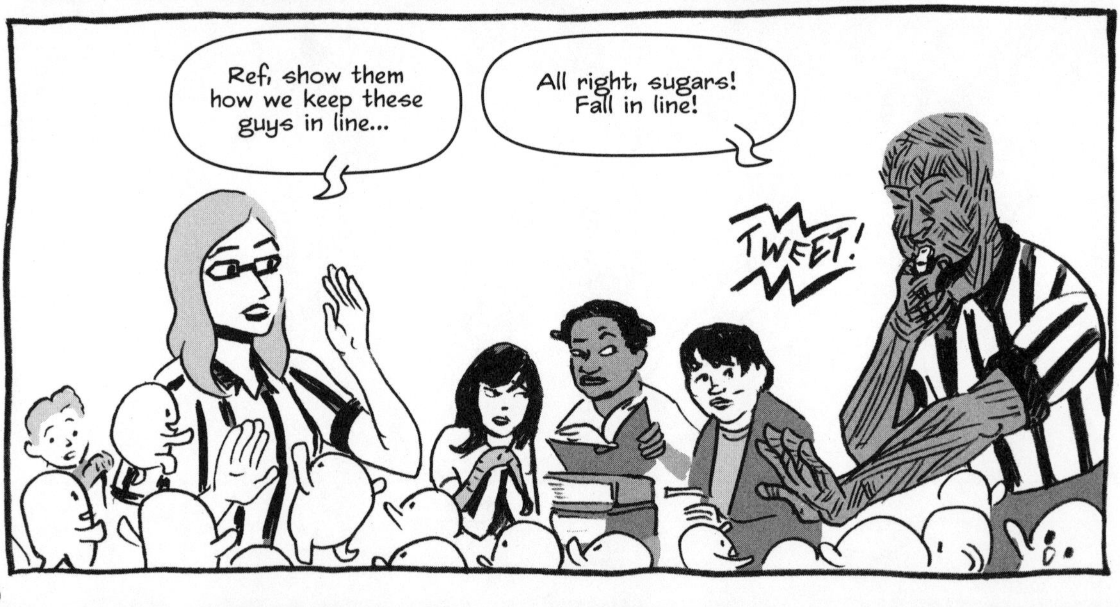
Ref, show them how we keep these guys in line...
All right, sugars! Fall in line!
TWEET!

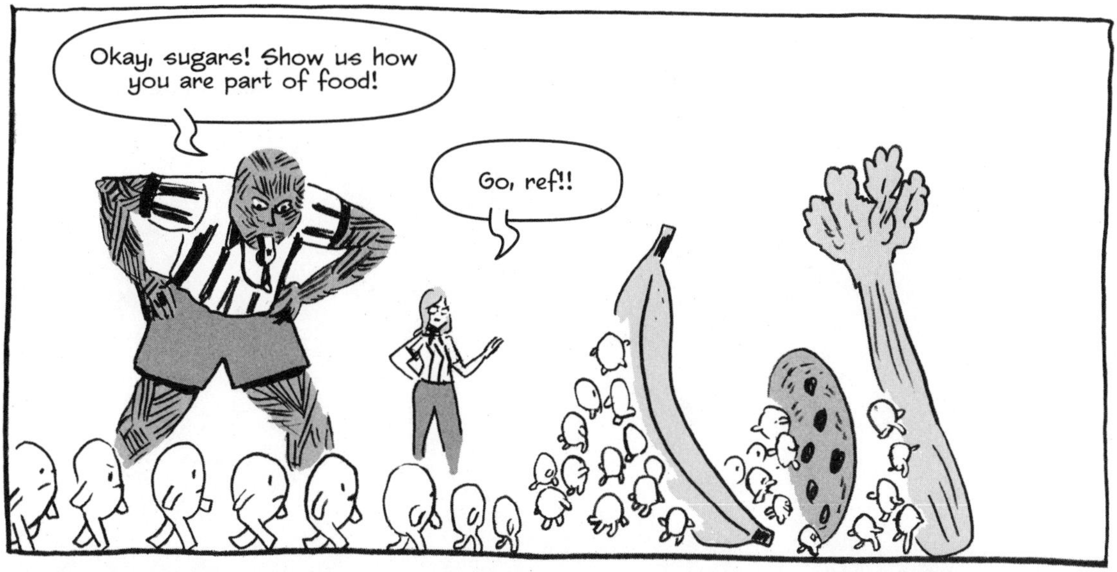
Okay, sugars! Show us how you are part of food!
Go, ref!!

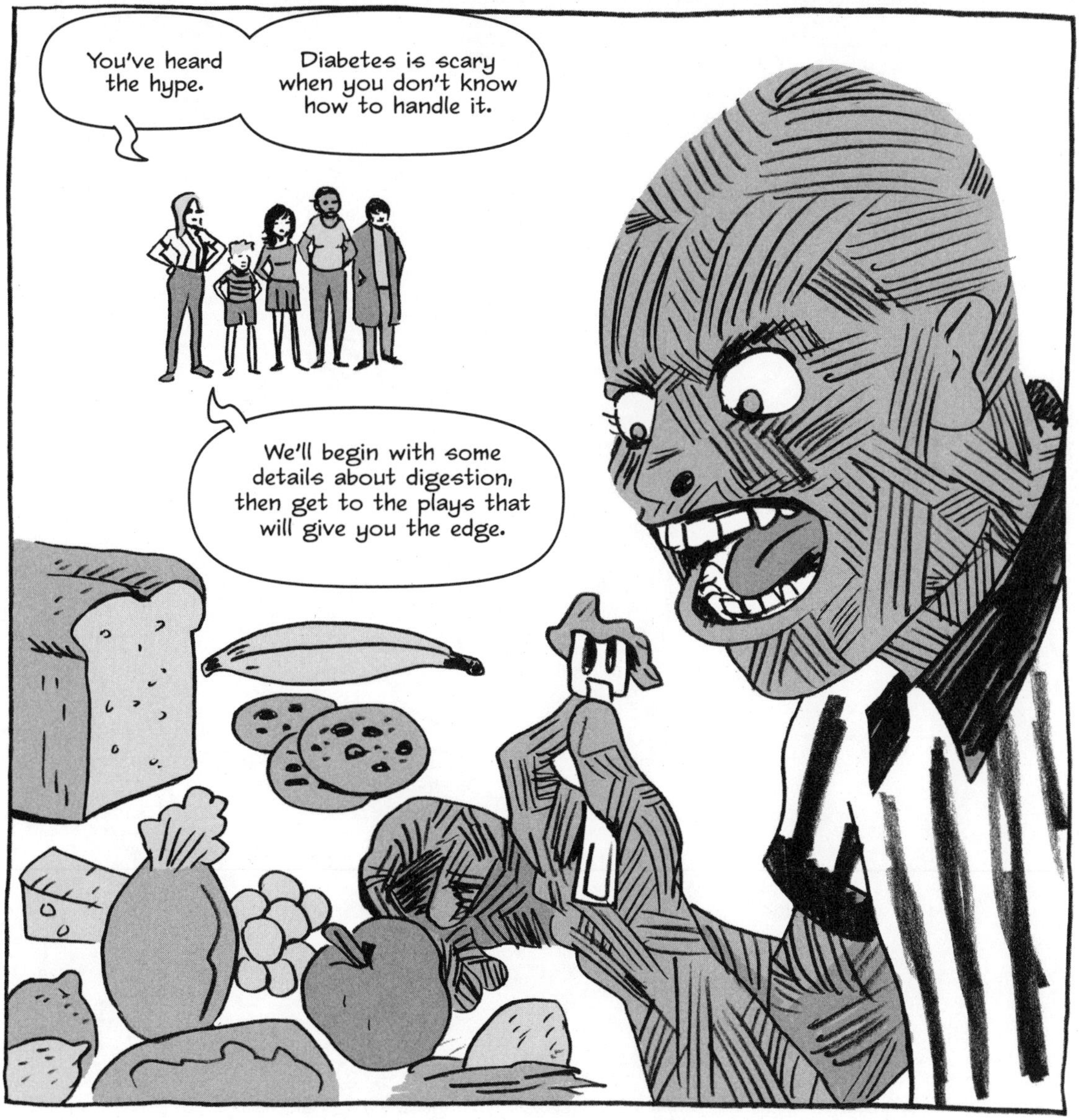
You've heard the hype.
Diabetes is scary when you don't know how to handle it.
We'll begin with some details about digestion, then get to the plays that will give you the edge.

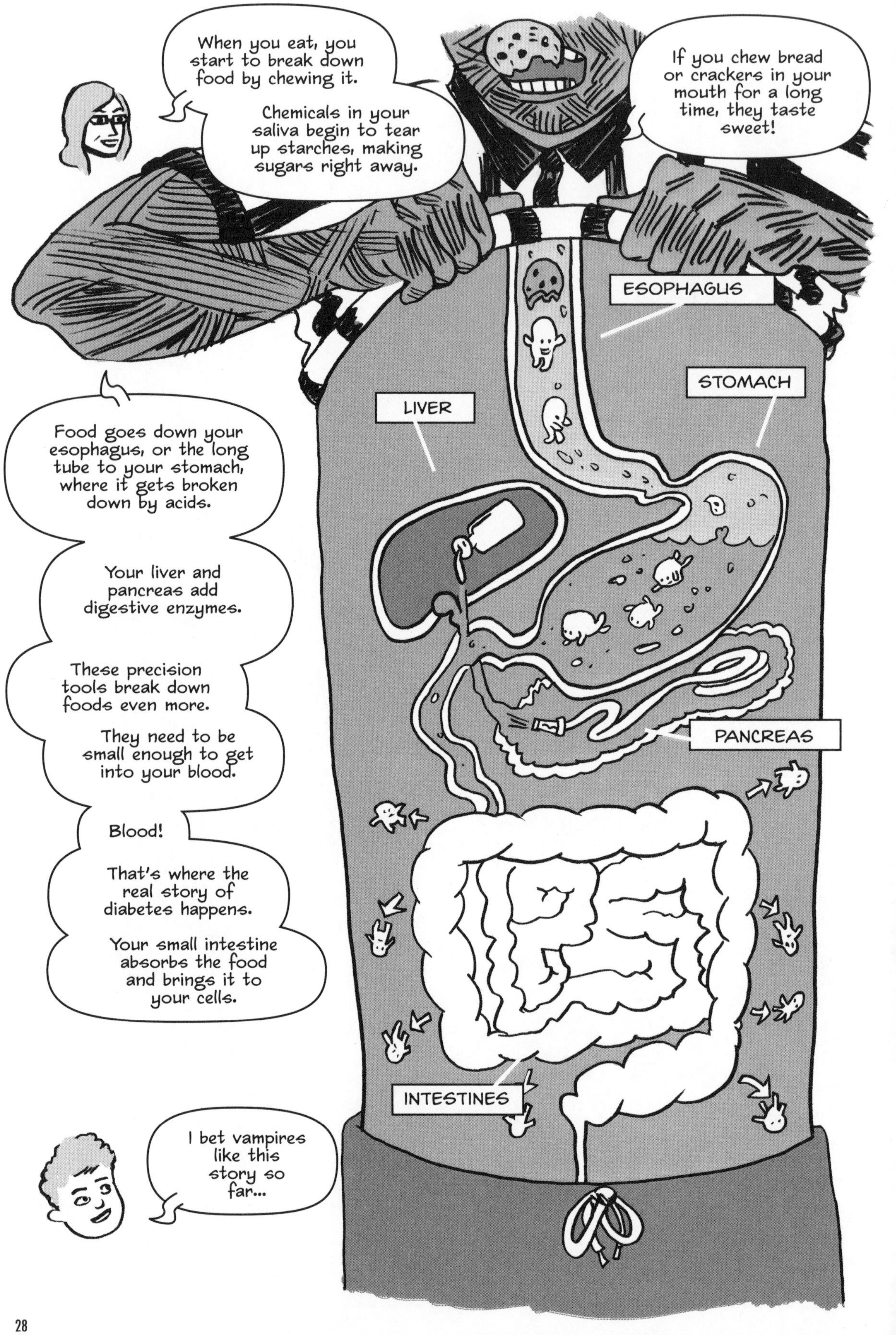
When you eat, you start to break down food by chewing it.
Chemicals in your saliva begin to tear up starches, making sugars right away.
If you chew bread or crackers in your mouth for a long time, they taste sweet!
ESOPHAGUS
STOMACH
LIVER
Food goes down your esophagus, or the long tube to your stomach, where it gets broken down by acids.
Your liver and pancreas add digestive enzymes.
These precision tools break down foods even more.
They need to be small enough to get into your blood.
Blood!
That's where the real story of diabetes happens.
Your small intestine absorbs the food and brings it to your cells.
PANCREAS
INTESTINES
I bet vampires like this story so far...

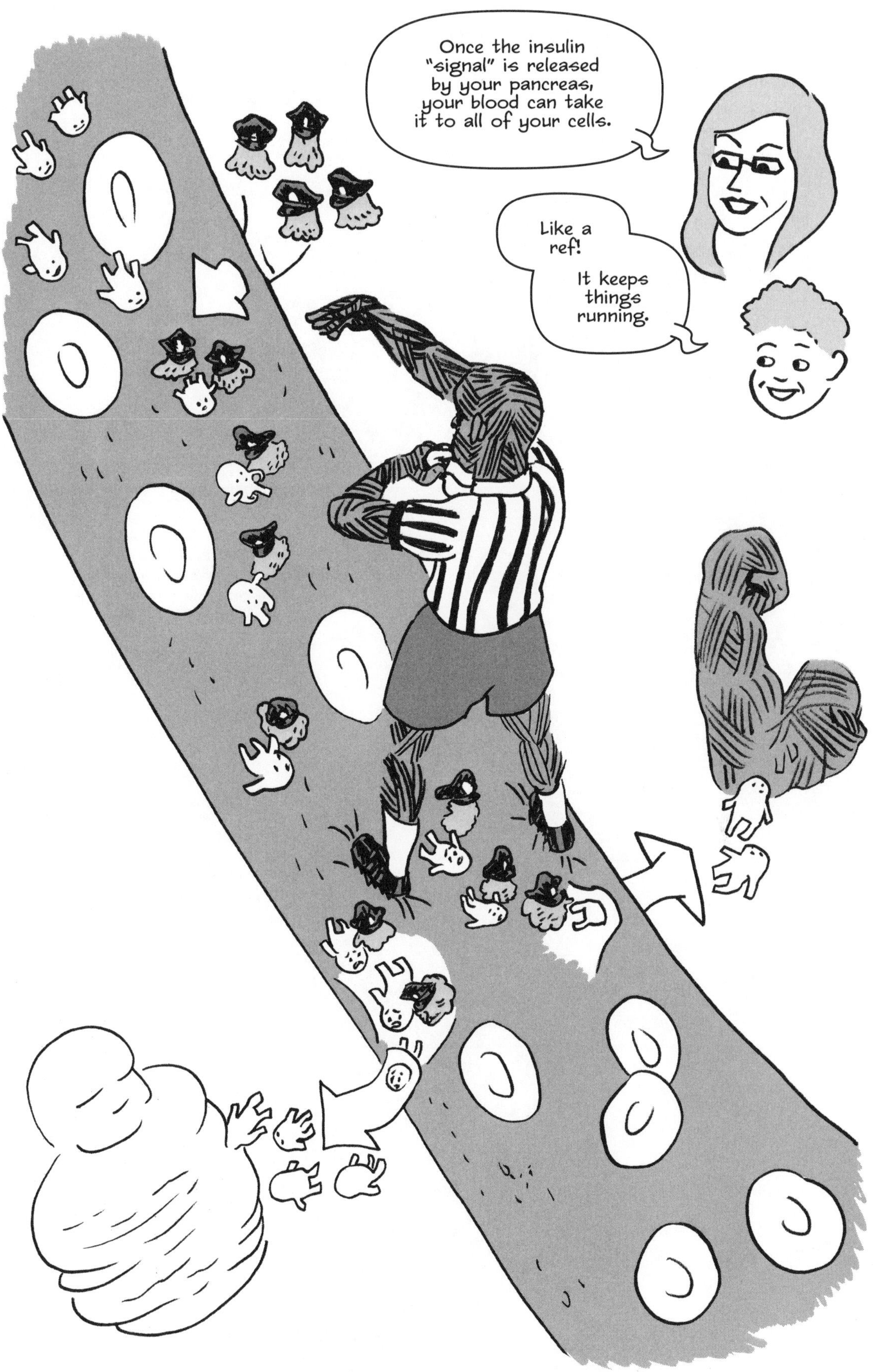

Once the insulin "signal" is released by your pancreas, your blood can take it to all of your cells.
Like a ref!
It keeps things running.

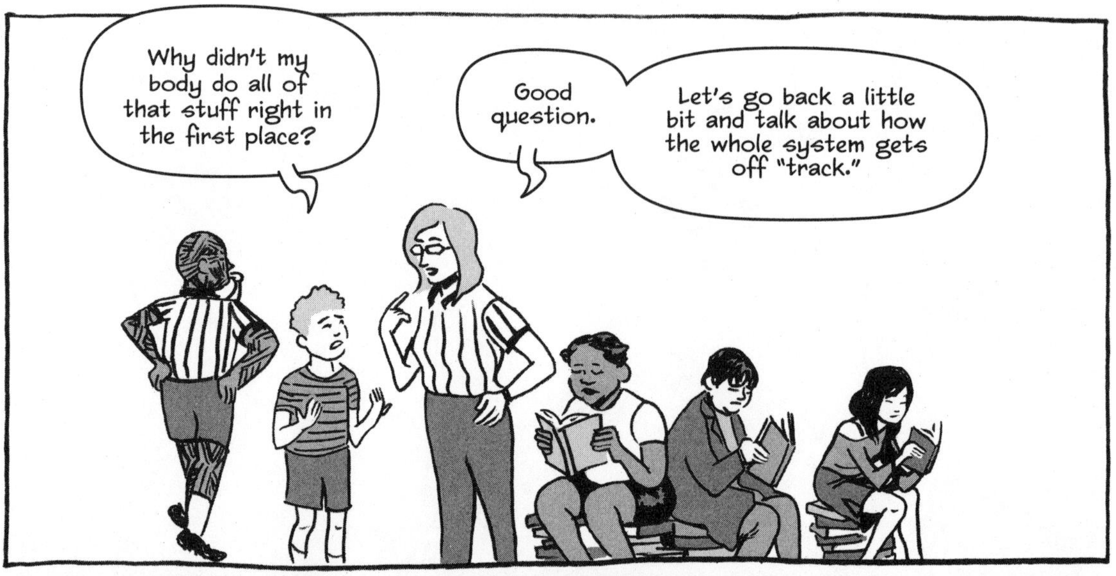
Why didn't my body do all of that stuff right in the first place?
Good question.
Let's go back a little bit and talk about how the whole system gets off "track."

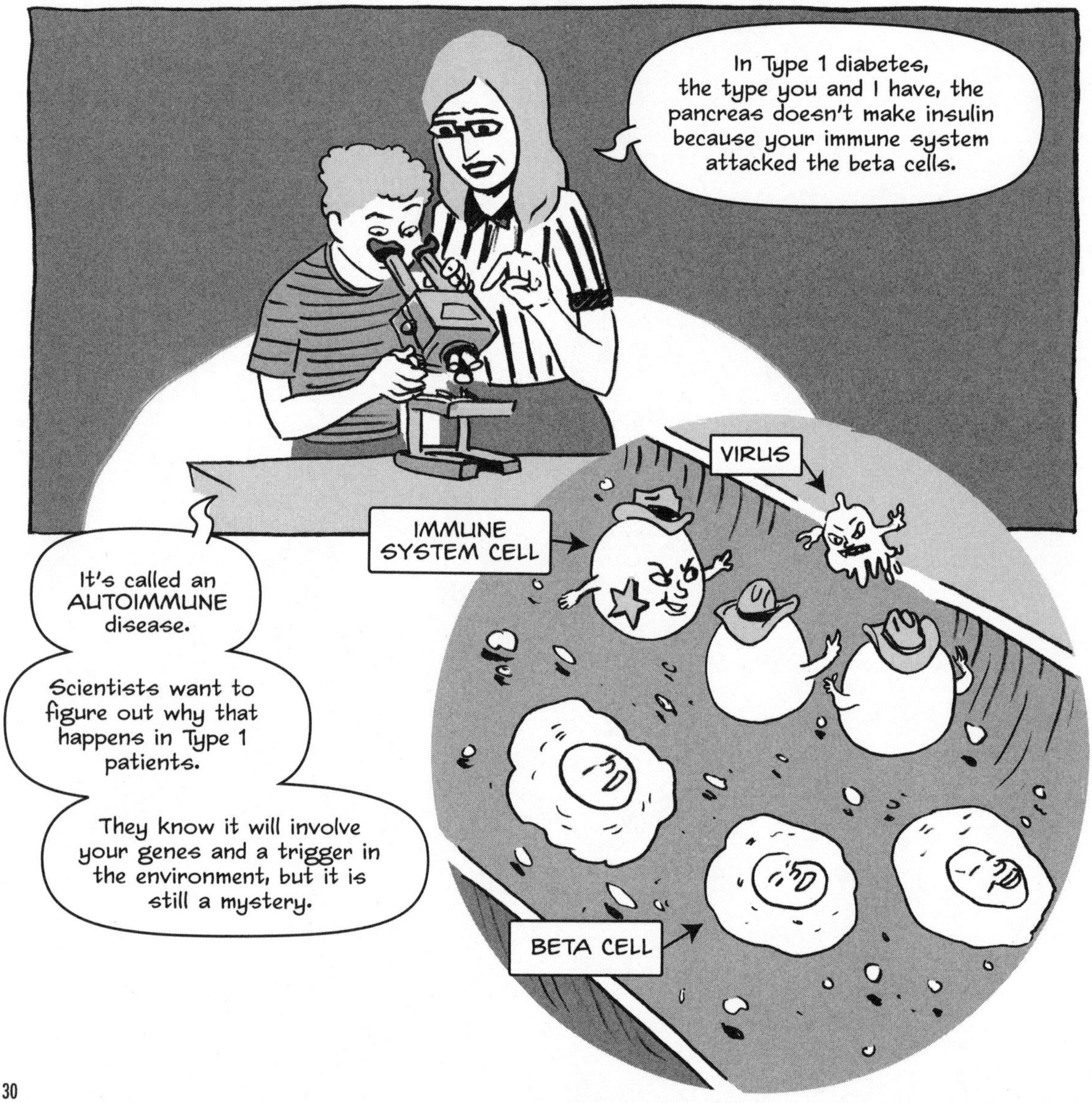
In Type 1 diabetes, the type you and I have, the pancreas doesn't make insulin because your immune system attacked the beta cells.
VIRUS
IMMUNE SYSTEM CELL
It's called an AUTOIMMUNE disease.
Scientists want to figure out why that happens in Type 1 patients.
They know it will involve your genes and a trigger in the environment, but it is still a mystery.
BETA CELL

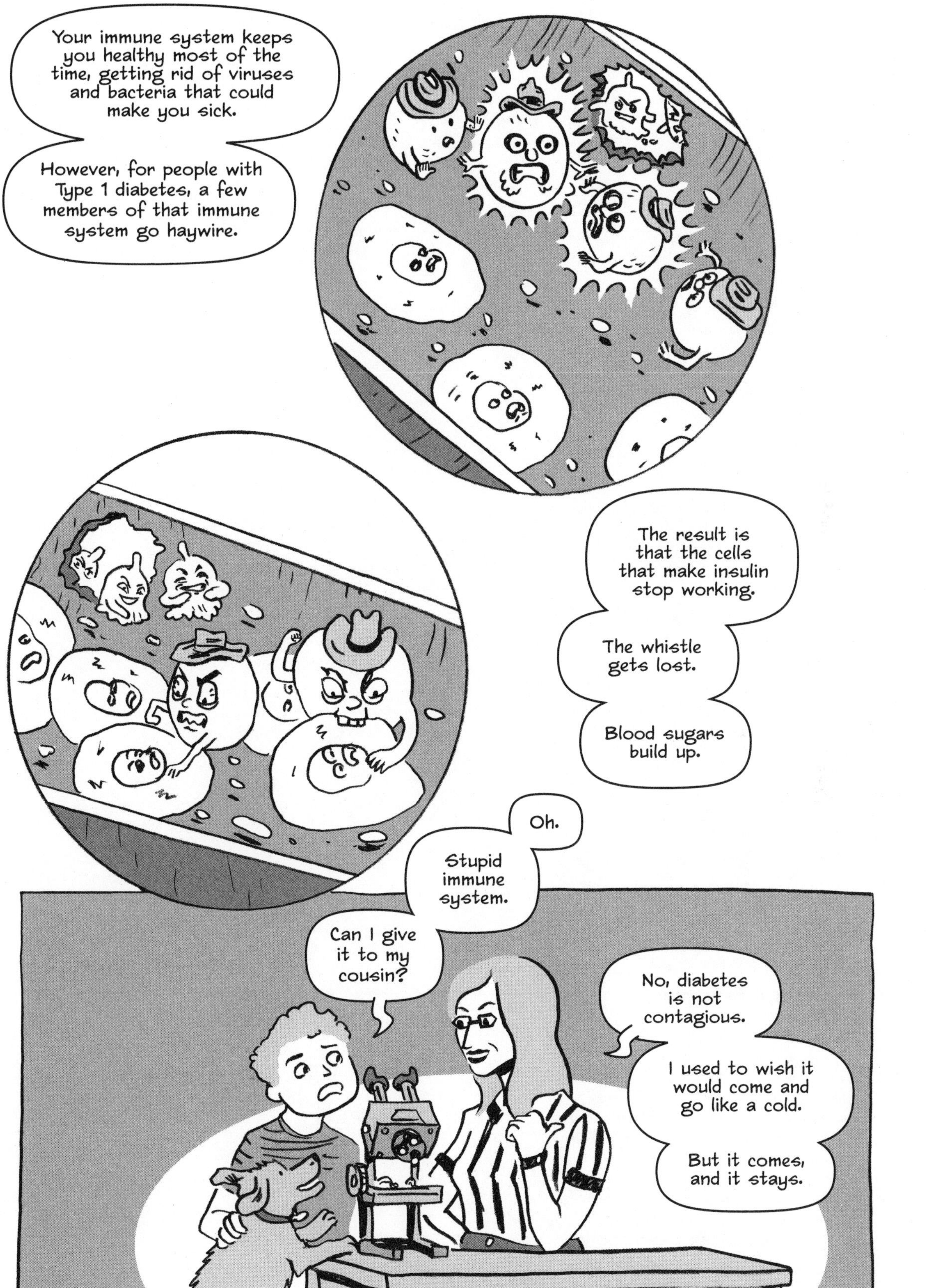
Your immune system keeps you healthy most of the time, getting rid of viruses and bacteria that could make you sick.
However, for people with Type 1 diabetes, a few members of that immune system go haywire.
The result is that the cells that make insulin stop working.
The whistle gets lost.
Blood sugars build up.
Oh.
Stupid immune system.
Can I give it to my cousin?
No, diabetes is not contagious.
I used to wish it would come and go like a cold.
But it comes, and it stays.

I know how you feel.
Your body isn't stupid, though.
It just lost a whistle.
Blocking the buildup of sugars with diet, exercise, and insulin is like getting the whistle back.

BANTING
Okay, so in order to balance my blood I have to know all about insulin.
I don't even know who figured out all this stuff.
Everyone knows about Pelé and Mia Hamm, but not whoever came up with insulin!

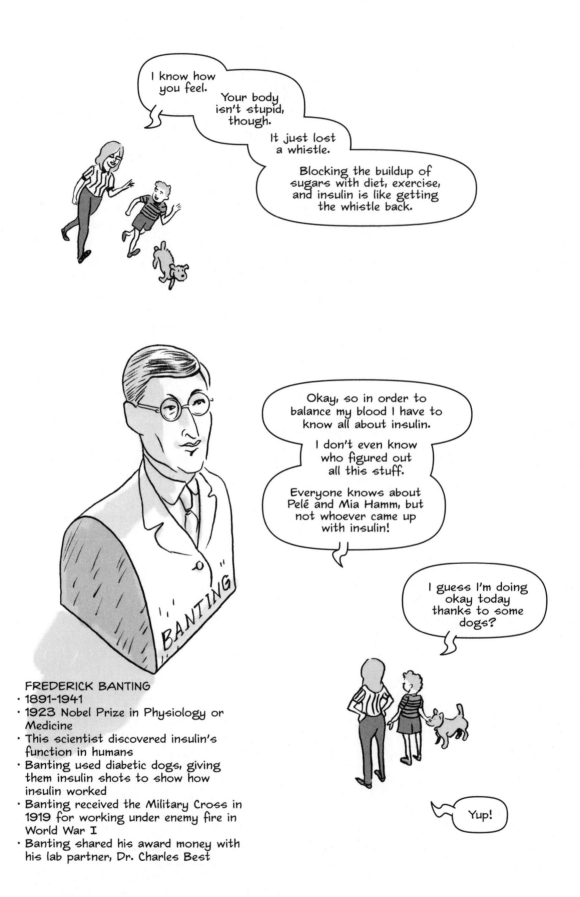

FREDERICK BANTING

- 1891–1941
- 1923 Nobel Prize in Physiology or Medicine
- This scientist discovered insulin's function in humans
- Banting used diabetic dogs, giving them insulin shots to show how insulin worked
- Banting received the Military Cross in 1919 for working under enemy fire in World War I
- Banting shared his award money with his lab partner, Dr. Charles Best

I guess I'm doing okay today thanks to some dogs?
Yup!

FREDERICK SANGER

- 1918–
- 1958 and 1980 Nobel Prize in Chemistry
- Figured out the sequence of the protein insulin, helping doctors begin to learn how to make human insulin for people with diabetes around the world
- Boating enthusiast
- Peace activist
- Declined a knighthood because he didn't like being called "sir"!

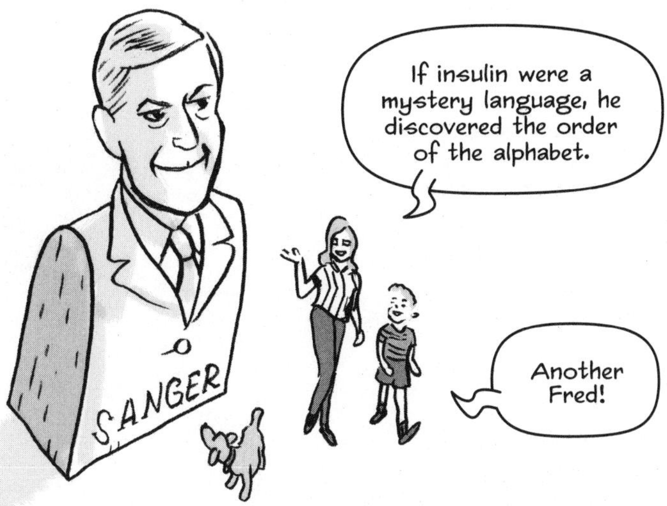

SANGER

> If insulin were a mystery language, he discovered the order of the alphabet.

> Another Fred!

DOROTHY CROWFOOT HODGKIN

- 1910–1994
- Was born in Egypt and spent many years in Sudan
- Started studying crystals when she was 10!
- In 1969, Dr. Hodgkin discovered the structure of the insulin molecule, using techniques that earned her the Nobel Prize in Chemistry
- Dr. Hodgkin used X-ray crystallography to discover the structure of complicated molecules like insulin and vitamin B_{12}

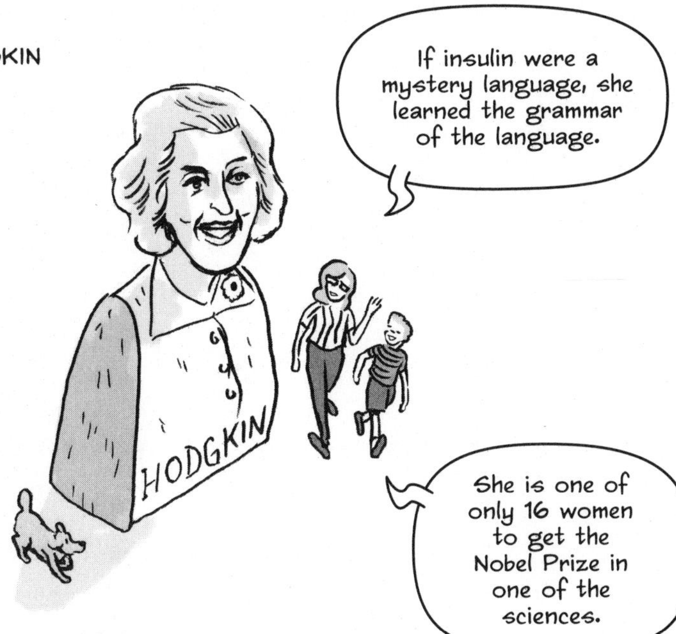

HODGKIN

> If insulin were a mystery language, she learned the grammar of the language.

> She is one of only 16 women to get the Nobel Prize in one of the sciences.

> Your first experience as a diabetic may have been finding out why you felt bad.

> When I was diagnosed, my vision was blurry, and I lost a lot of weight.

> My visit to the doctor was a tough day.

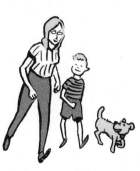

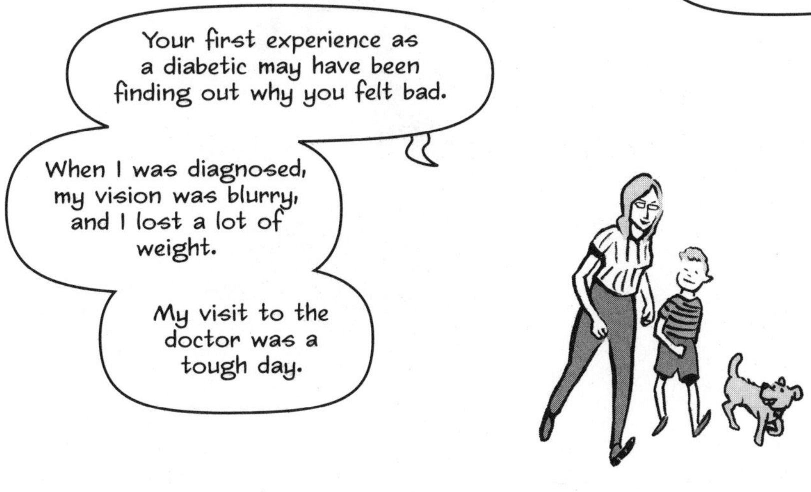

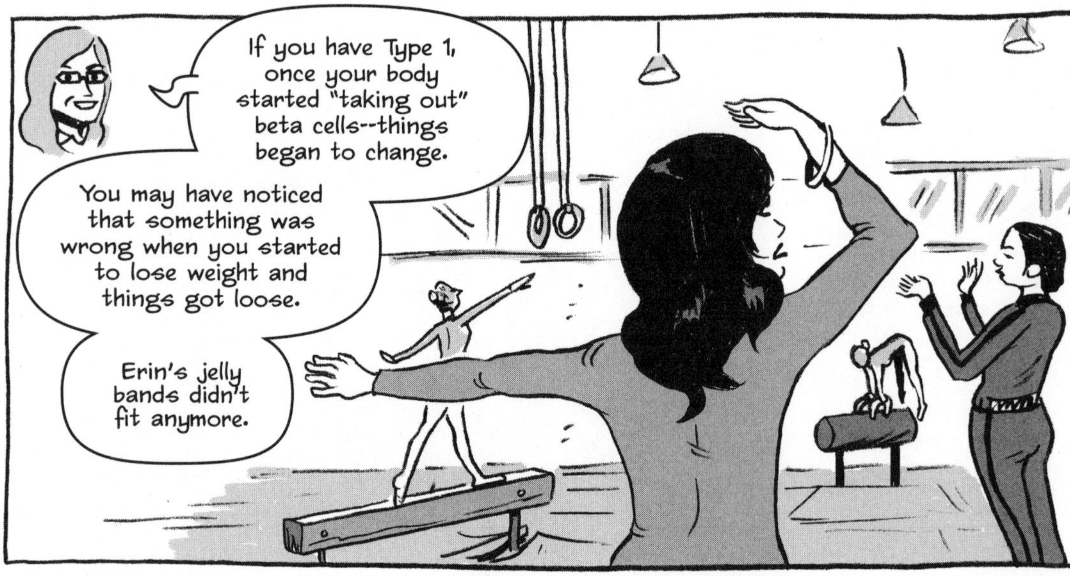
If you have Type 1, once your body started "taking out" beta cells--things began to change.
You may have noticed that something was wrong when you started to lose weight and things got loose.
Erin's jelly bands didn't fit anymore.

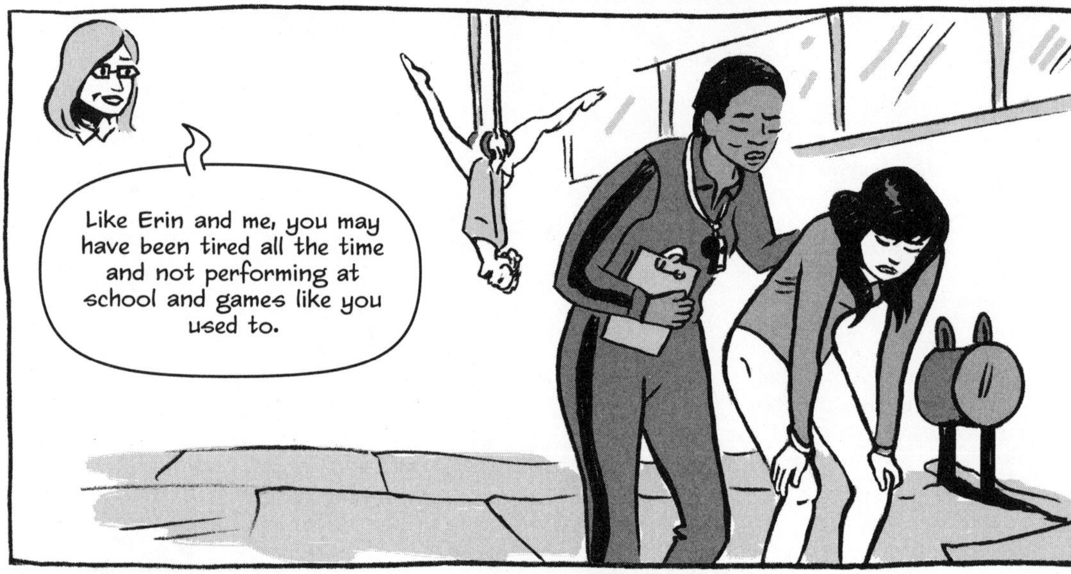
Like Erin and me, you may have been tired all the time and not performing at school and games like you used to.

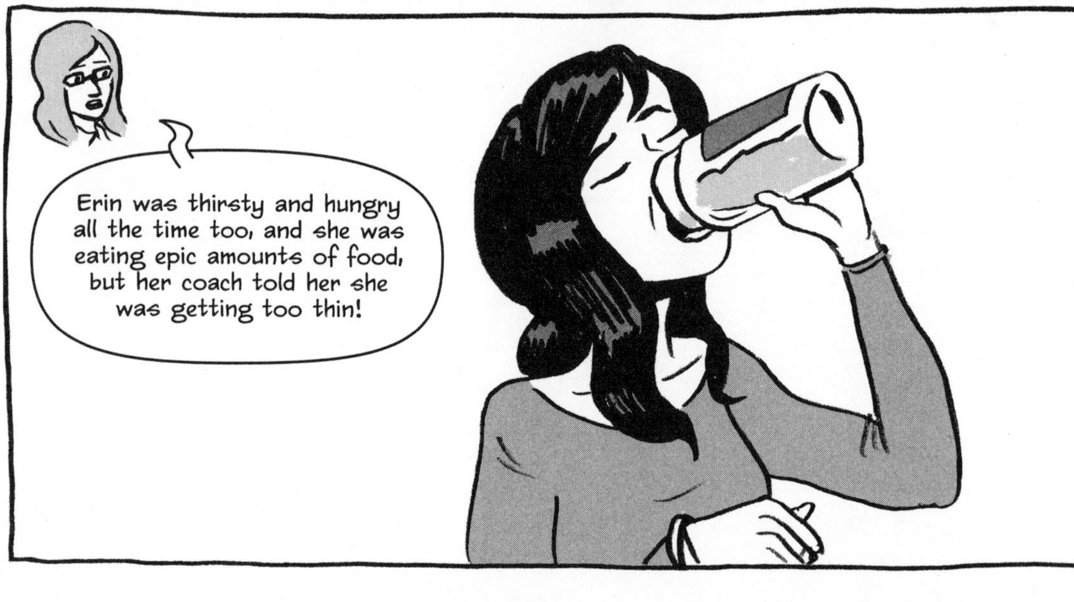
Erin was thirsty and hungry all the time too, and she was eating epic amounts of food, but her coach told her she was getting too thin!

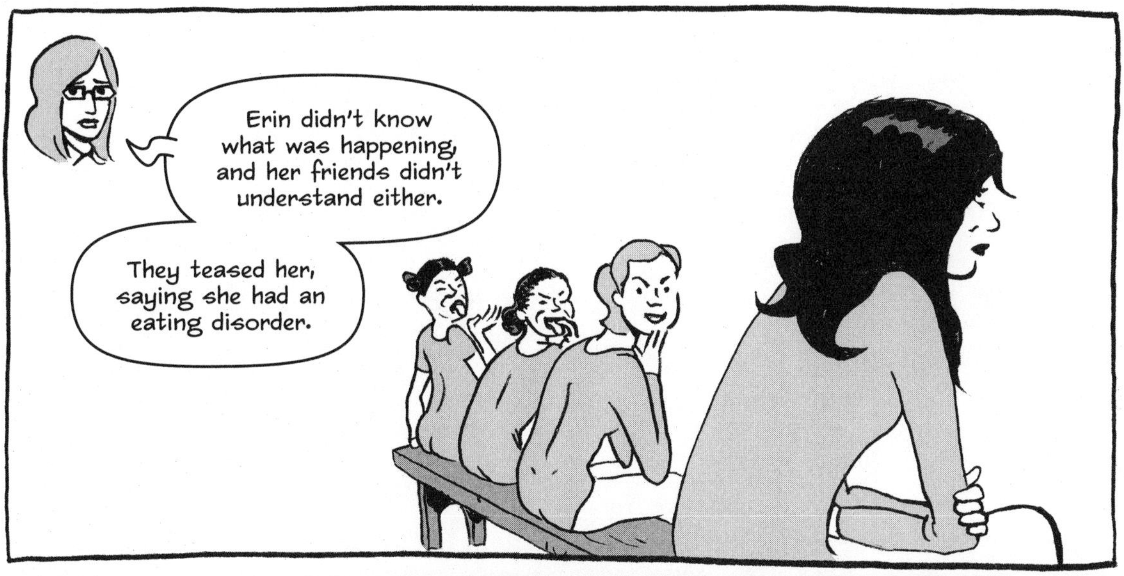
Erin didn't know what was happening, and her friends didn't understand either.
They teased her, saying she had an eating disorder.

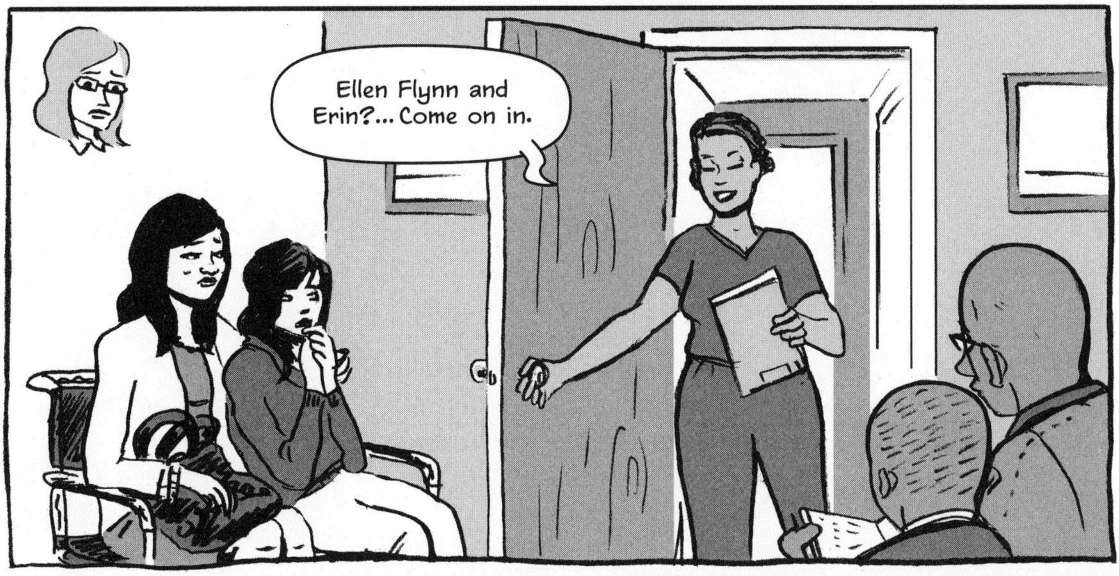
Ellen Flynn and Erin?... Come on in.

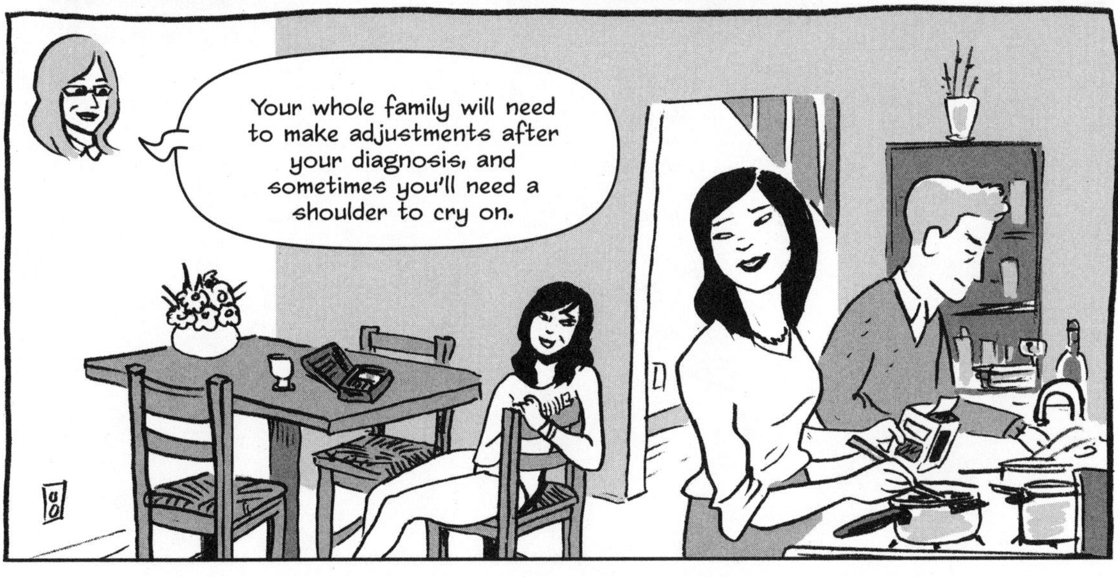
Your whole family will need to make adjustments after your diagnosis, and sometimes you'll need a shoulder to cry on.

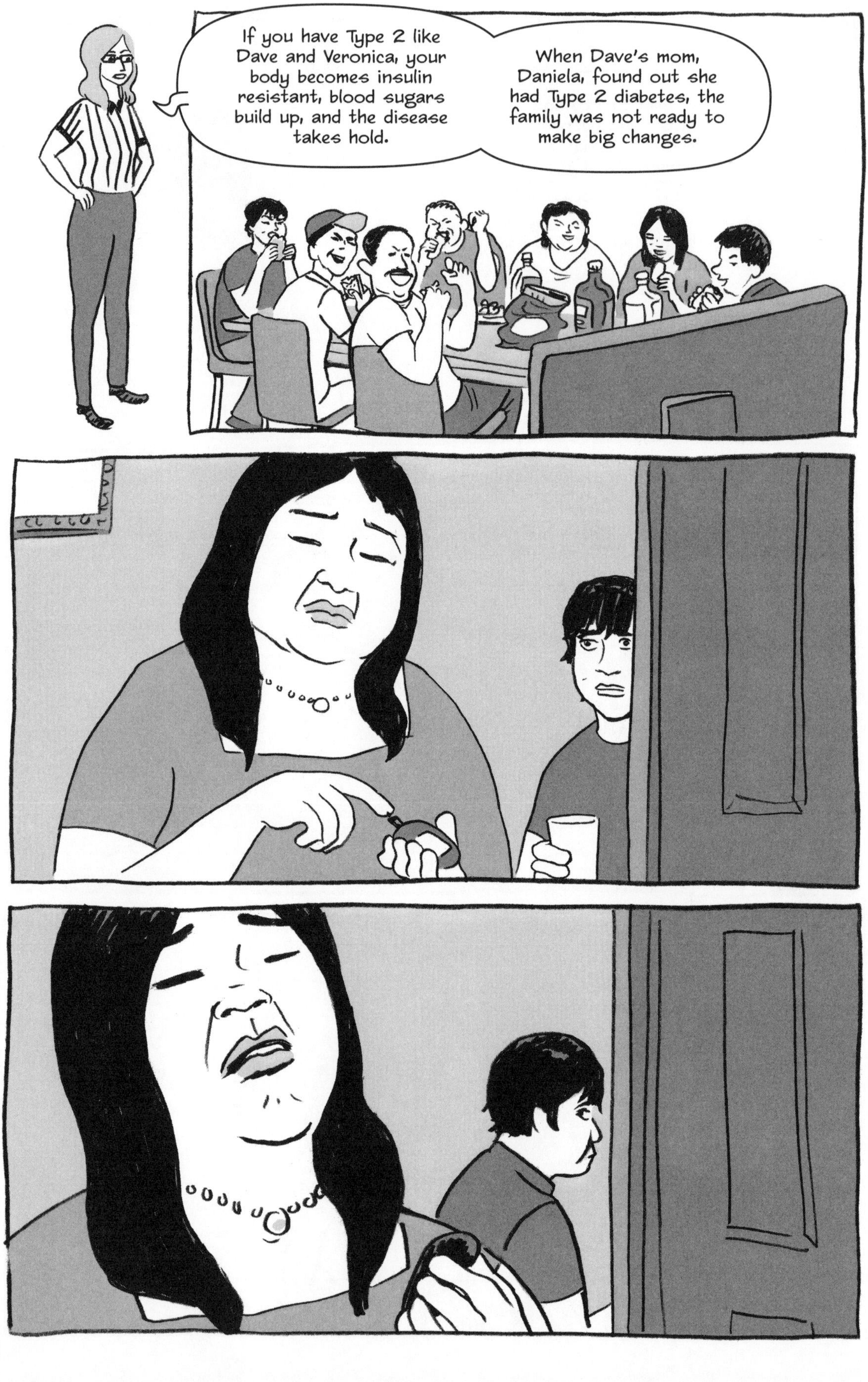
If you have Type 2 like Dave and Veronica, your body becomes insulin resistant, blood sugars build up, and the disease takes hold.
When Dave's mom, Daniela, found out she had Type 2 diabetes, the family was not ready to make big changes.

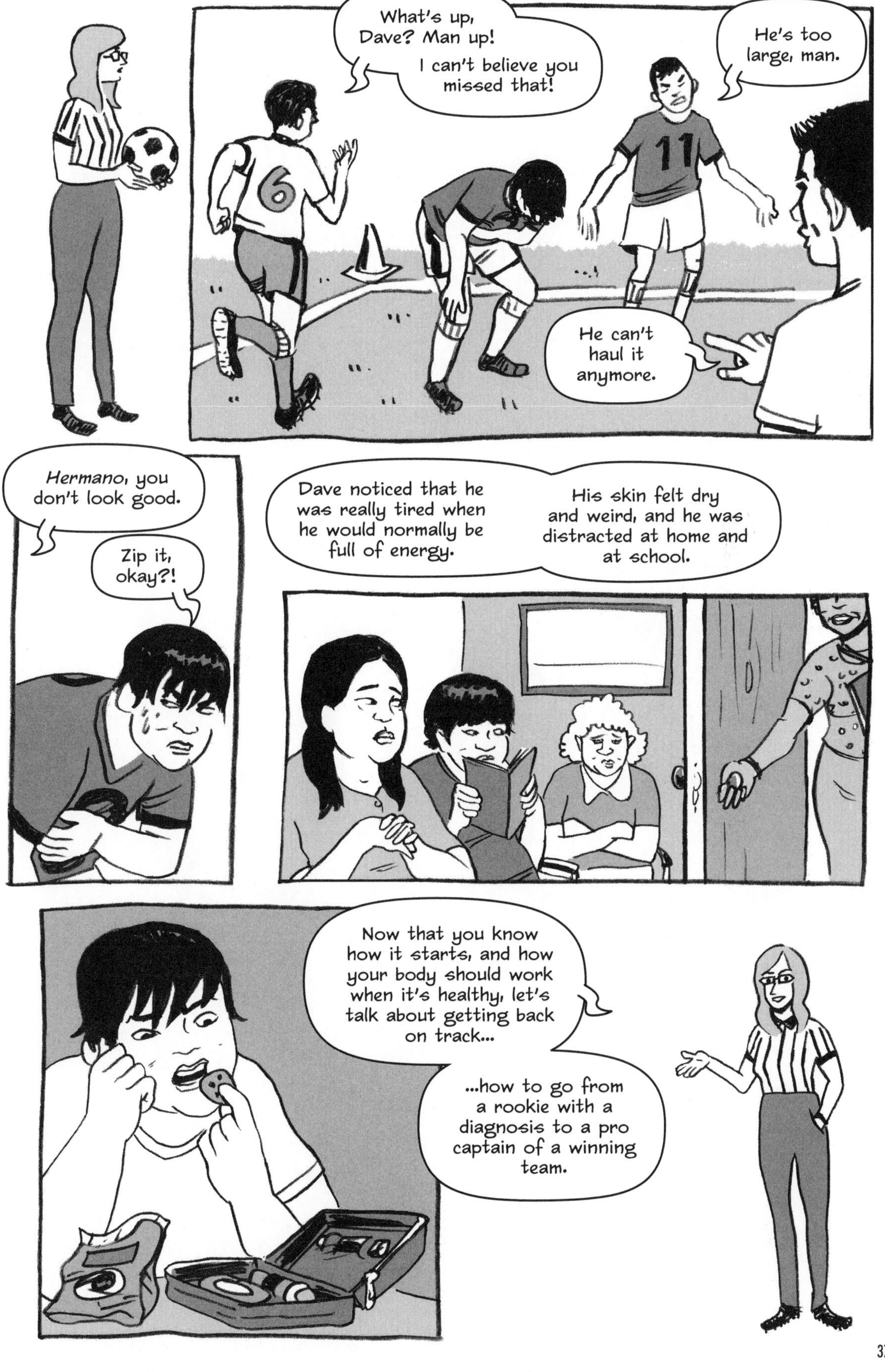
What's up, Dave? Man up!
I can't believe you missed that!
He's too large, man.
He can't haul it anymore.
Hermano, you don't look good.
Zip it, okay?!
Dave noticed that he was really tired when he would normally be full of energy.
His skin felt dry and weird, and he was distracted at home and at school.
Now that you know how it starts, and how your body should work when it's healthy, let's talk about getting back on track...
...how to go from a rookie with a diagnosis to a pro captain of a winning team.
11
6

PART TWO: YOUR TEAM

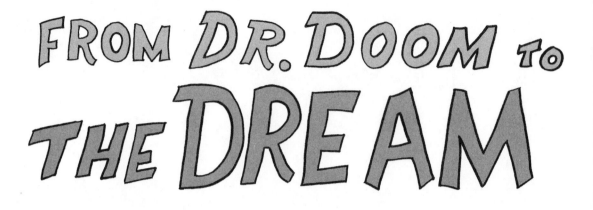

FROM DR. DOOM to THE DREAM

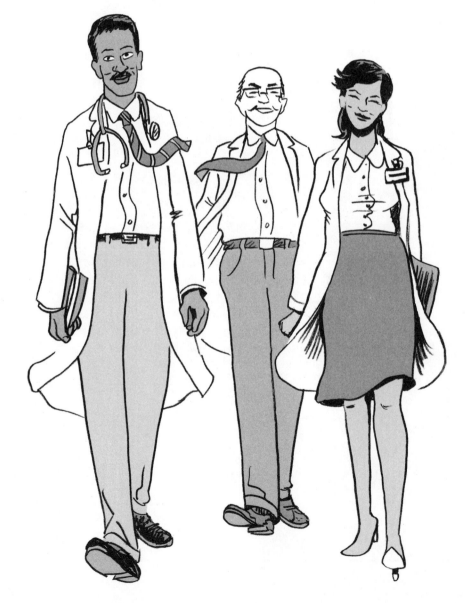

TEAM

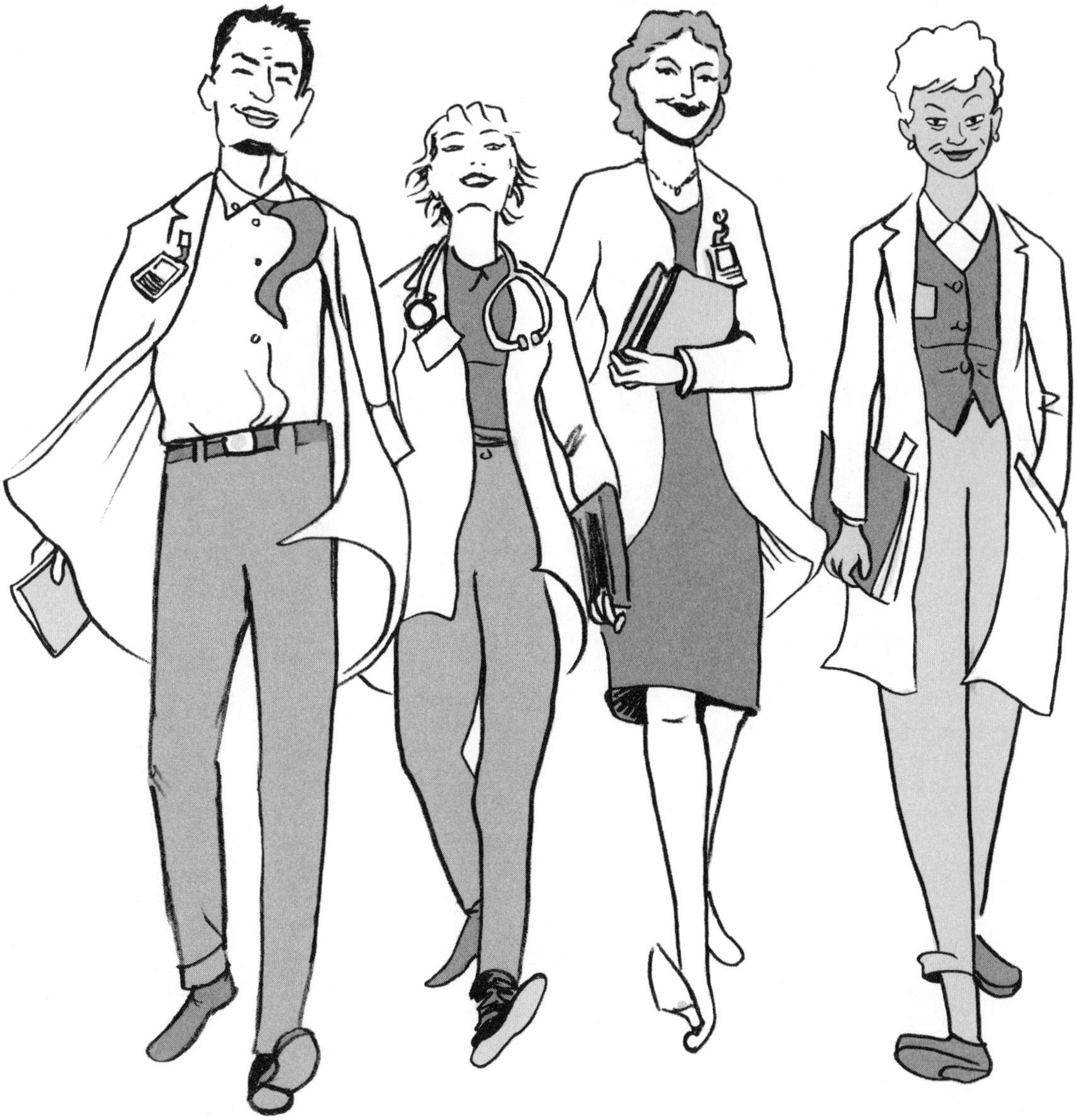

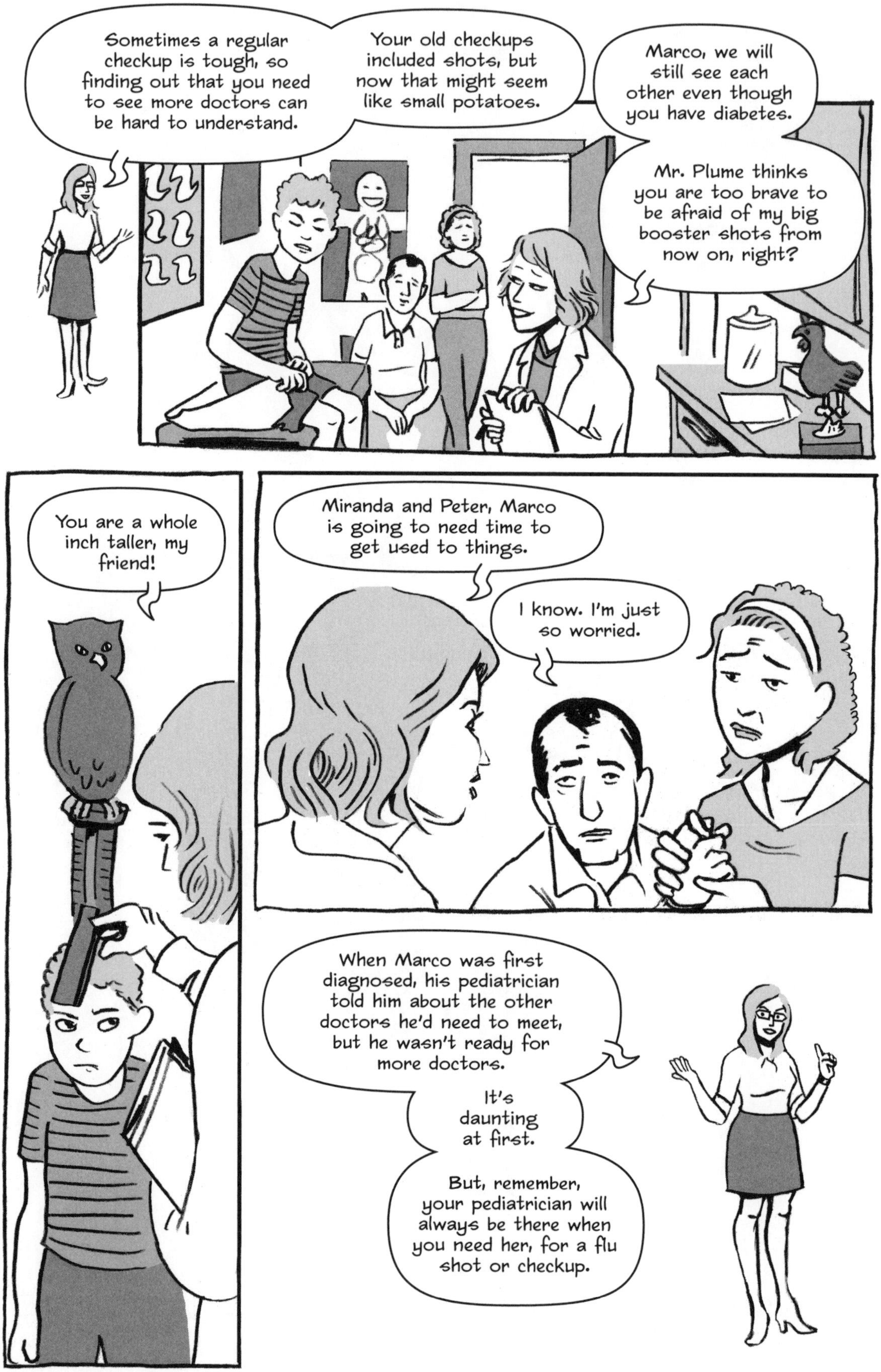
Sometimes a regular checkup is tough, so finding out that you need to see more doctors can be hard to understand.
Your old checkups included shots, but now that might seem like small potatoes.
Marco, we will still see each other even though you have diabetes.
Mr. Plume thinks you are too brave to be afraid of my big booster shots from now on, right?
You are a whole inch taller, my friend!
Miranda and Peter, Marco is going to need time to get used to things.
I know. I'm just so worried.
When Marco was first diagnosed, his pediatrician told him about the other doctors he'd need to meet, but he wasn't ready for more doctors.
It's daunting at first.
But, remember, your pediatrician will always be there when you need her, for a flu shot or checkup.

YOUR PEDIATRICIAN OR INTERNIST

Main Job:
Pediatricians are your first stop for monitoring your growth and health. It is probably your pediatrician who noticed your symptoms.

Years of Training: 10+.

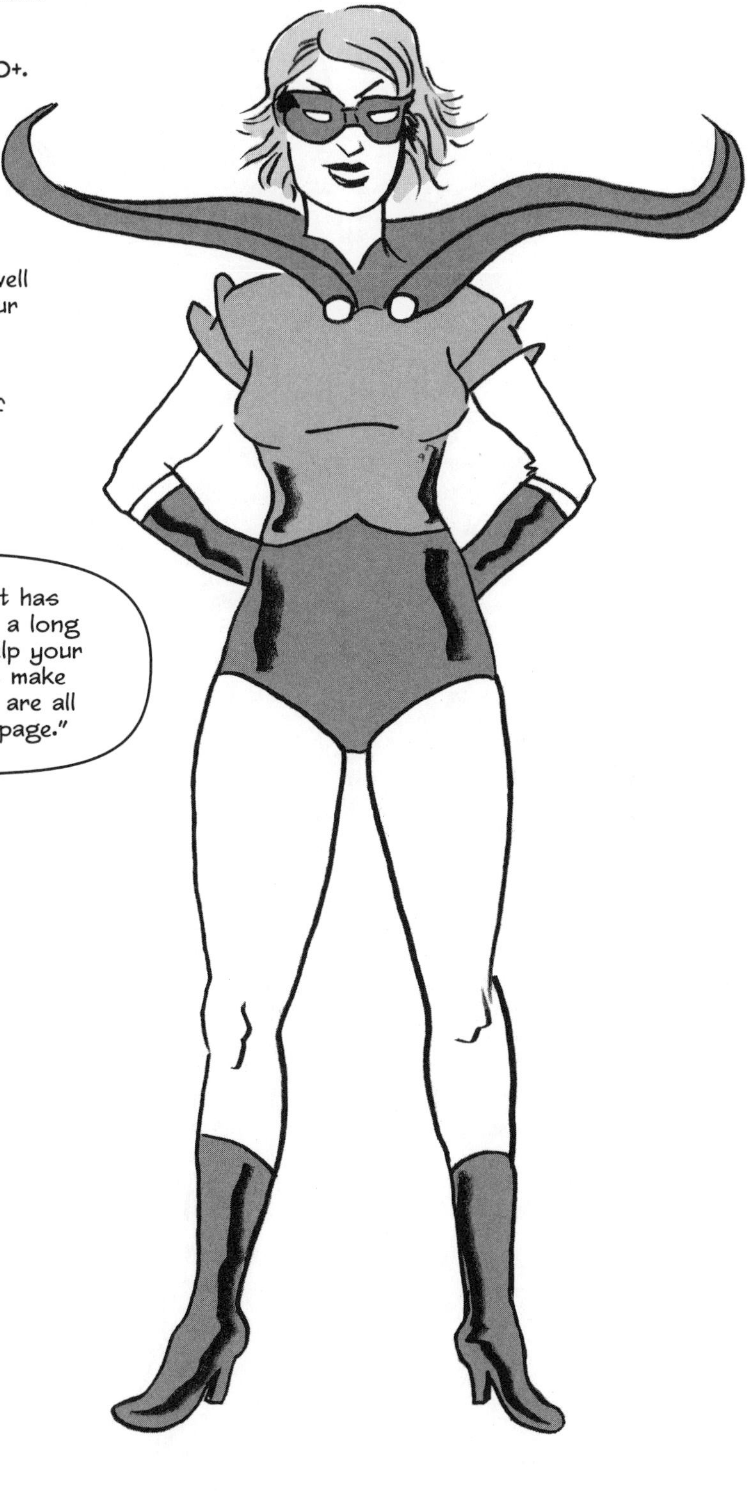

Special Ops:
Keeping the big picture in mind, as well as answering all your parents' questions!

Frequency of Visits:
Once a year, more if illness occurs.

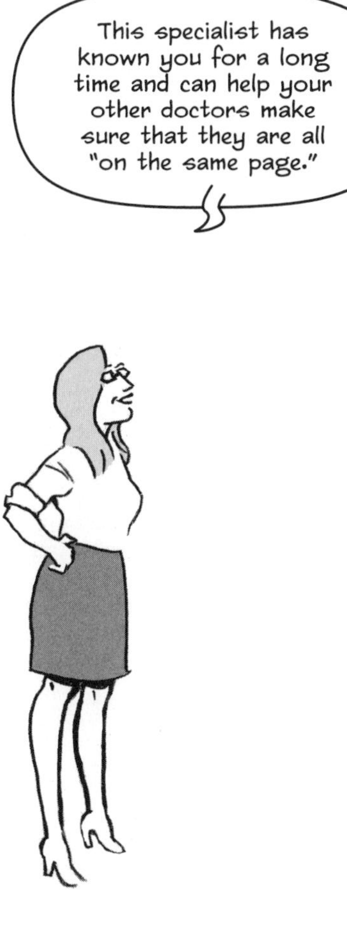
This specialist has known you for a long time and can help your other doctors make sure that they are all "on the same page."

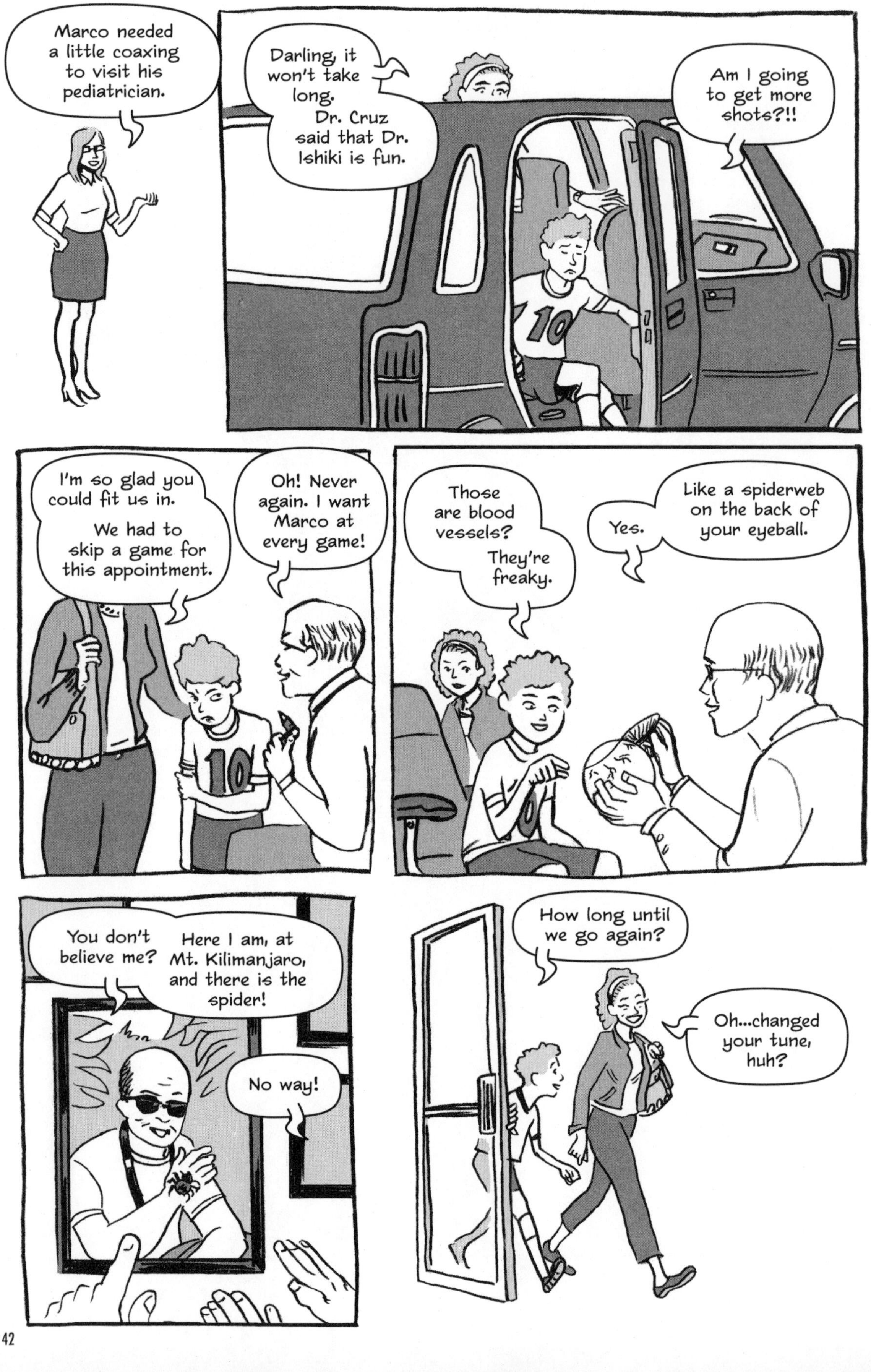
Marco needed a little coaxing to visit his pediatrician.
Darling, it won't take long.
Dr. Cruz said that Dr. Ishiki is fun.
Am I going to get more shots?!!
I'm so glad you could fit us in.
We had to skip a game for this appointment.
Oh! Never again. I want Marco at every game!
Those are blood vessels?
They're freaky.
Yes.
Like a spiderweb on the back of your eyeball.
You don't believe me?
Here I am, at Mt. Kilimanjaro, and there is the spider!
No way!
How long until we go again?
Oh...changed your tune, huh?

YOUR ENDOCRINOLOGIST

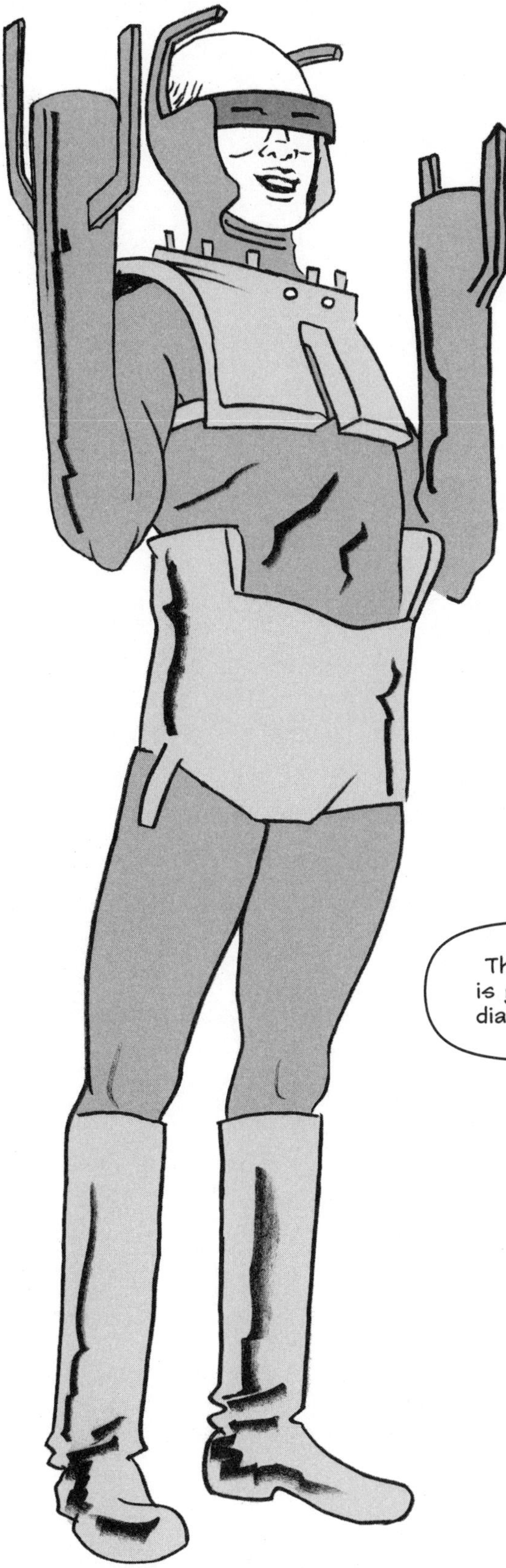

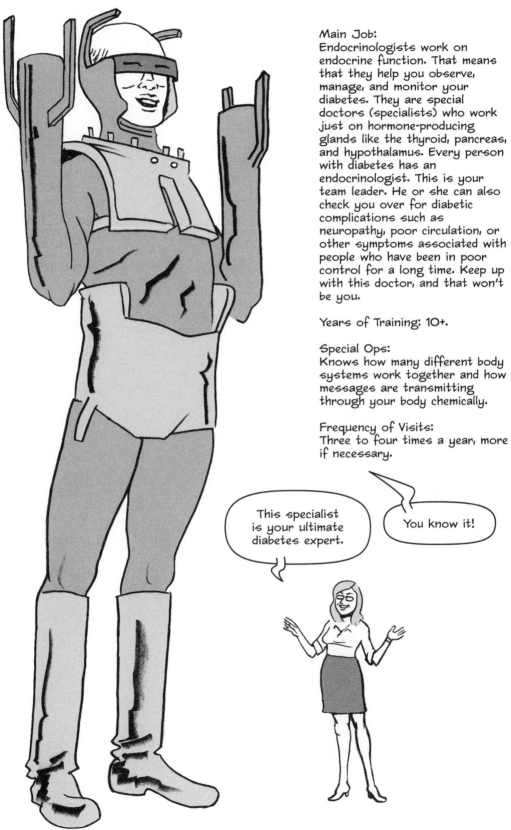

Main Job:
Endocrinologists work on endocrine function. That means that they help you observe, manage, and monitor your diabetes. They are special doctors (specialists) who work just on hormone-producing glands like the thyroid, pancreas, and hypothalamus. Every person with diabetes has an endocrinologist. This is your team leader. He or she can also check you over for diabetic complications such as neuropathy, poor circulation, or other symptoms associated with people who have been in poor control for a long time. Keep up with this doctor, and that won't be you.

Years of Training: 10+.

Special Ops:
Knows how many different body systems work together and how messages are transmitting through your body chemically.

Frequency of Visits:
Three to four times a year, more if necessary.

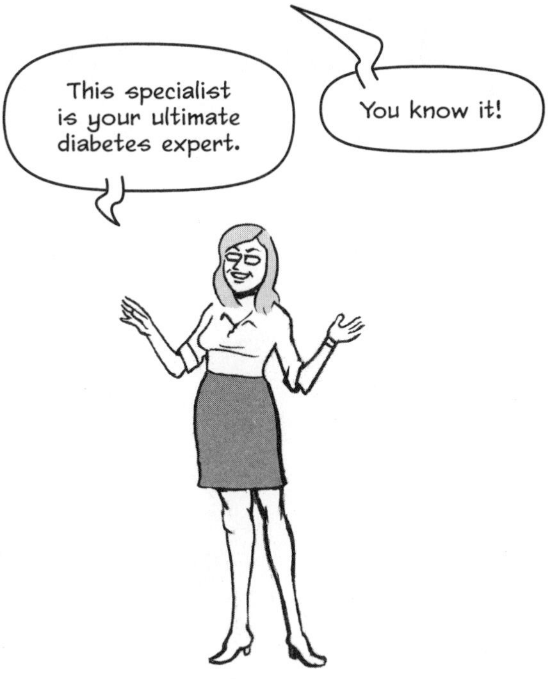
This specialist is your ultimate diabetes expert.
You know it!

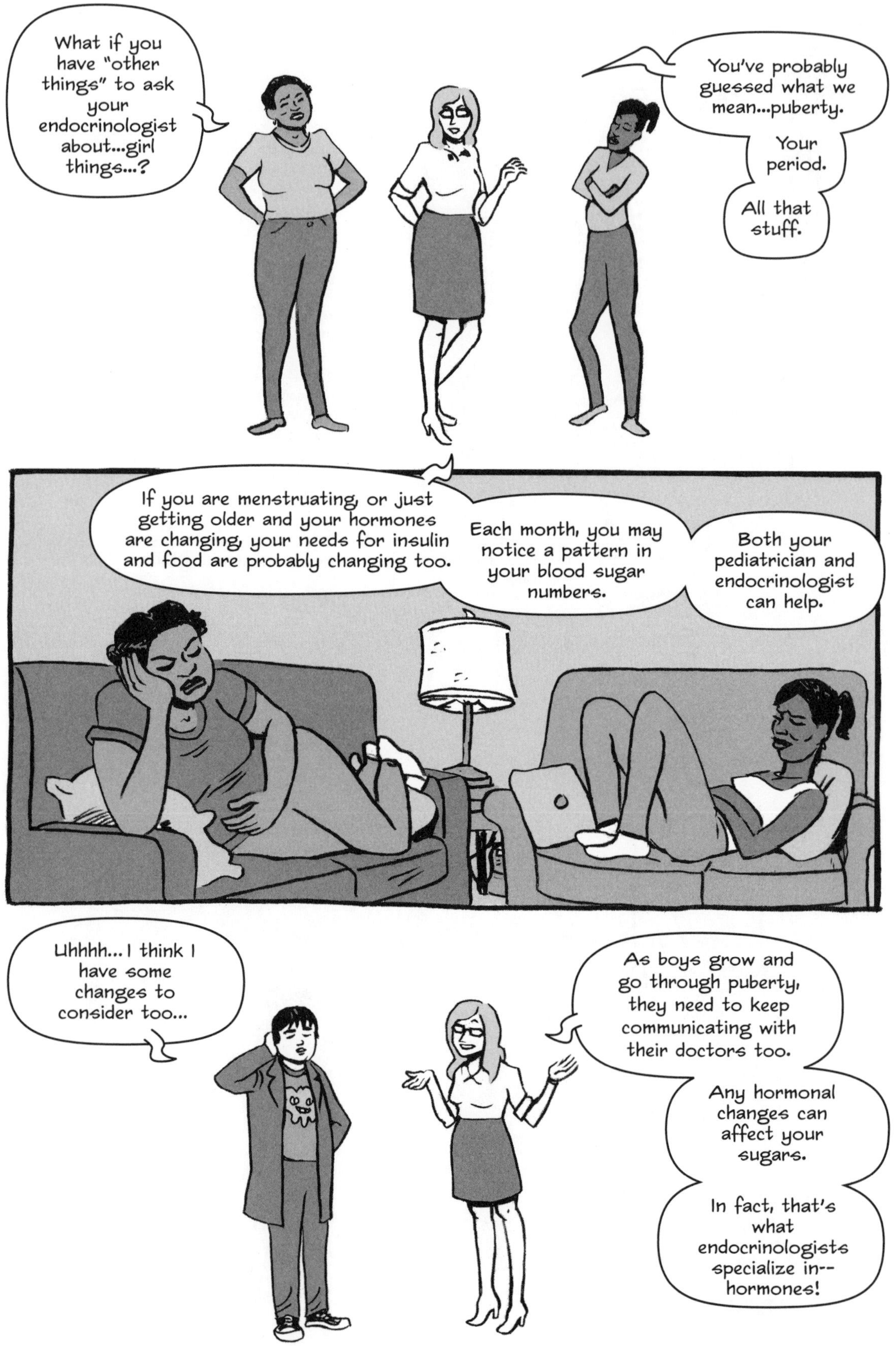

What if you have "other things" to ask your endocrinologist about...girl things...?
You've probably guessed what we mean...puberty.
Your period.
All that stuff.
If you are menstruating, or just getting older and your hormones are changing, your needs for insulin and food are probably changing too.
Each month, you may notice a pattern in your blood sugar numbers.
Both your pediatrician and endocrinologist can help.
Uhhhh... I think I have some changes to consider too...
As boys grow and go through puberty, they need to keep communicating with their doctors too.
Any hormonal changes can affect your sugars.
In fact, that's what endocrinologists specialize in--hormones!

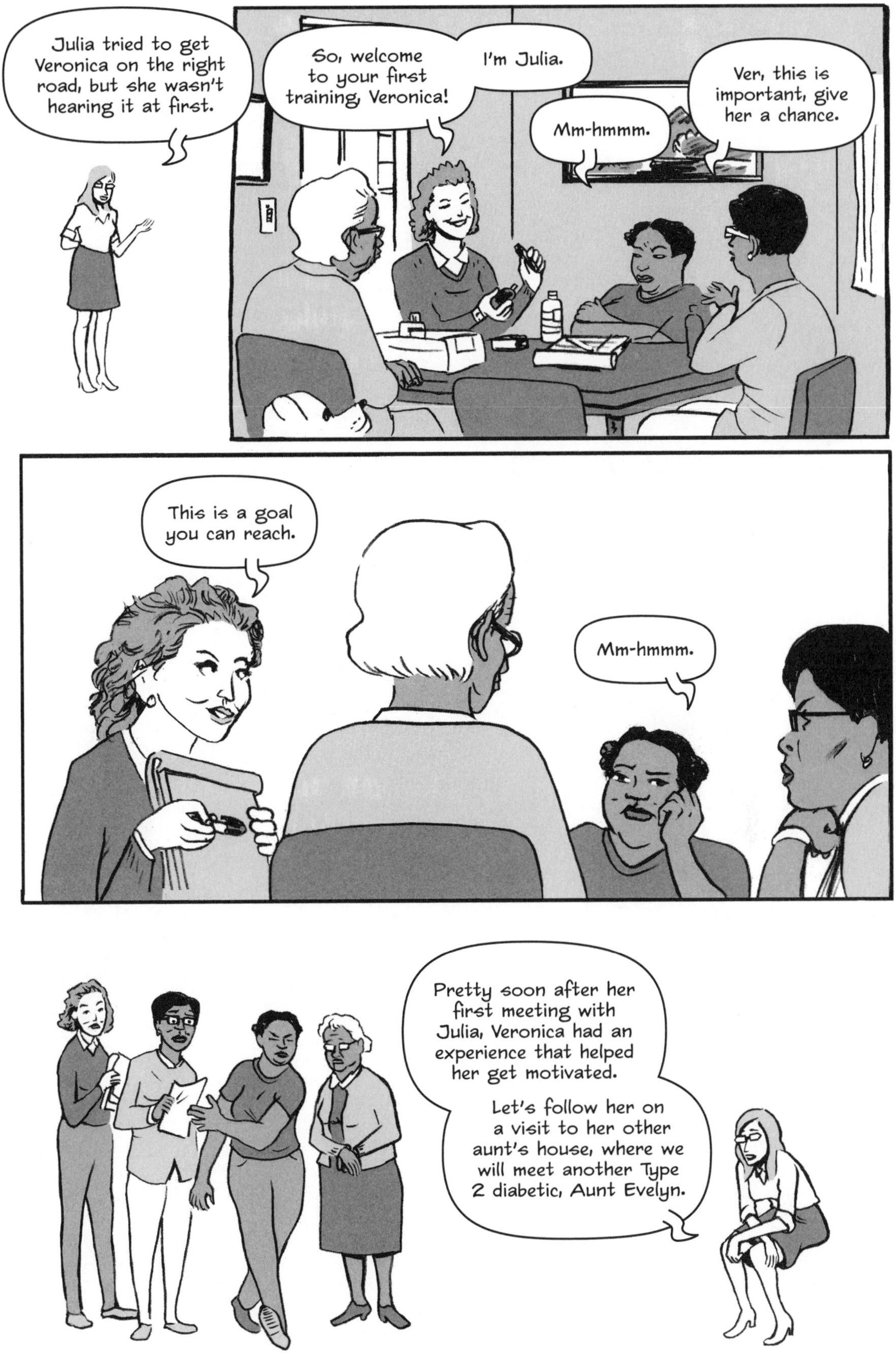

Julia tried to get Veronica on the right road, but she wasn't hearing it at first.
So, welcome to your first training, Veronica!
I'm Julia.
Mm-hmmm.
Ver, this is important, give her a chance.
This is a goal you can reach.
Mm-hmmm.
Pretty soon after her first meeting with Julia, Veronica had an experience that helped her get motivated.
Let's follow her on a visit to her other aunt's house, where we will meet another Type 2 diabetic, Aunt Evelyn.

YOUR CERTIFIED DIABETES NURSE EDUCATOR (CDE)

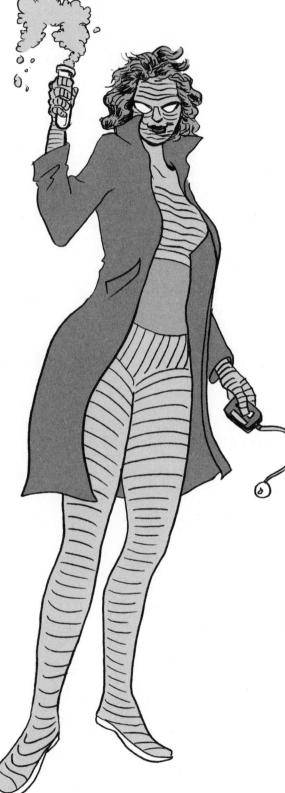

Main Job:
Diabetes educators are health care professionals who focus on educating people who have or are at risk of having diabetes. Diabetes educators apply in-depth knowledge and skills in the biological and social sciences, communication, counseling, and education to provide self-management education and training.

Years of Training:
Often 6+. Educators begin by going to nursing school, then many go on to get certified diabetes educator credentials, and some become board certified in advanced diabetes management (BC-ADM).

Special Ops:
Their specialty is making diabetes make sense for you.

Frequency of Visits:
Anytime you are trying new self-care techniques or new equipment.

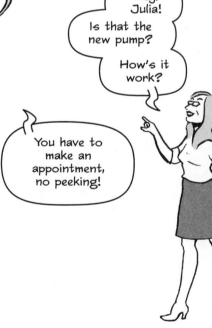

Hey, Julia!

Is that the new pump?

How's it work?

You have to make an appointment, no peeking!

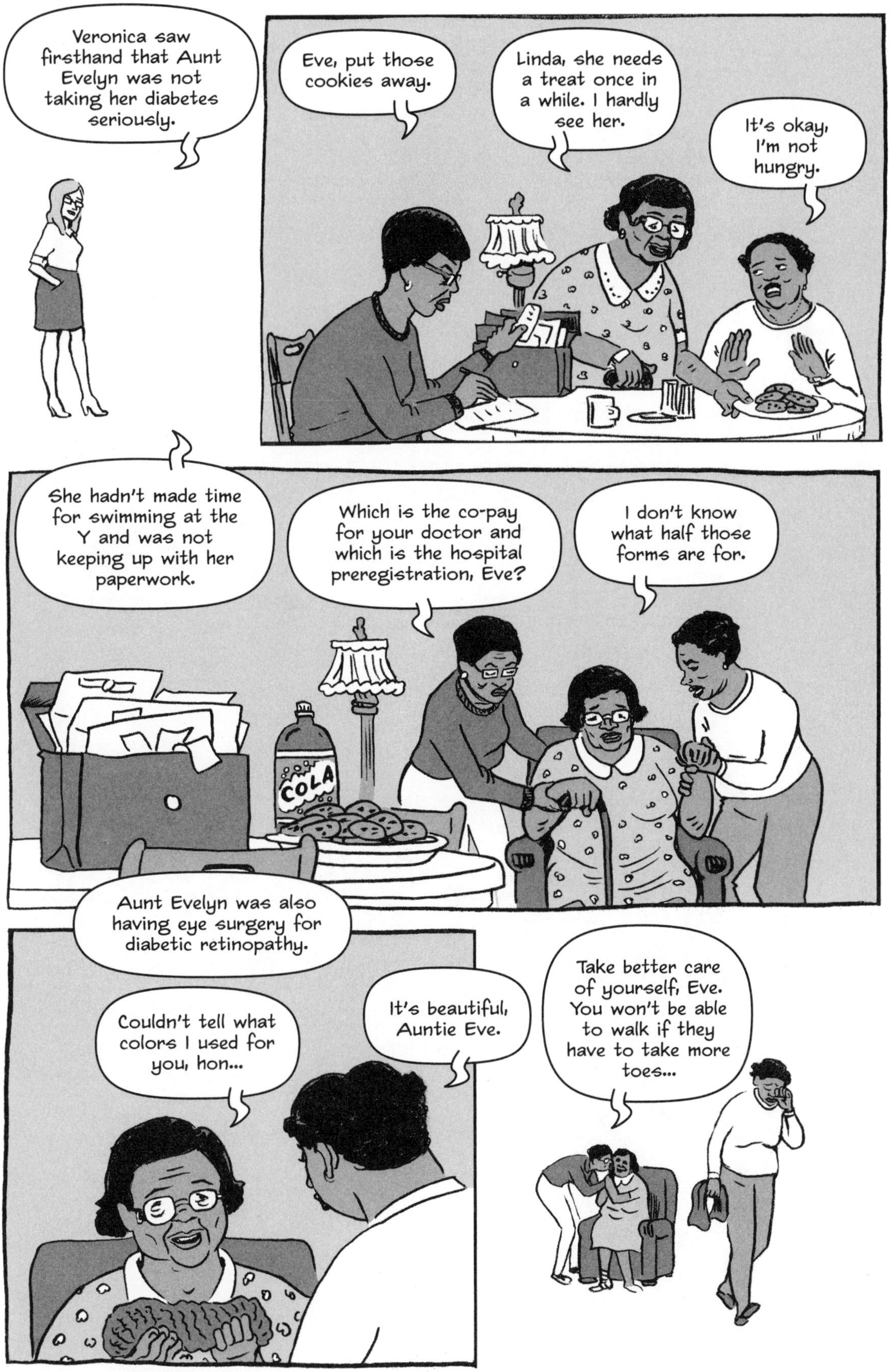
Veronica saw firsthand that Aunt Evelyn was not taking her diabetes seriously.
Eve, put those cookies away.
Linda, she needs a treat once in a while. I hardly see her.
It's okay, I'm not hungry.
She hadn't made time for swimming at the Y and was not keeping up with her paperwork.
Which is the co-pay for your doctor and which is the hospital preregistration, Eve?
I don't know what half those forms are for.
COLA
Aunt Evelyn was also having eye surgery for diabetic retinopathy.
Couldn't tell what colors I used for you, hon...
It's beautiful, Auntie Eve.
Take better care of yourself, Eve. You won't be able to walk if they have to take more toes...

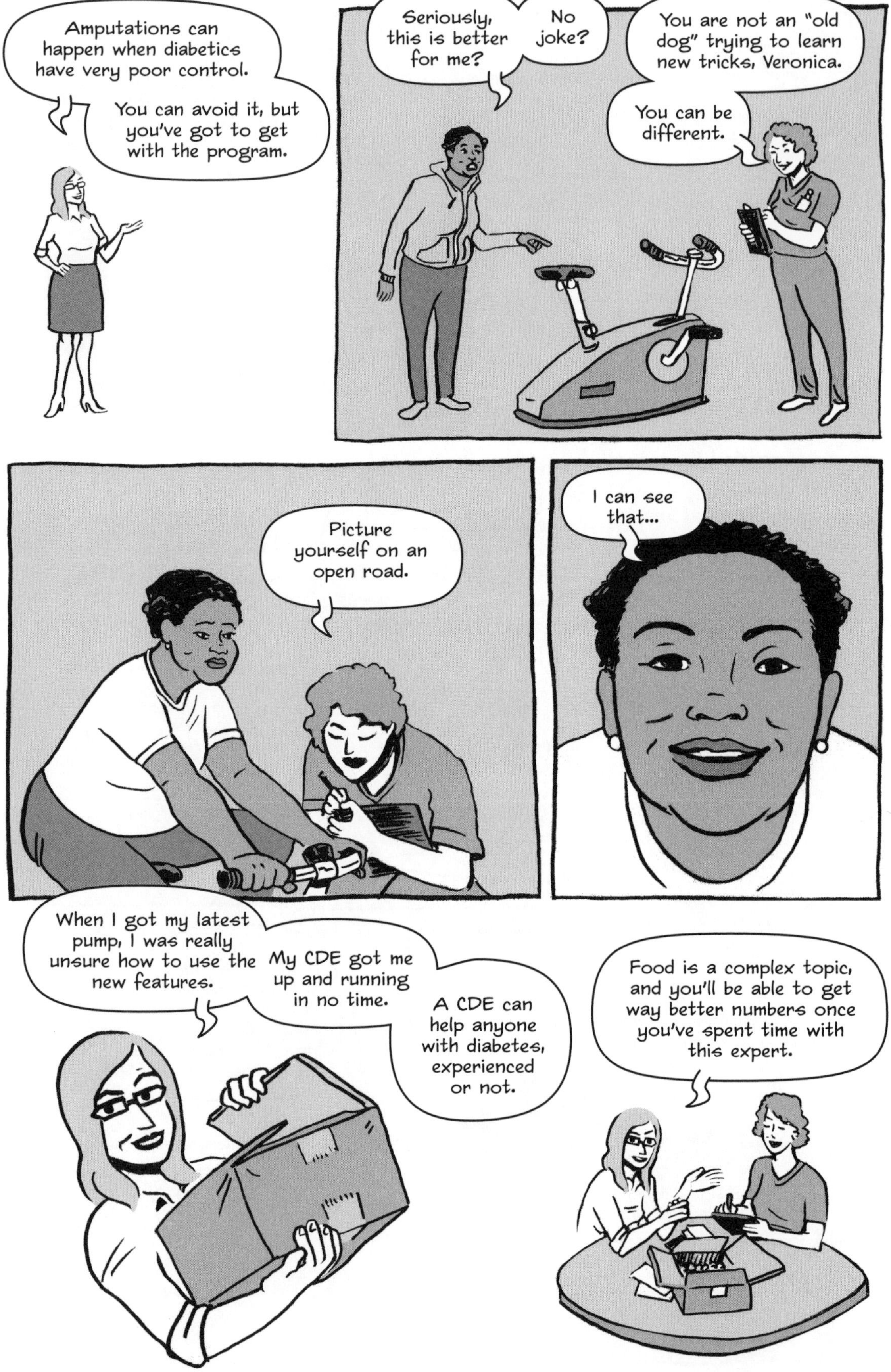
Amputations can happen when diabetics have very poor control.
You can avoid it, but you've got to get with the program.
Seriously, this is better for me?
No joke?
You are not an "old dog" trying to learn new tricks, Veronica.
You can be different.
Picture yourself on an open road.
I can see that...
When I got my latest pump, I was really unsure how to use the new features.
My CDE got me up and running in no time.
A CDE can help anyone with diabetes, experienced or not.
Food is a complex topic, and you'll be able to get way better numbers once you've spent time with this expert.

YOUR CERTIFIED NUTRITION SPECIALIST (CNS)

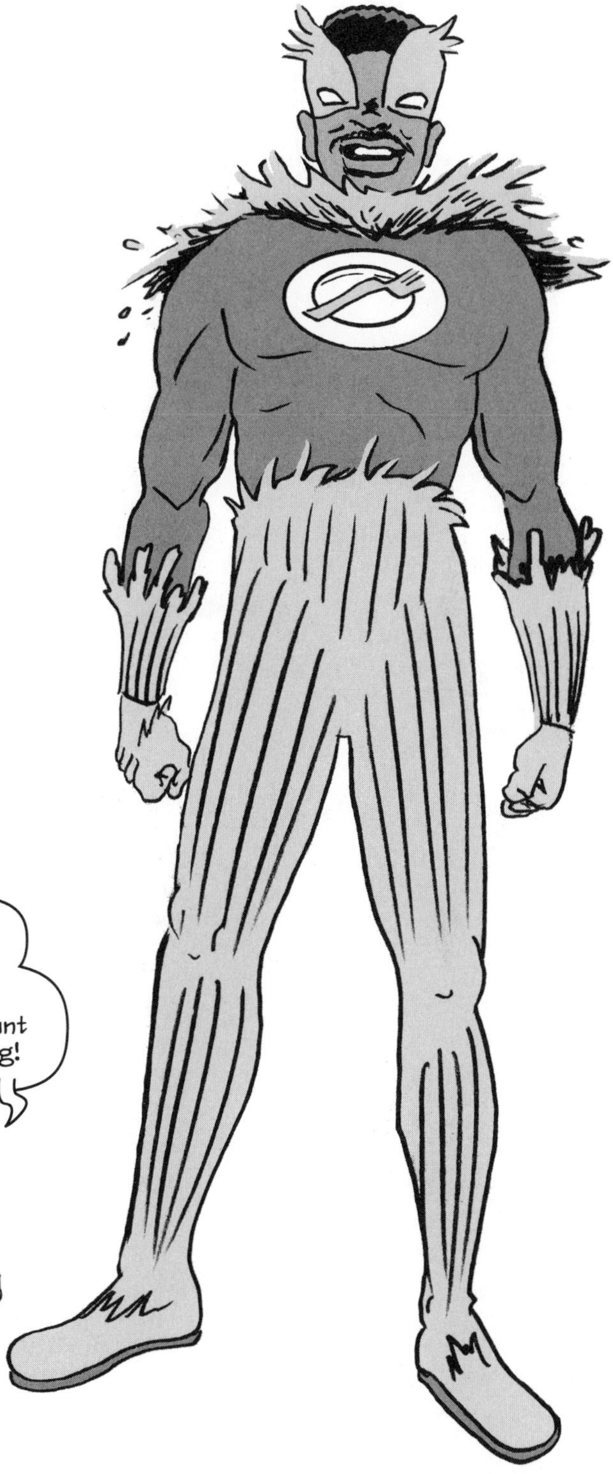

Main Job:
Food is one of the most important parts of managing diabetes. These specialists can help you find the right foods and help you learn to adjust your diet.

Years of Training:
6+. Although nutritionists may specialize in different foods and populations, they usually have a four-year degree in nutrition science, a master's or PhD in nutrition, and additional certification and licensing.

Special Ops:
If you are what you eat, they help you eat the best you can!

Frequency of Visits:
Usually several after diagnosis, then following major changes in diet or weight or new sports routines.

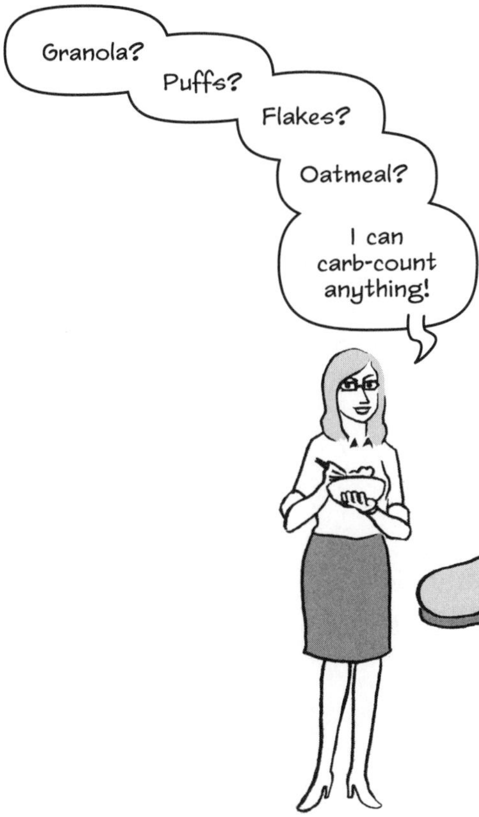
Granola?
Puffs?
Flakes?
Oatmeal?
I can carb-count anything!

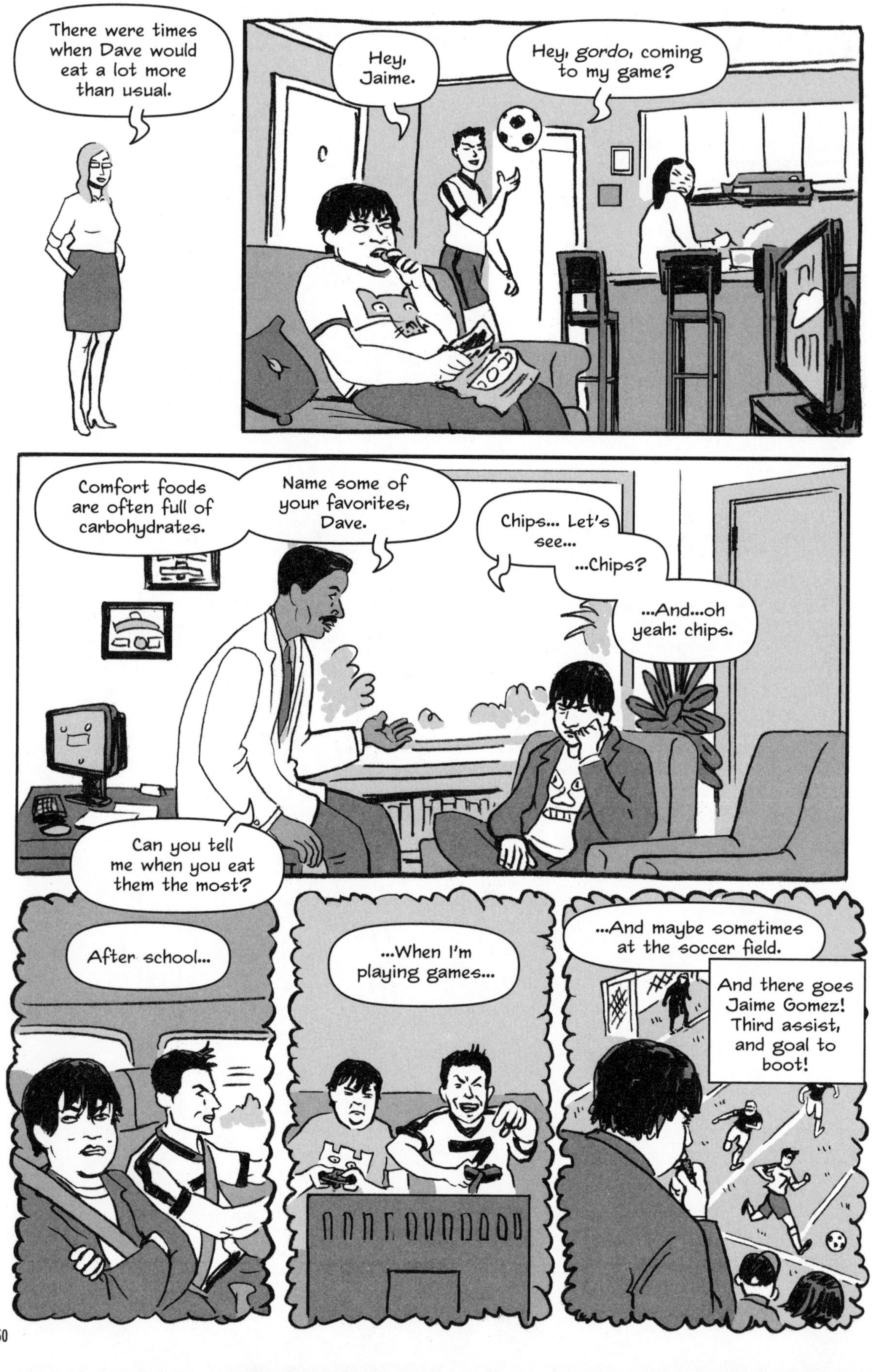

There were times when Dave would eat a lot more than usual.
Hey, Jaime.
Hey, *gordo*, coming to my game?
Comfort foods are often full of carbohydrates.
Name some of your favorites, Dave.
Chips... Let's see...
...Chips?
...And...oh yeah: chips.
Can you tell me when you eat them the most?
After school...
...When I'm playing games...
...And maybe sometimes at the soccer field.
And there goes Jaime Gomez! Third assist, and goal to boot!

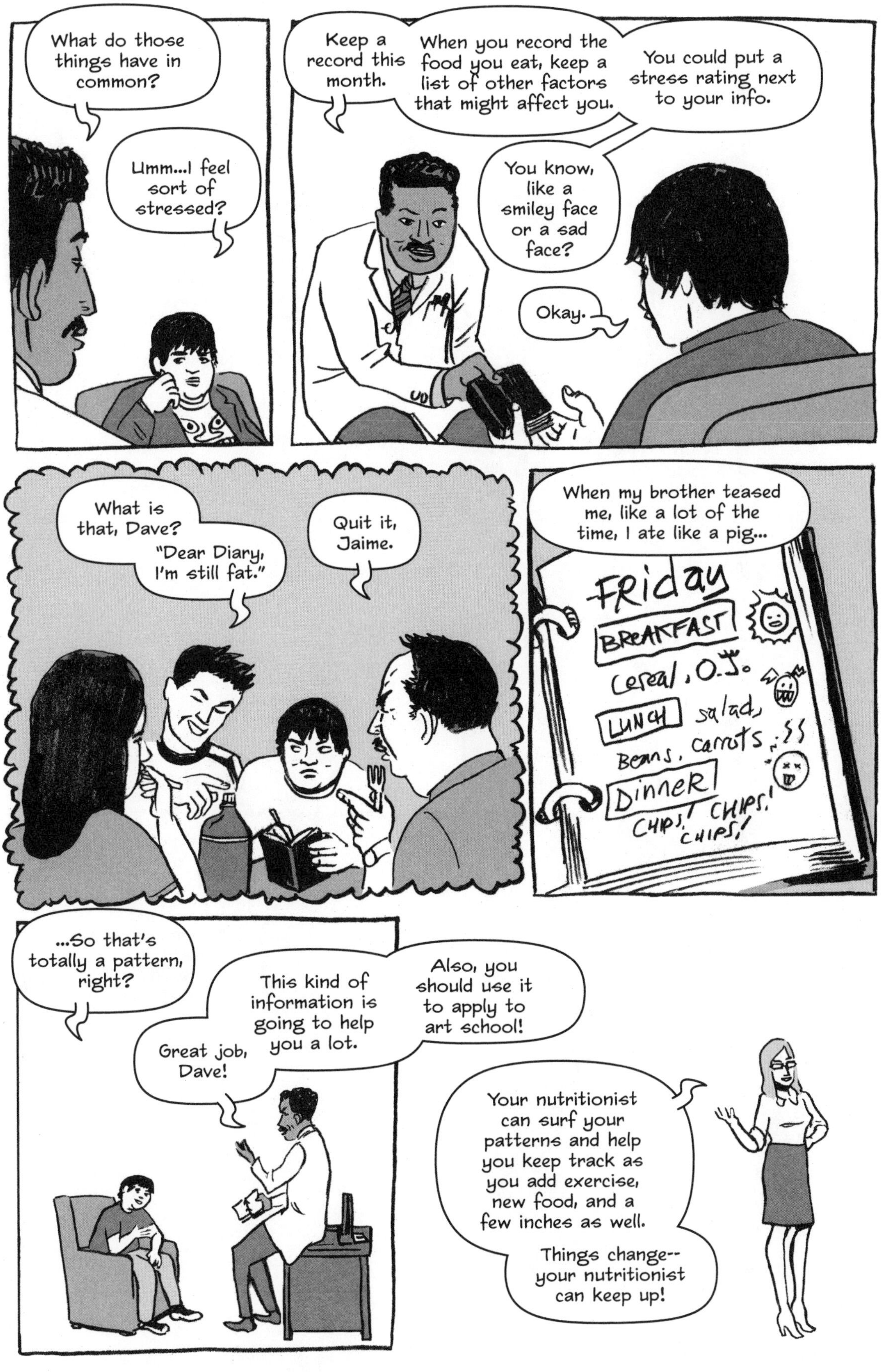

What do those things have in common?
Umm...I feel sort of stressed?
Keep a record this month.
When you record the food you eat, keep a list of other factors that might affect you.
You could put a stress rating next to your info.
You know, like a smiley face or a sad face?
Okay.
What is that, Dave?
"Dear Diary, I'm still fat."
Quit it, Jaime.
When my brother teased me, like a lot of the time, I ate like a pig...
Friday
BREAKFAST
cereal, O.J.
LUNCH salad, Beans, carrots
Dinner
CHIPS! CHIPS! CHIPS!
...So that's totally a pattern, right?
Great job, Dave!
This kind of information is going to help you a lot.
Also, you should use it to apply to art school!
Your nutritionist can surf your patterns and help you keep track as you add exercise, new food, and a few inches as well.
Things change--your nutritionist can keep up!

YOUR OPHTHALMOLOGIST

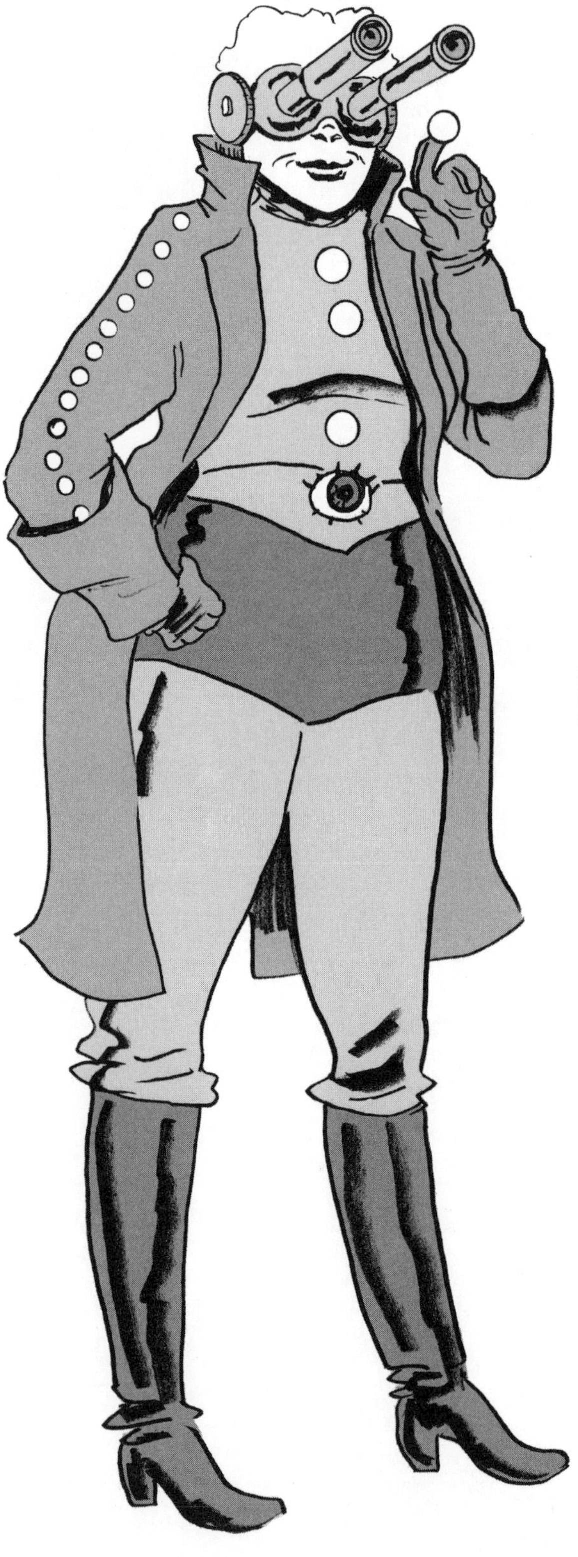

Main Job:
Diabetics have to monitor the small capillaries in the backs of their eyes (retinas). These can indicate your overall health and are susceptible to damage due to prolonged high blood sugars. Your ophthalmologist will look for glaucoma, retinopathy, and any other eyeball issues you may have.

Years of Training: 8+.

Special Ops:
No problem checking if you need glasses too!

Frequency of Visits:
Every year.

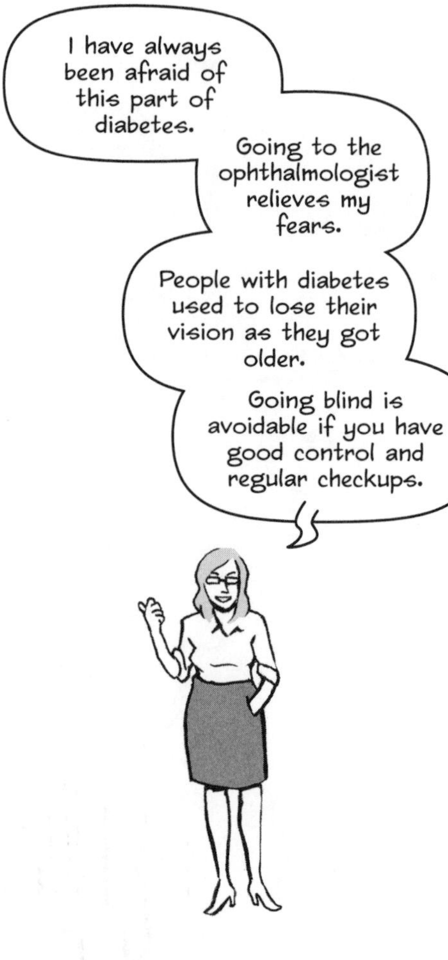
I have always been afraid of this part of diabetes.
Going to the ophthalmologist relieves my fears.
People with diabetes used to lose their vision as they got older.
Going blind is avoidable if you have good control and regular checkups.

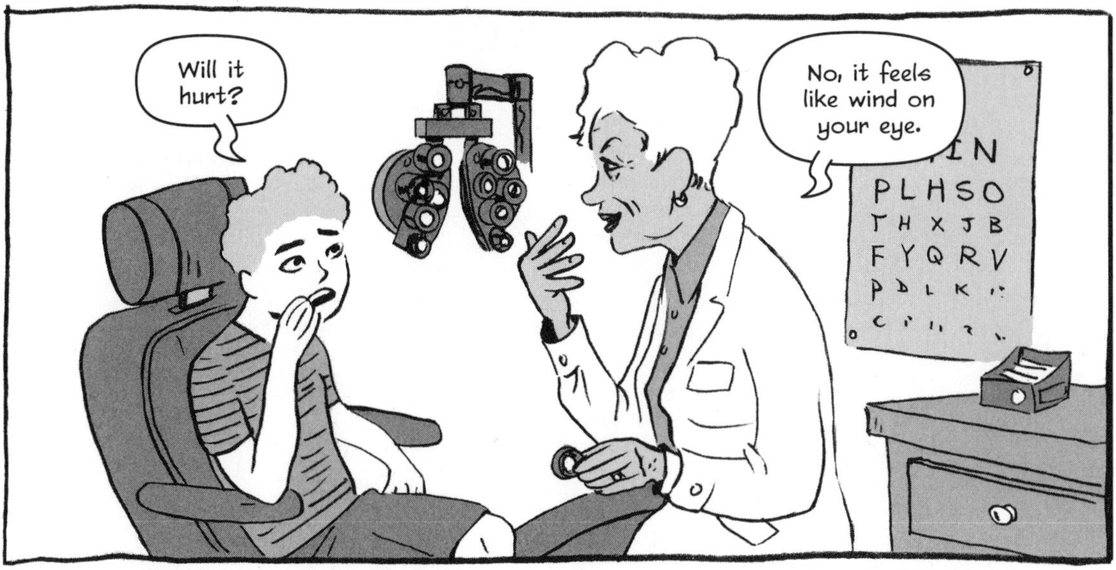
Will it hurt?
No, it feels like wind on your eye.
PLHSO
THXJB
FYQRV

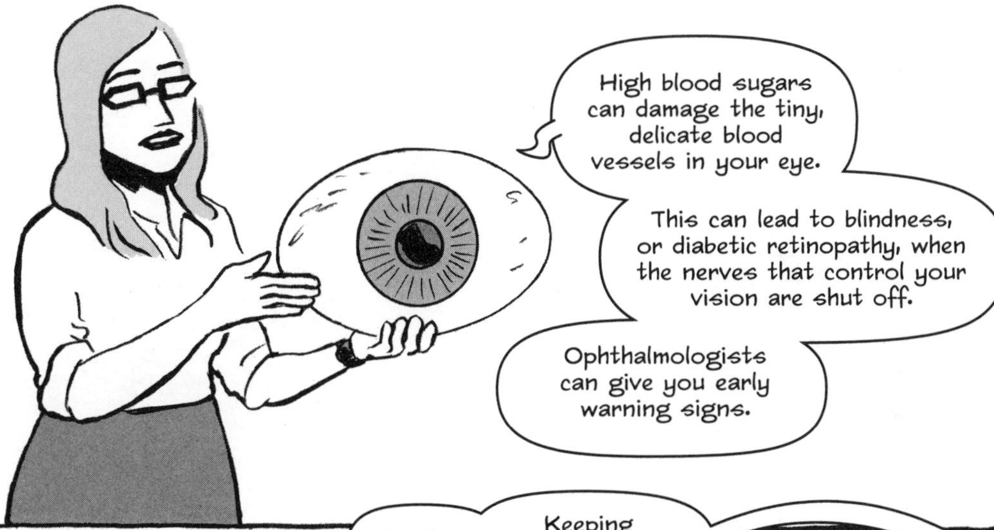
High blood sugars can damage the tiny, delicate blood vessels in your eye.
This can lead to blindness, or diabetic retinopathy, when the nerves that control your vision are shut off.
Ophthalmologists can give you early warning signs.

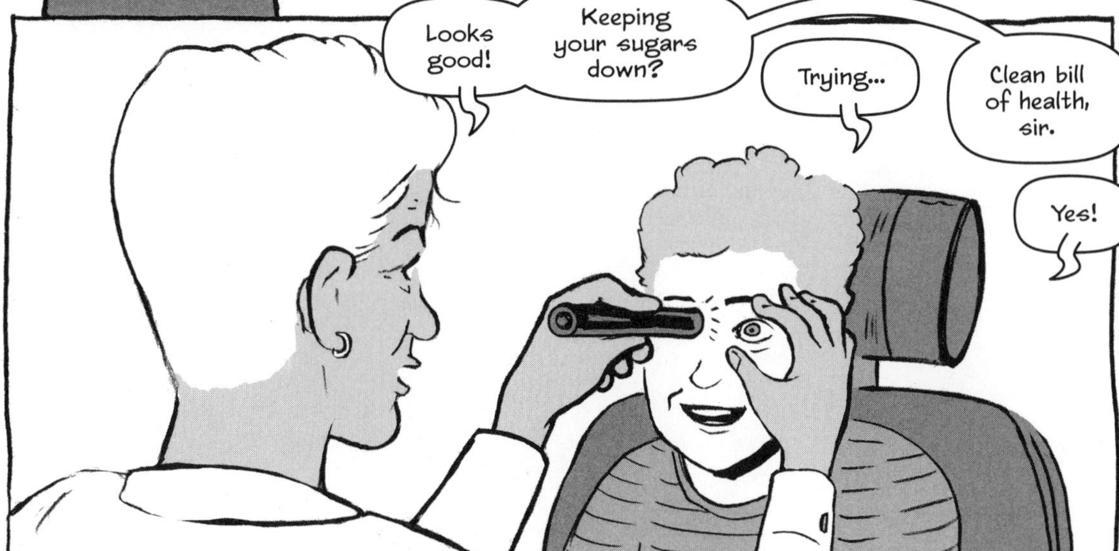
Looks good!
Keeping your sugars down?
Trying...
Clean bill of health, sir.
Yes!

CARING FOR YOUR FEET

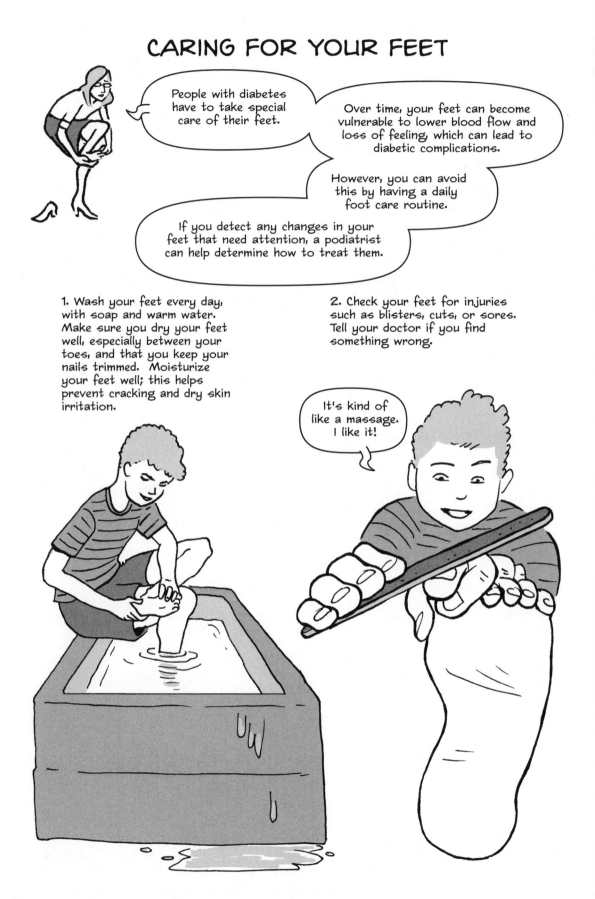

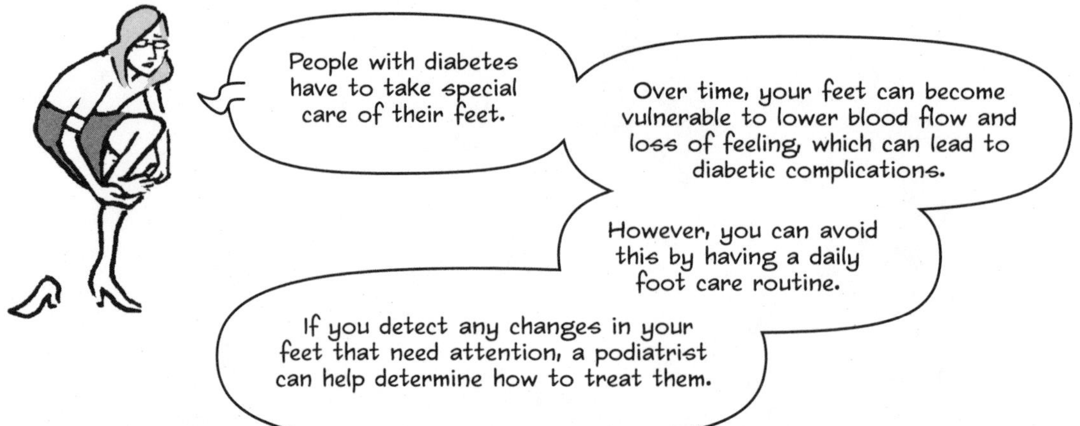
People with diabetes have to take special care of their feet.
Over time, your feet can become vulnerable to lower blood flow and loss of feeling, which can lead to diabetic complications.
However, you can avoid this by having a daily foot care routine.
If you detect any changes in your feet that need attention, a podiatrist can help determine how to treat them.

1. Wash your feet every day, with soap and warm water. Make sure you dry your feet well, especially between your toes, and that you keep your nails trimmed. Moisturize your feet well; this helps prevent cracking and dry skin irritation.

2. Check your feet for injuries such as blisters, cuts, or sores. Tell your doctor if you find something wrong.

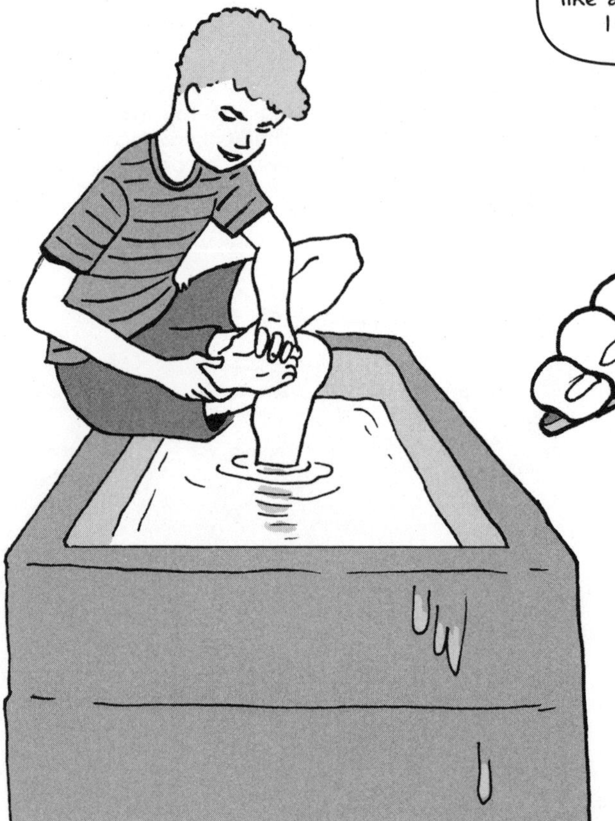

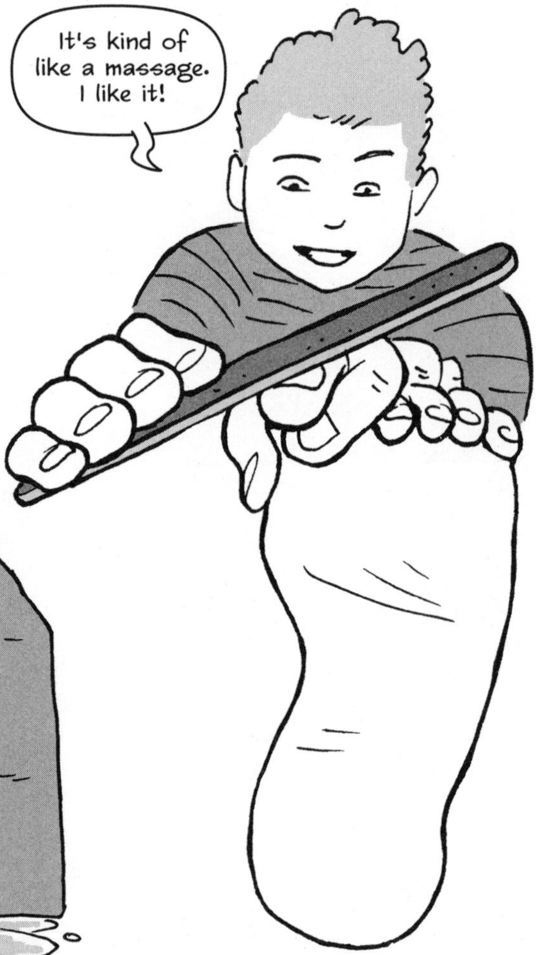
It's kind of like a massage. I like it!

3. Always change your socks!
Take care of your feet by keeping
them toasty and clean in well-
fitting socks and shoes.

4. Being barefoot can lead to
injuries, so be sure to wear
shoes, or water shoes,
whenever you are out and
about. Keep your feet
protected by checking shoes
for cracks or punctures from
rocks and nails.

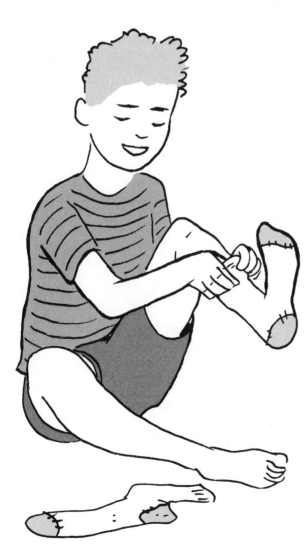

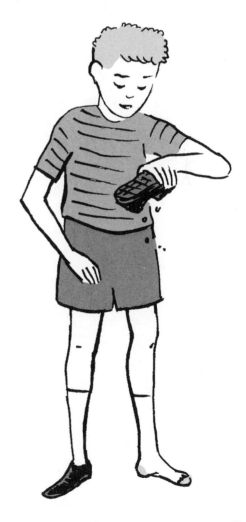

YOUR EXERCISE PHYSIOLOGIST

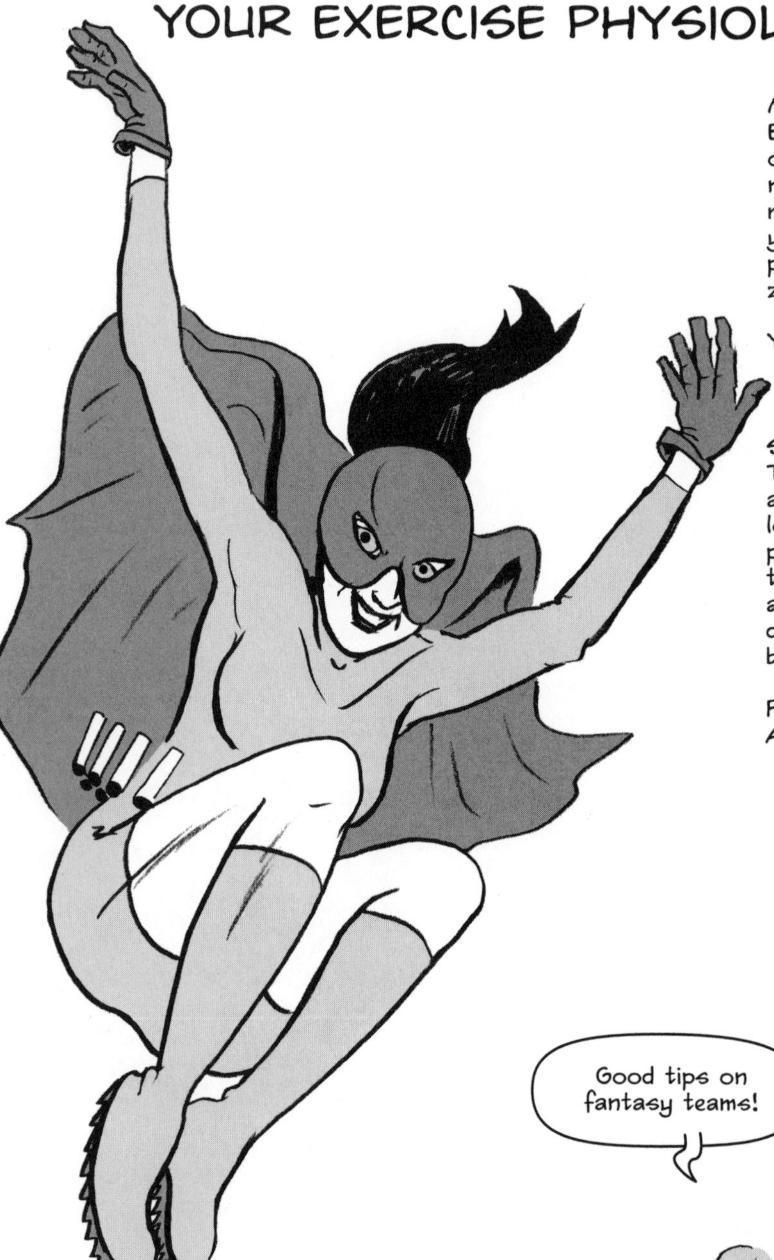

Main Job:
Exercise is a critical part of your program. You need a fun, healthy routine in order to keep your health intact. This person will get you from zero to hero in no time.

Years of Training: 8+.

Special Ops:
This specialist can make all the difference in your long-term care if you are planning to be involved in team sports. A fit and active life can keep diabetes complications at bay.

Frequency of Visits:
As needed.

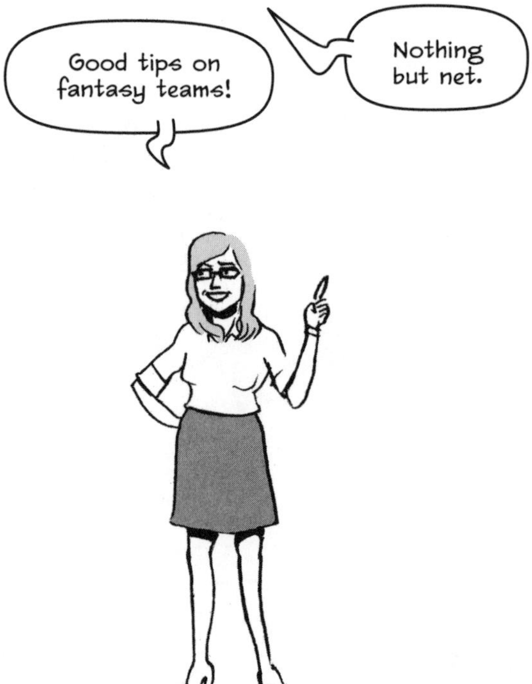
Good tips on fantasy teams!
Nothing but net.

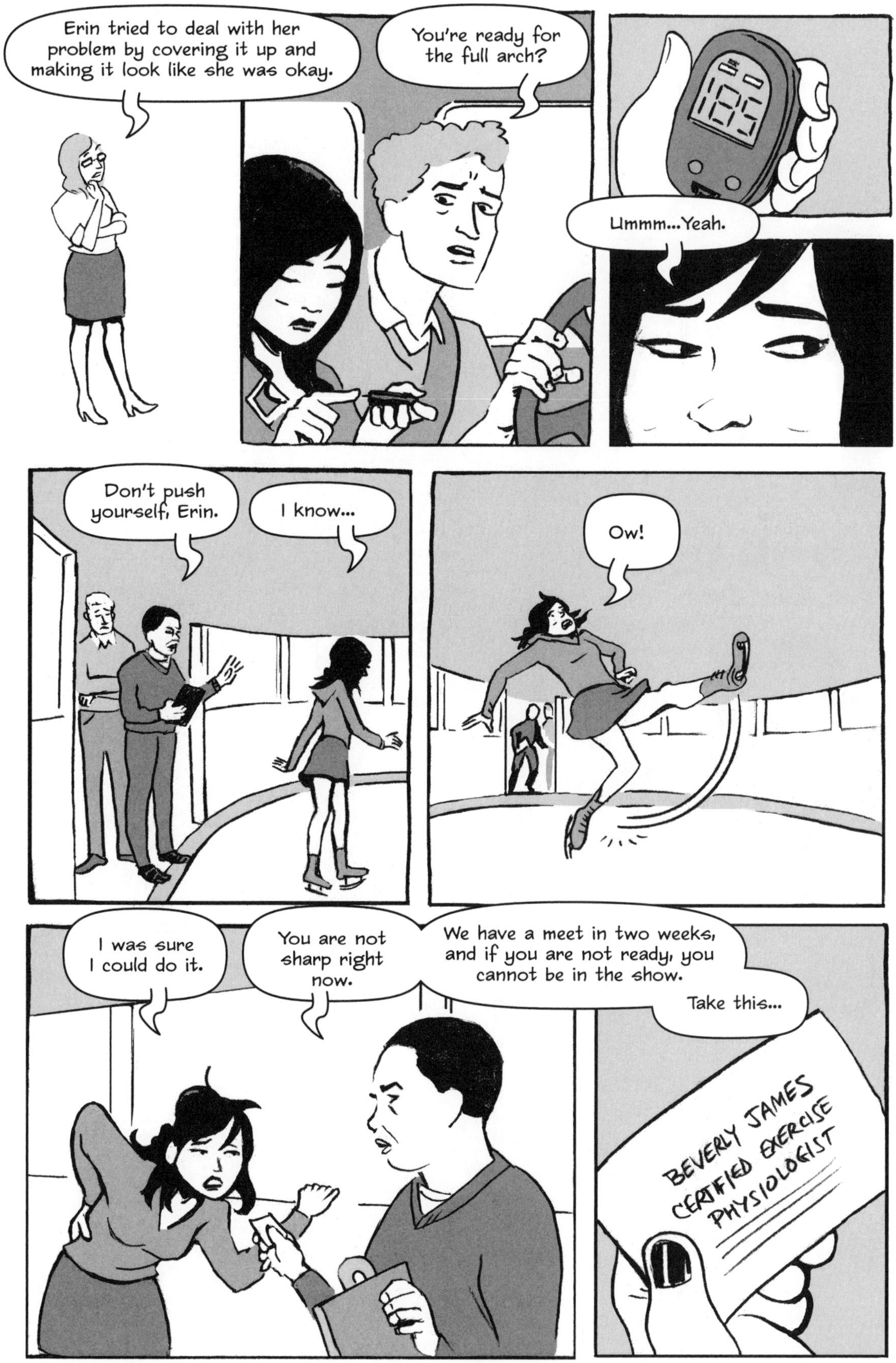
Erin tried to deal with her problem by covering it up and making it look like she was okay.
You're ready for the full arch?
Ummm...Yeah.
Don't push yourself, Erin.
I know...
Ow!
I was sure I could do it.
You are not sharp right now.
We have a meet in two weeks, and if you are not ready, you cannot be in the show.
Take this...
BEVERLY JAMES
CERTIFIED EXERCISE PHYSIOLOGIST

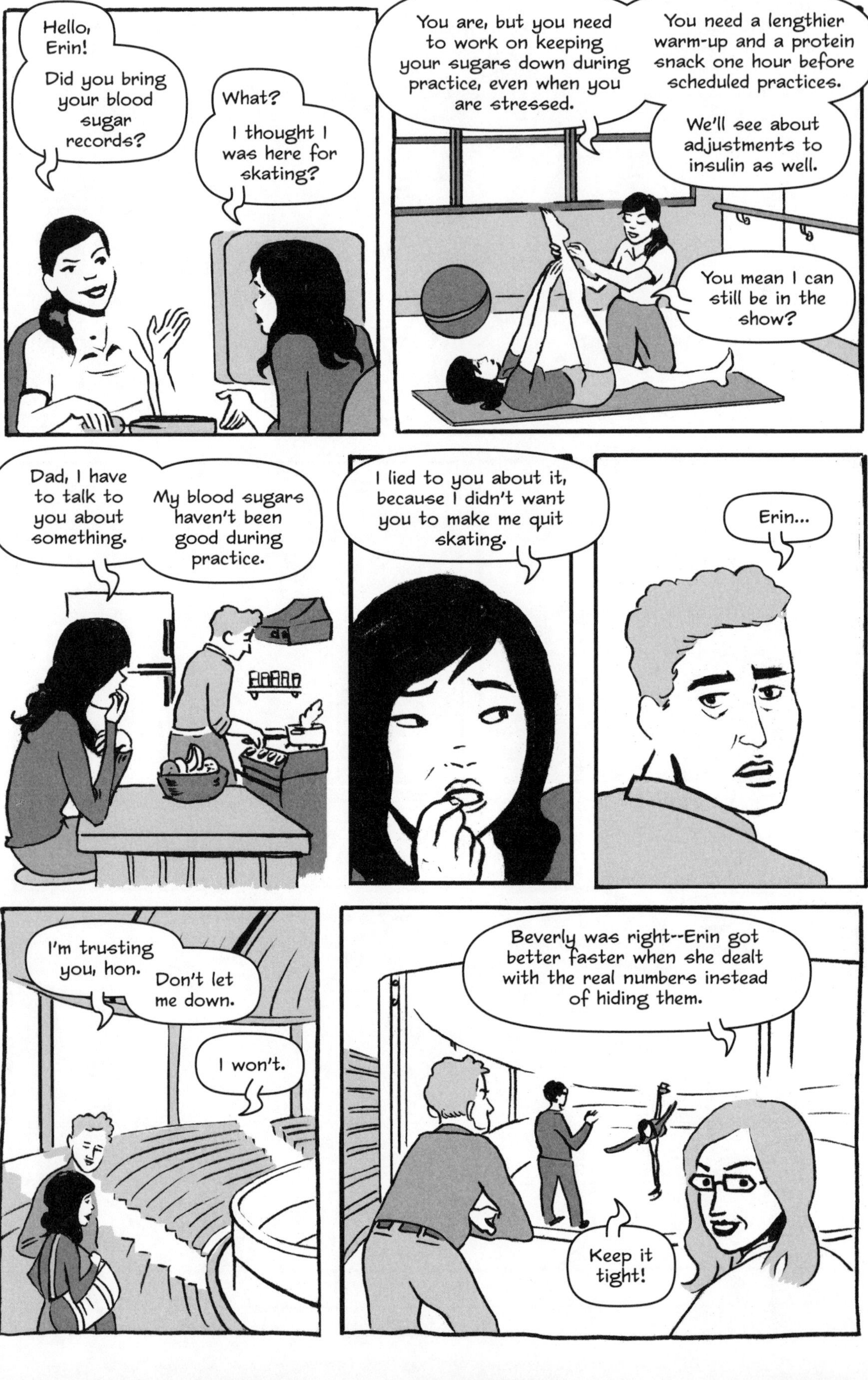
Hello, Erin!
Did you bring your blood sugar records?
What?
I thought I was here for skating?
You are, but you need to work on keeping your sugars down during practice, even when you are stressed.
You need a lengthier warm-up and a protein snack one hour before scheduled practices.
We'll see about adjustments to insulin as well.
You mean I can still be in the show?
Dad, I have to talk to you about something.
My blood sugars haven't been good during practice.
I lied to you about it, because I didn't want you to make me quit skating.
Erin...
I'm trusting you, hon.
Don't let me down.
I won't.
Beverly was right--Erin got better faster when she dealt with the real numbers instead of hiding them.
Keep it tight!

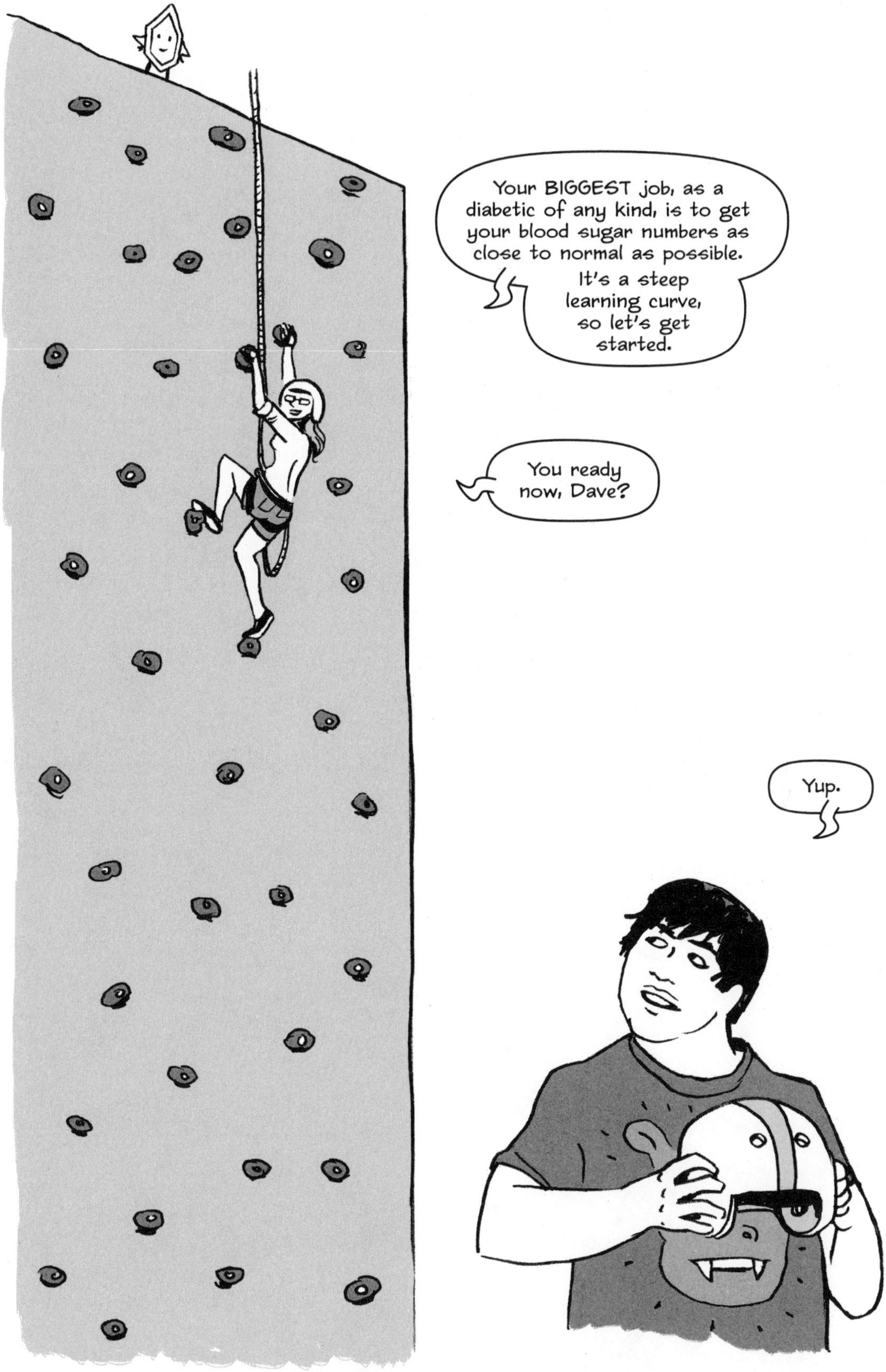
Your BIGGEST job, as a diabetic of any kind, is to get your blood sugar numbers as close to normal as possible.
It's a steep learning curve, so let's get started.
You ready now, Dave?
Yup.

PART THREE: HOW TO GET IN THE GAME

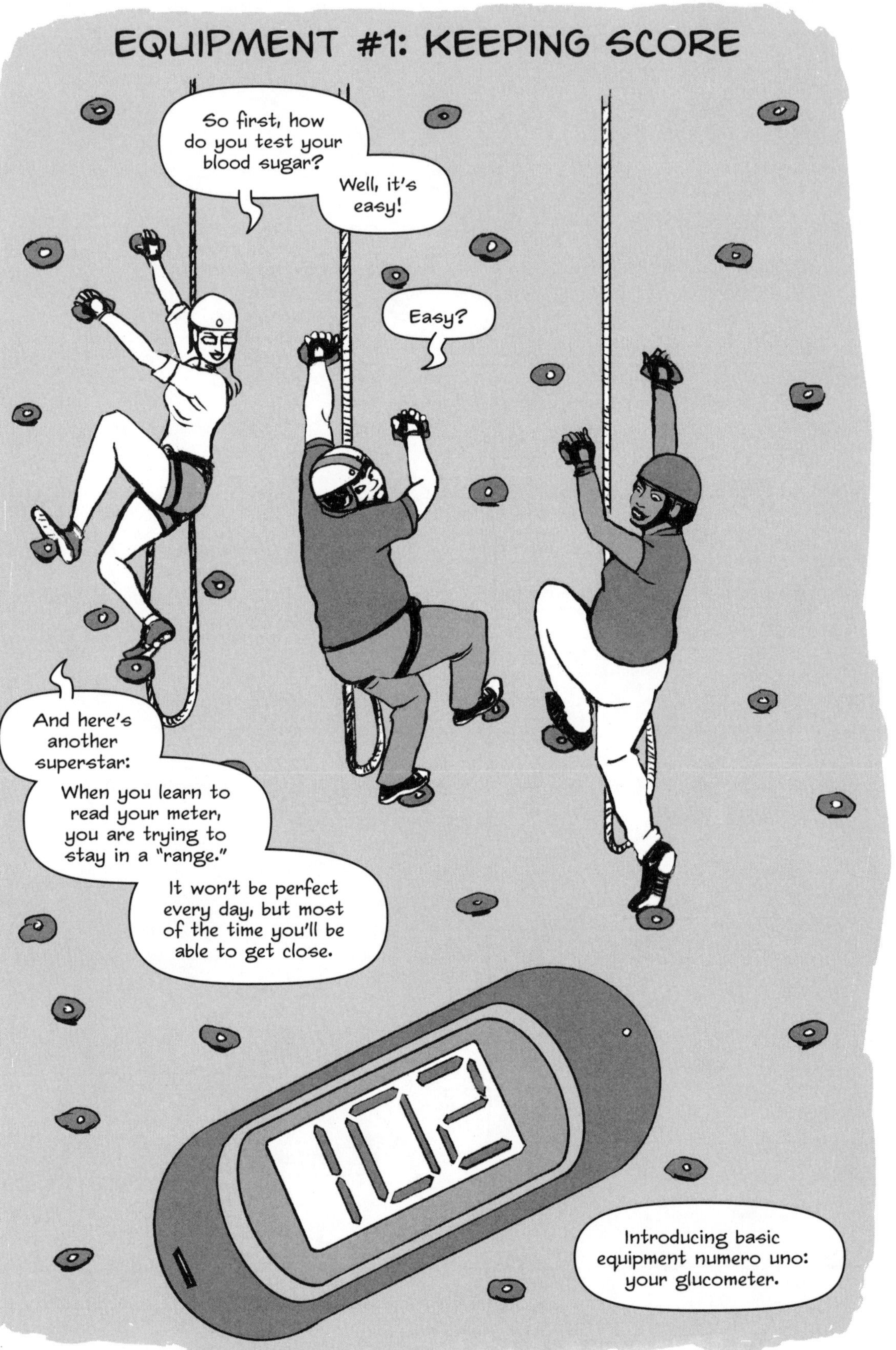
EQUIPMENT #1: KEEPING SCORE
So first, how do you test your blood sugar?
Well, it's easy!
Easy?
And here's another superstar:
When you learn to read your meter, you are trying to stay in a "range."
It won't be perfect every day, but most of the time you'll be able to get close.
102
Introducing basic equipment numero uno: your glucometer.

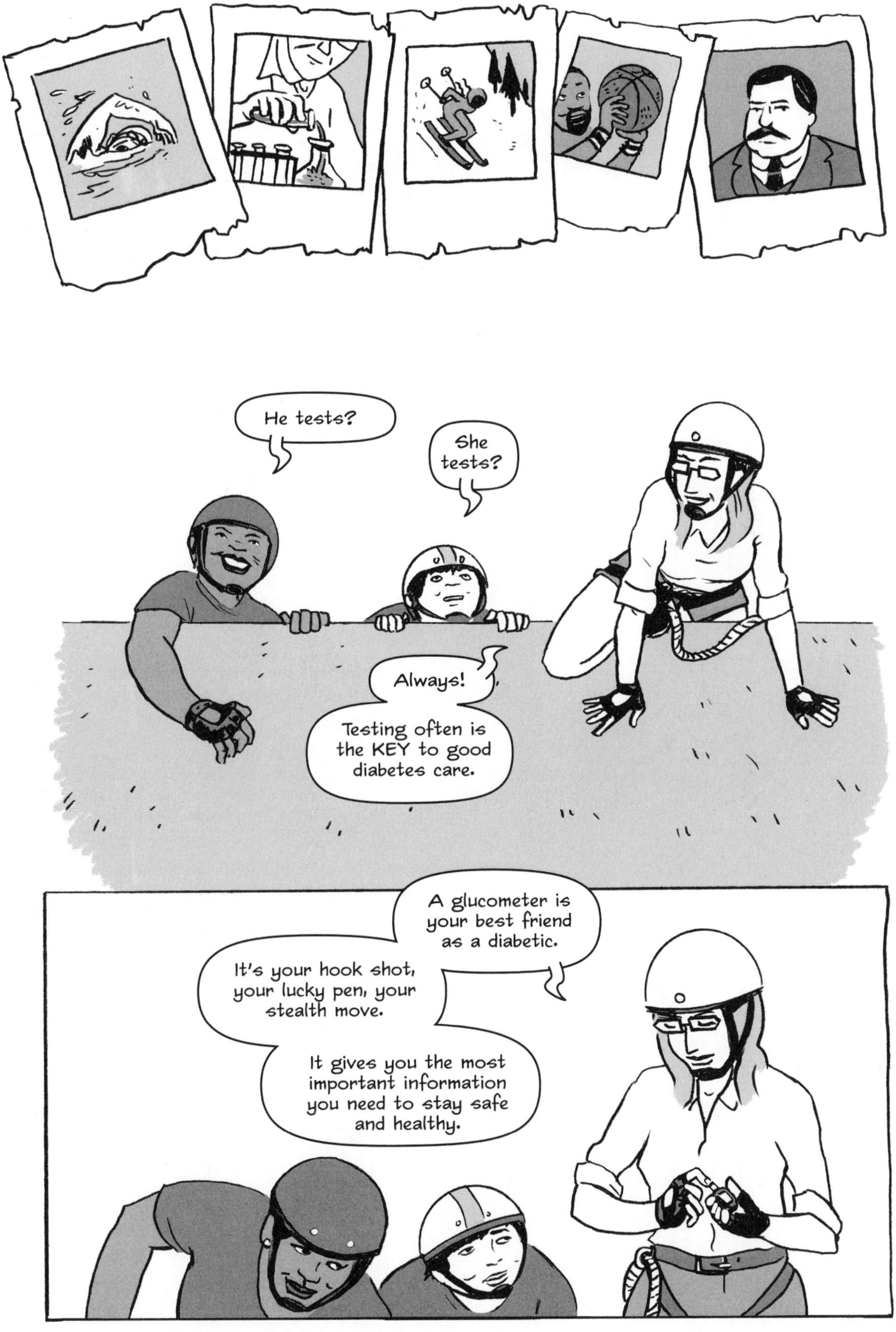
He tests?
She tests?
Always!
Testing often is the KEY to good diabetes care.
A glucometer is your best friend as a diabetic.
It's your hook shot, your lucky pen, your stealth move.
It gives you the most important information you need to stay safe and healthy.

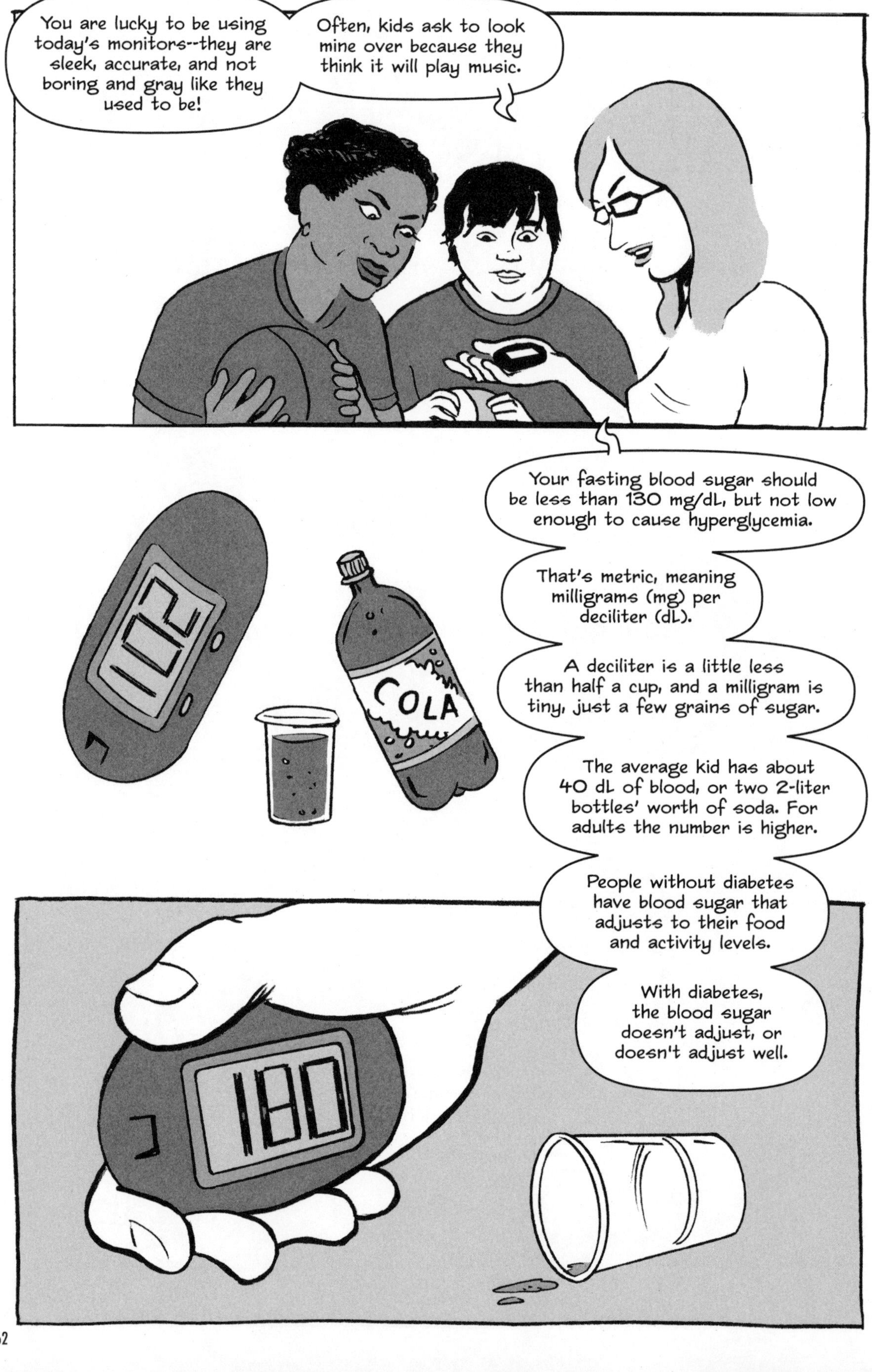
You are lucky to be using today's monitors--they are sleek, accurate, and not boring and gray like they used to be!
Often, kids ask to look mine over because they think it will play music.
Your fasting blood sugar should be less than 130 mg/dL, but not low enough to cause hyperglycemia.
That's metric, meaning milligrams (mg) per deciliter (dL).
A deciliter is a little less than half a cup, and a milligram is tiny, just a few grains of sugar.
The average kid has about 40 dL of blood, or two 2-liter bottles' worth of soda. For adults the number is higher.
People without diabetes have blood sugar that adjusts to their food and activity levels.
With diabetes, the blood sugar doesn't adjust, or doesn't adjust well.
COLA
180

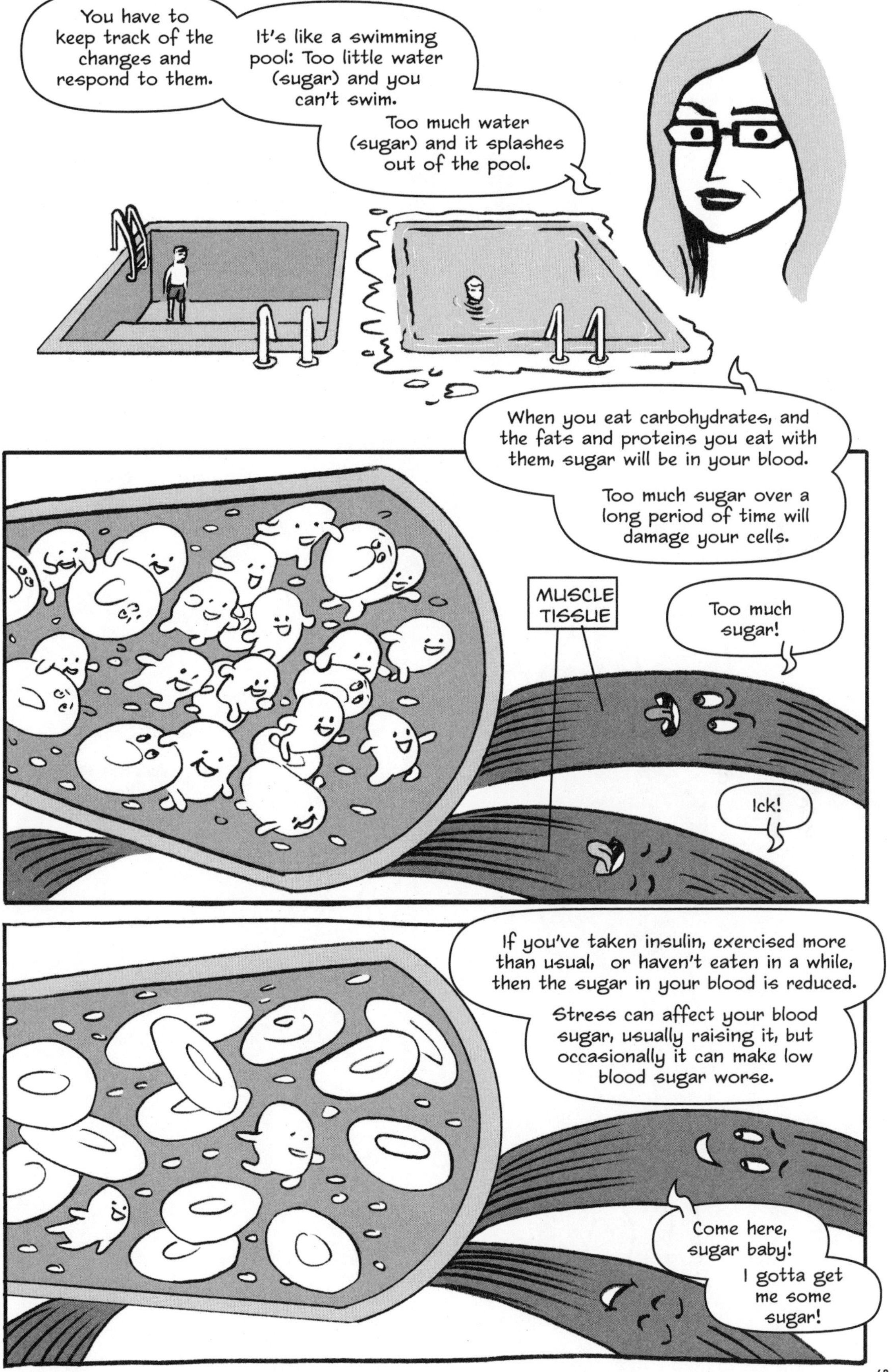
You have to keep track of the changes and respond to them.
It's like a swimming pool: Too little water (sugar) and you can't swim.
Too much water (sugar) and it splashes out of the pool.
When you eat carbohydrates, and the fats and proteins you eat with them, sugar will be in your blood.
Too much sugar over a long period of time will damage your cells.
MUSCLE TISSUE
Too much sugar!
Ick!
If you've taken insulin, exercised more than usual, or haven't eaten in a while, then the sugar in your blood is reduced.
Stress can affect your blood sugar, usually raising it, but occasionally it can make low blood sugar worse.
Come here, sugar baby!
I gotta get me some sugar!

HYPOGLYCEMIA

- Dizziness
- Tingling or numb feelings in your mouth
- Vision problems
- Disorientation
- Weakness
- Headaches

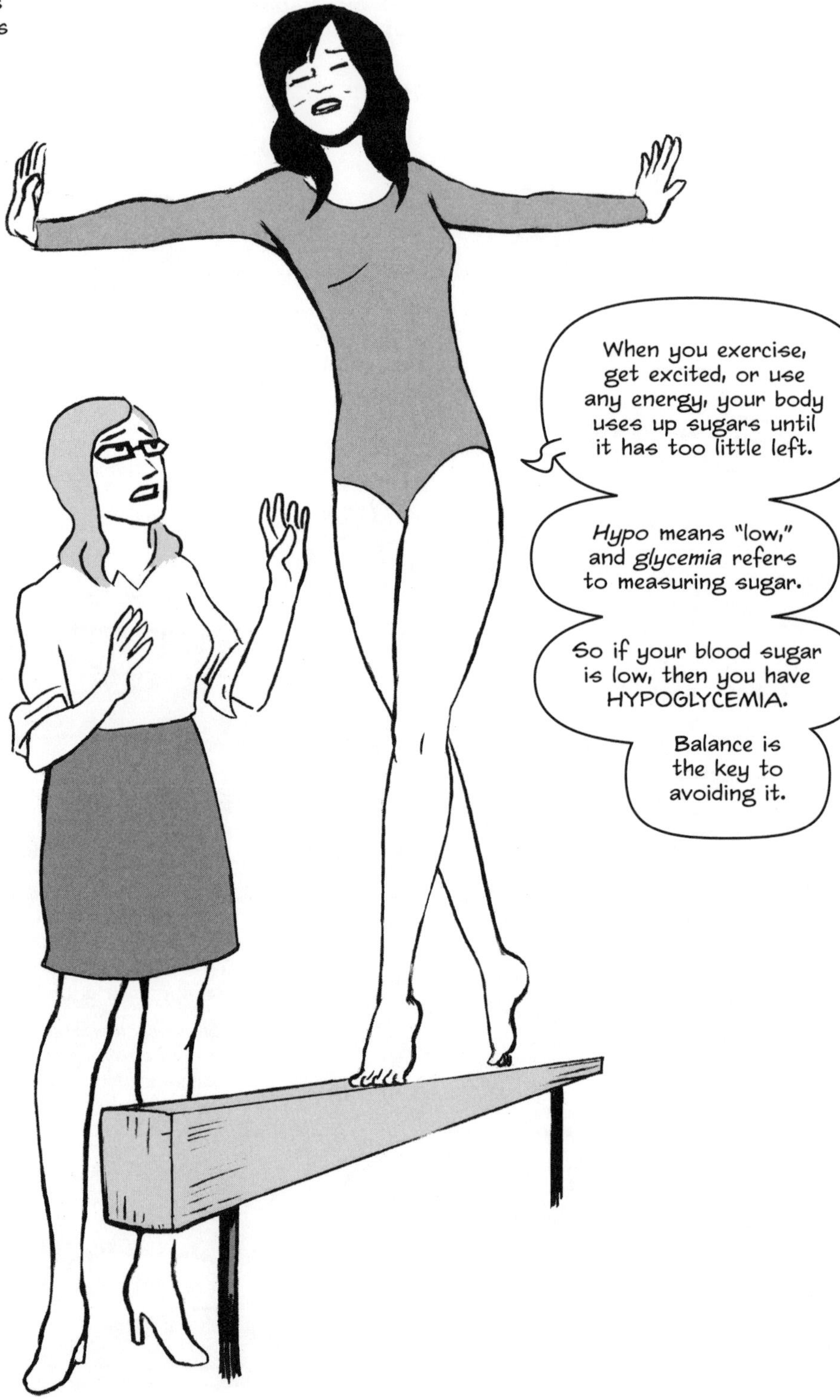

When you exercise, get excited, or use any energy, your body uses up sugars until it has too little left.
Hypo means "low," and *glycemia* refers to measuring sugar.
So if your blood sugar is low, then you have HYPOGLYCEMIA.
Balance is the key to avoiding it.

HYPERGLYCEMIA

- Sluggish
- Irritated
- Dehydrated
- Thirsty

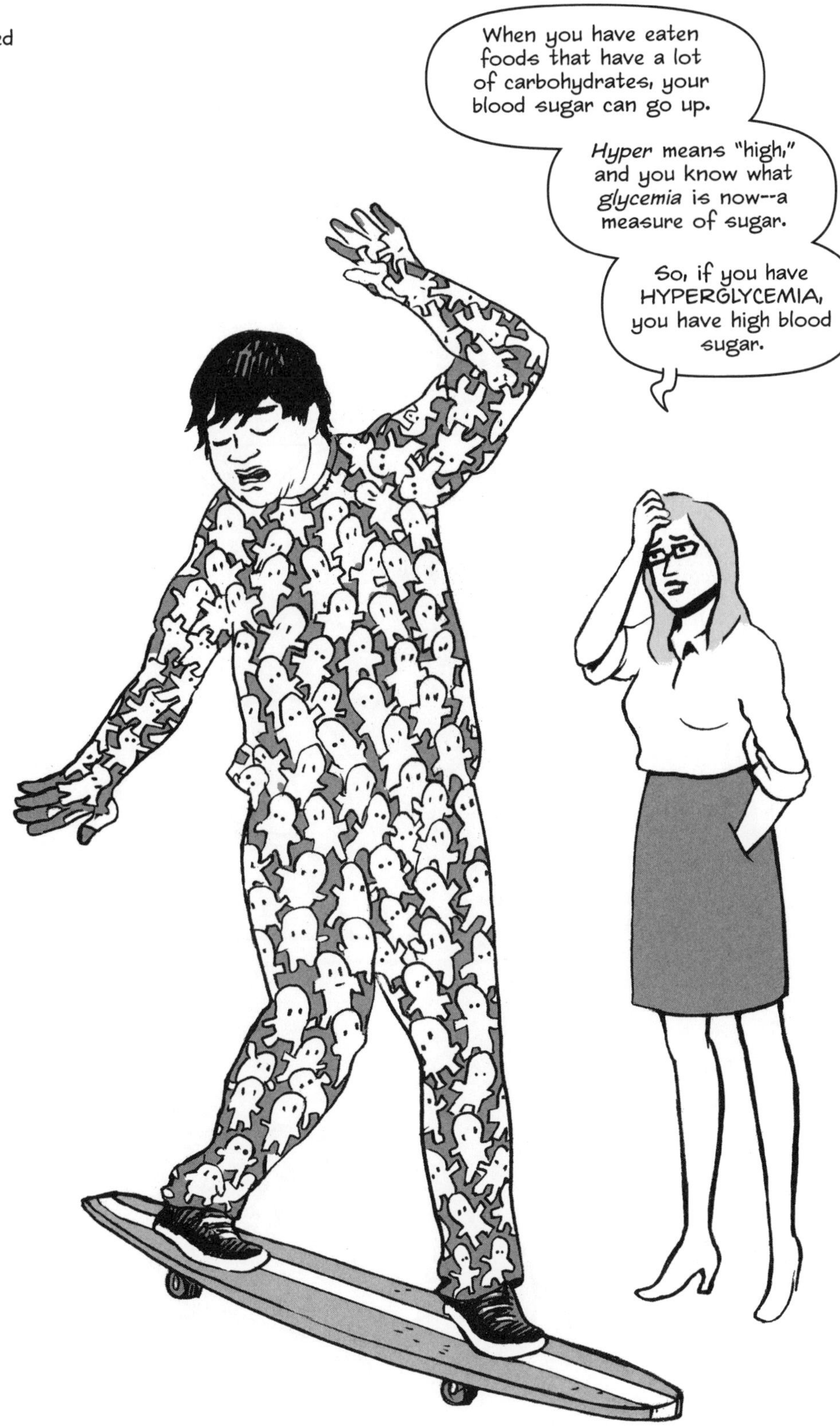
When you have eaten foods that have a lot of carbohydrates, your blood sugar can go up.
Hyper means "high," and you know what *glycemia* is now--a measure of sugar.
So, if you have HYPERGLYCEMIA, you have high blood sugar.

LOWS AND HIGHS

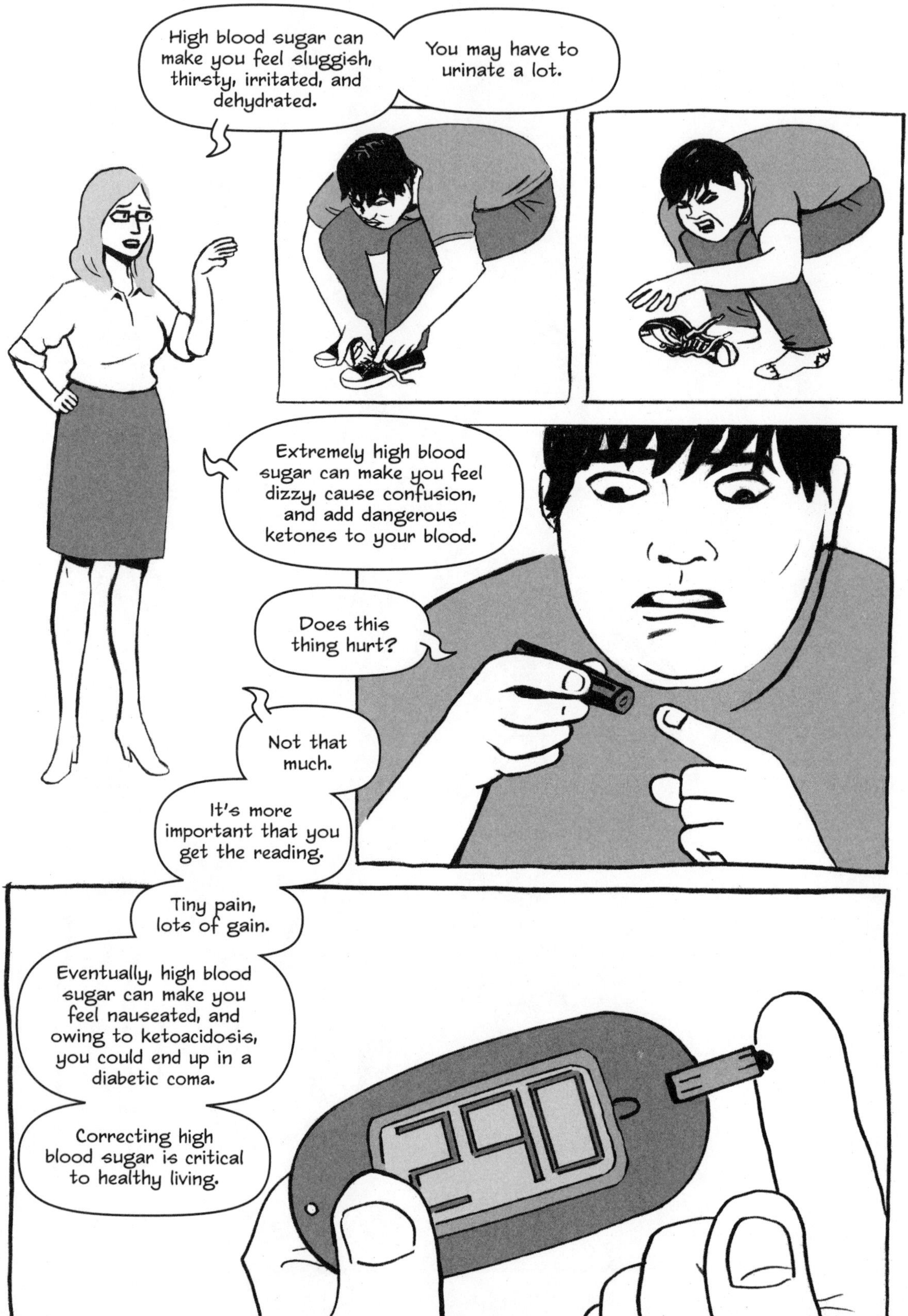
High blood sugar can make you feel sluggish, thirsty, irritated, and dehydrated.
You may have to urinate a lot.
Extremely high blood sugar can make you feel dizzy, cause confusion, and add dangerous ketones to your blood.
Does this thing hurt?
Not that much.
It's more important that you get the reading.
Tiny pain, lots of gain.
Eventually, high blood sugar can make you feel nauseated, and owing to ketoacidosis, you could end up in a diabetic coma.
Correcting high blood sugar is critical to healthy living.

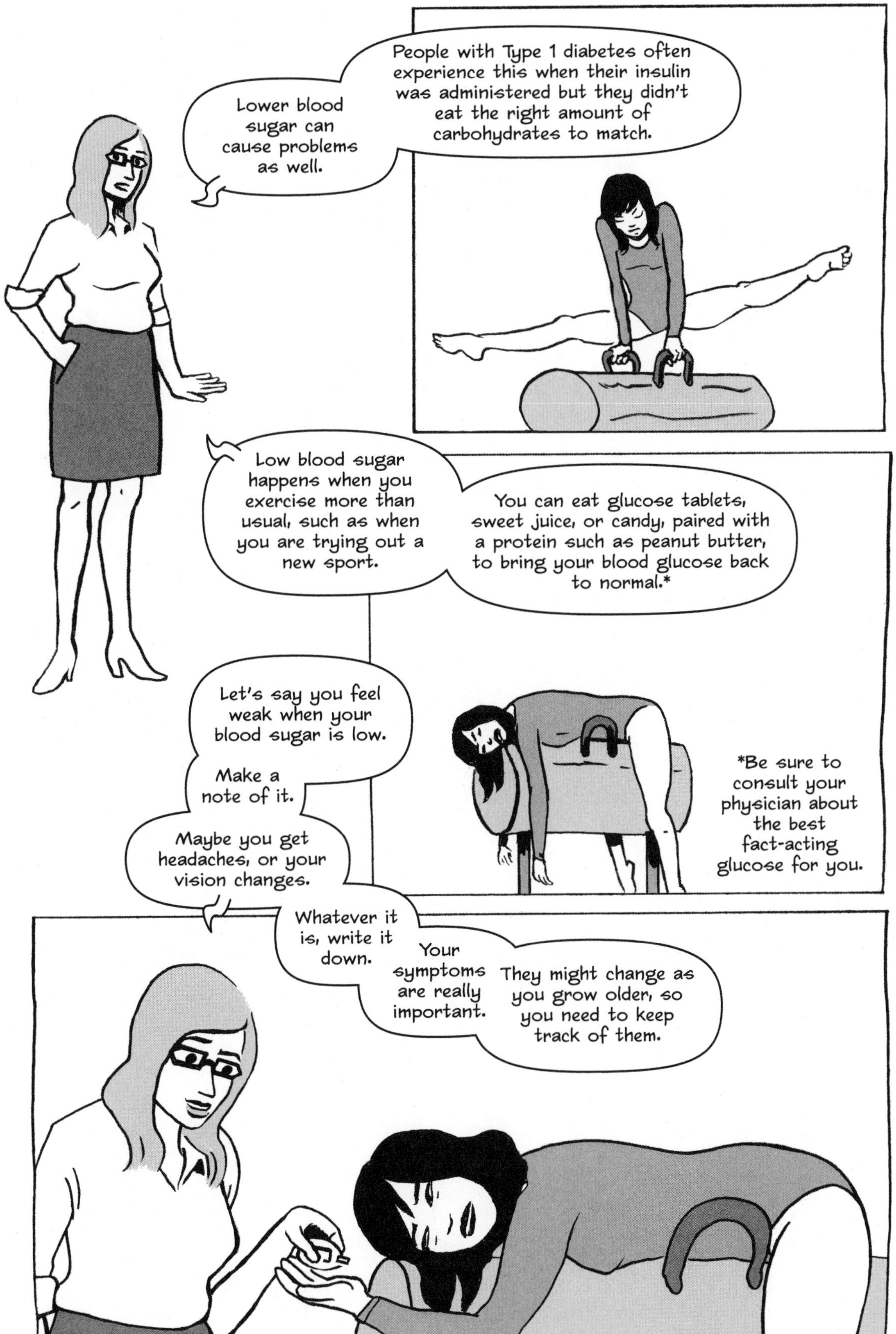
Lower blood sugar can cause problems as well.
People with Type 1 diabetes often experience this when their insulin was administered but they didn't eat the right amount of carbohydrates to match.
Low blood sugar happens when you exercise more than usual, such as when you are trying out a new sport.
You can eat glucose tablets, sweet juice, or candy, paired with a protein such as peanut butter, to bring your blood glucose back to normal.*
Let's say you feel weak when your blood sugar is low.
Make a note of it.
Maybe you get headaches, or your vision changes.
*Be sure to consult your physician about the best fact-acting glucose for you.
Whatever it is, write it down.
Your symptoms are really important.
They might change as you grow older, so you need to keep track of them.

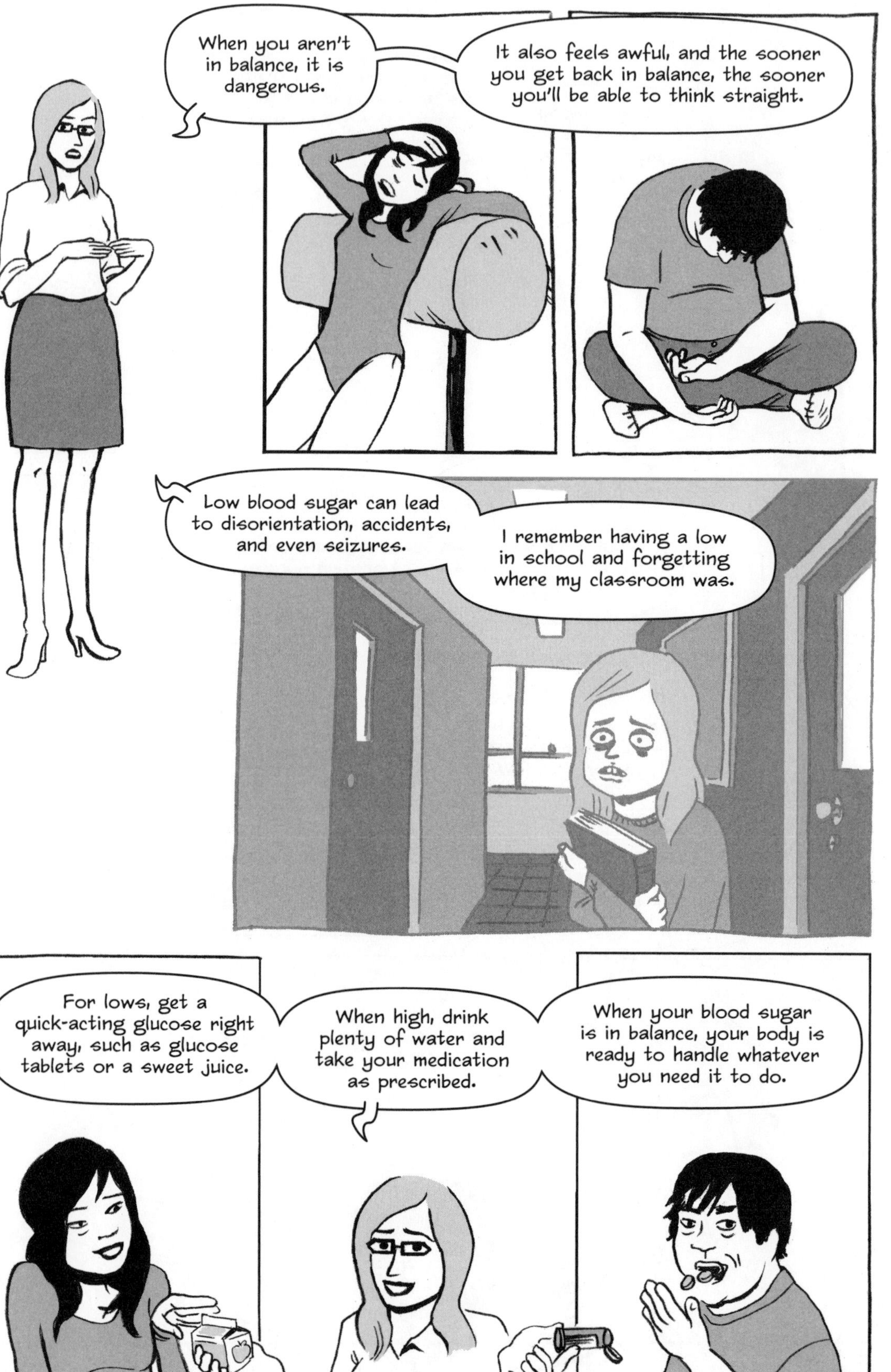
When you aren't in balance, it is dangerous.
It also feels awful, and the sooner you get back in balance, the sooner you'll be able to think straight.
Low blood sugar can lead to disorientation, accidents, and even seizures.
I remember having a low in school and forgetting where my classroom was.
For lows, get a quick-acting glucose right away, such as glucose tablets or a sweet juice.
When high, drink plenty of water and take your medication as prescribed.
When your blood sugar is in balance, your body is ready to handle whatever you need it to do.

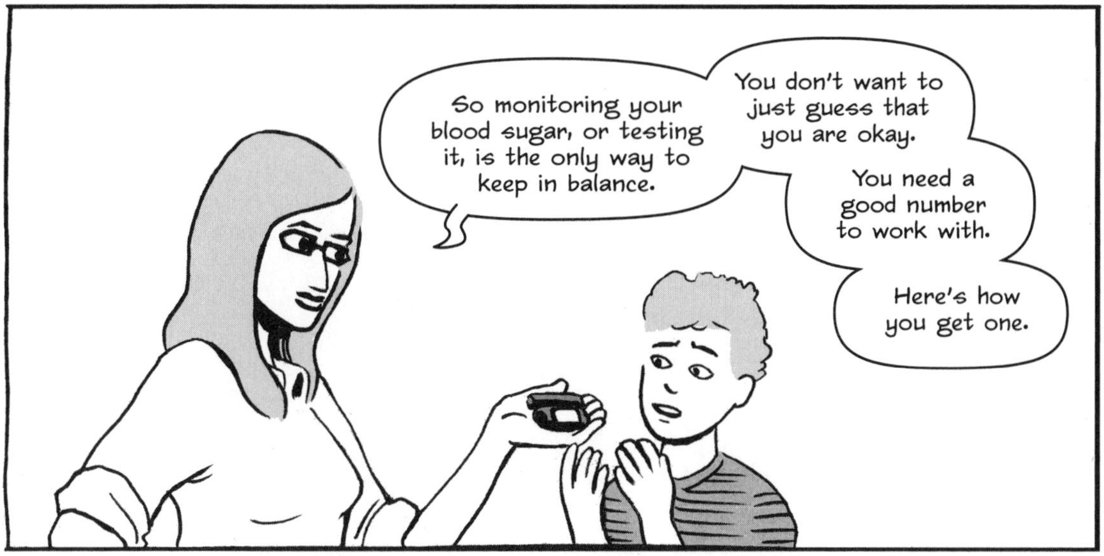
So monitoring your blood sugar, or testing it, is the only way to keep in balance.
You don't want to just guess that you are okay.
You need a good number to work with.
Here's how you get one.

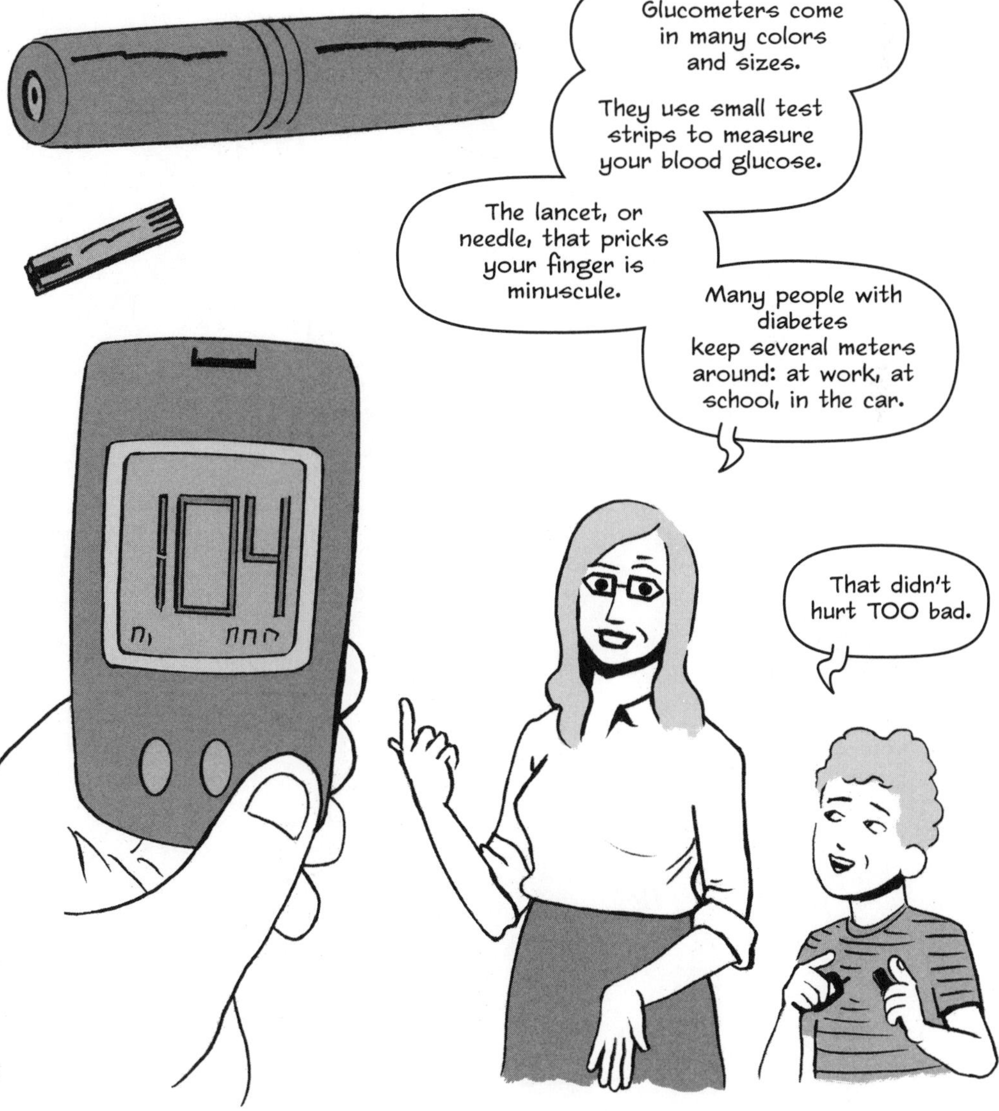
Glucometers come in many colors and sizes.
They use small test strips to measure your blood glucose.
The lancet, or needle, that pricks your finger is minuscule.
Many people with diabetes keep several meters around: at work, at school, in the car.
104
That didn't hurt TOO bad.

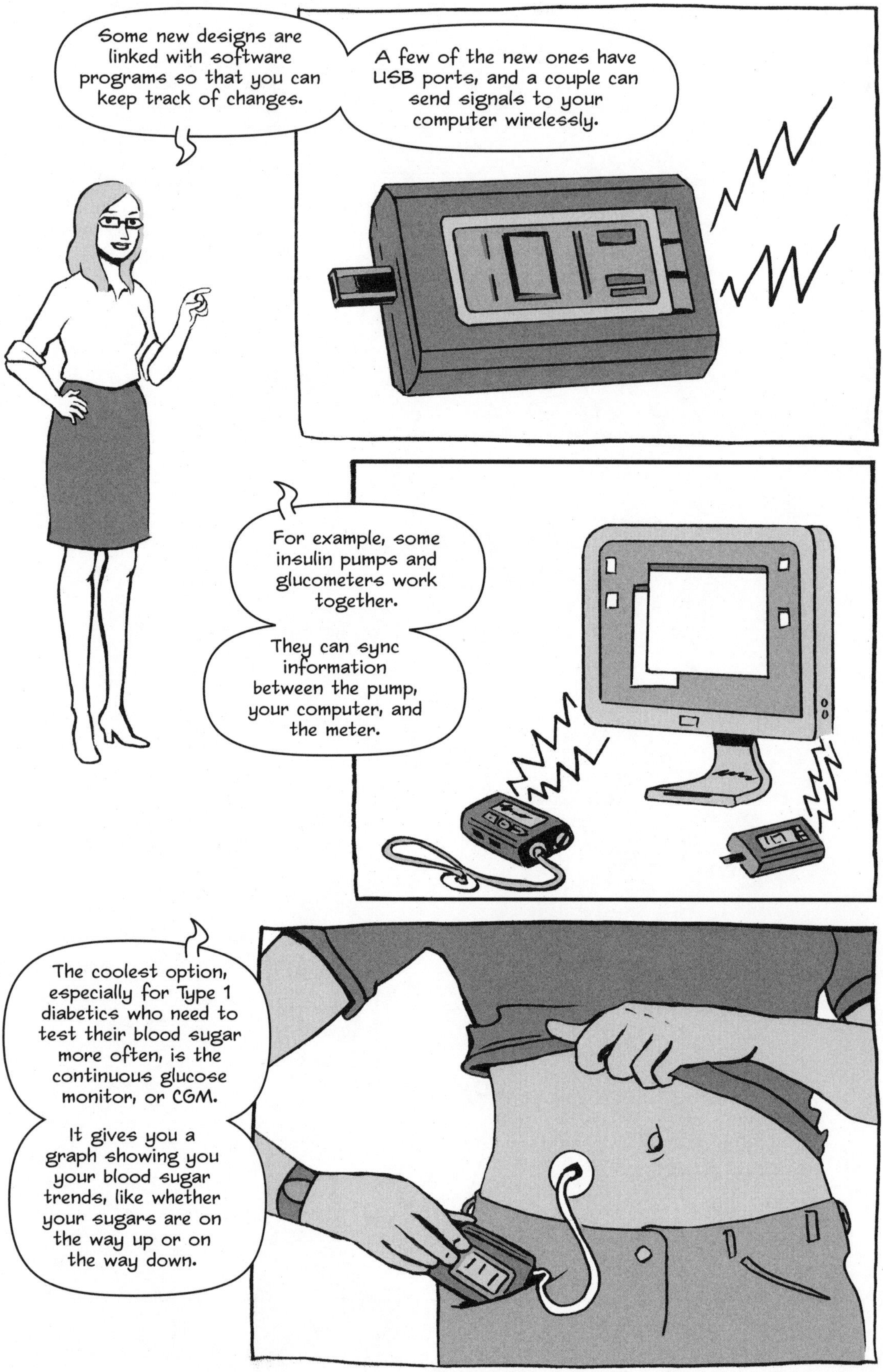

Some new designs are linked with software programs so that you can keep track of changes.
A few of the new ones have USB ports, and a couple can send signals to your computer wirelessly.
For example, some insulin pumps and glucometers work together.
They can sync information between the pump, your computer, and the meter.
The coolest option, especially for Type 1 diabetics who need to test their blood sugar more often, is the continuous glucose monitor, or CGM.
It gives you a graph showing you your blood sugar trends, like whether your sugars are on the way up or on the way down.

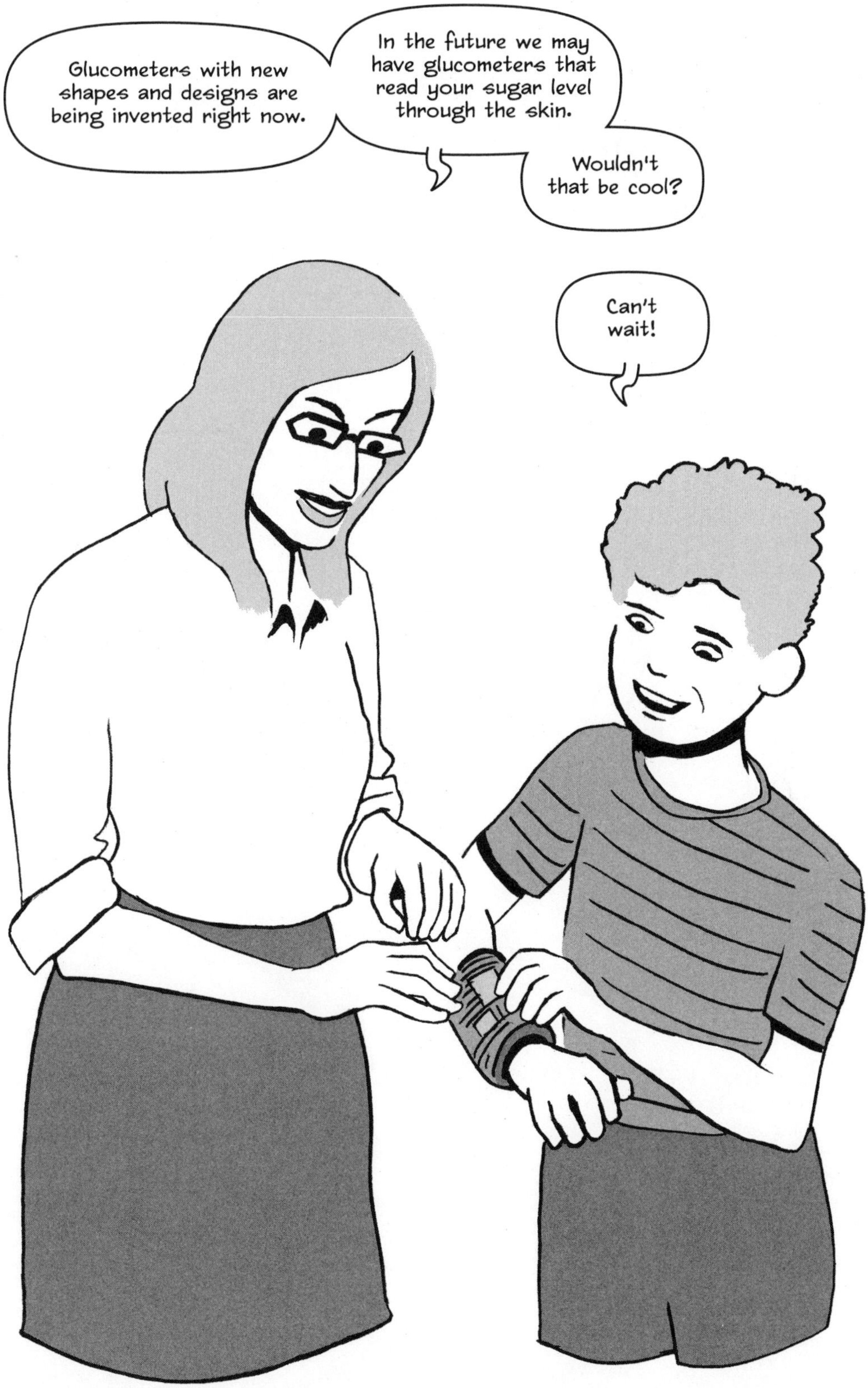
Glucometers with new shapes and designs are being invented right now.
In the future we may have glucometers that read your sugar level through the skin.
Wouldn't that be cool?
Can't wait!

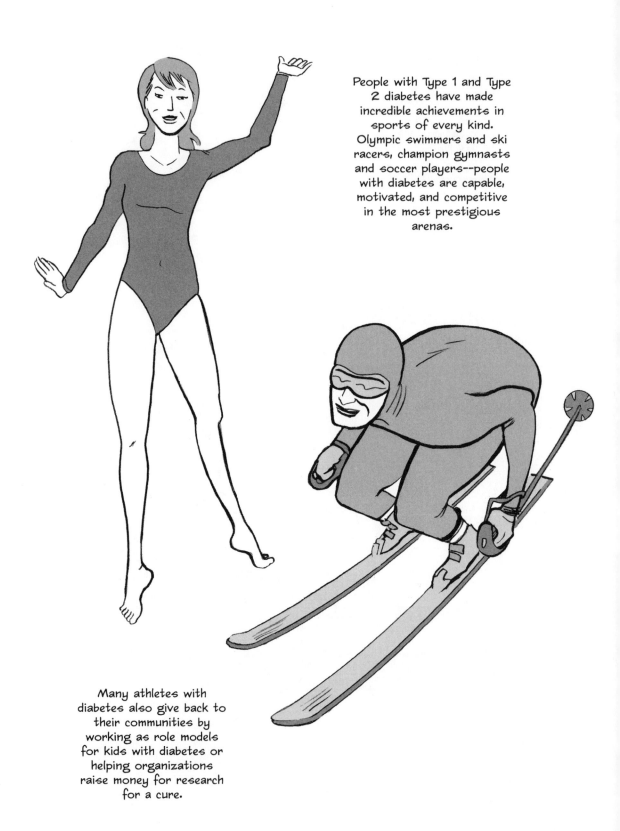

People with Type 1 and Type 2 diabetes have made incredible achievements in sports of every kind. Olympic swimmers and ski racers, champion gymnasts and soccer players--people with diabetes are capable, motivated, and competitive in the most prestigious arenas.

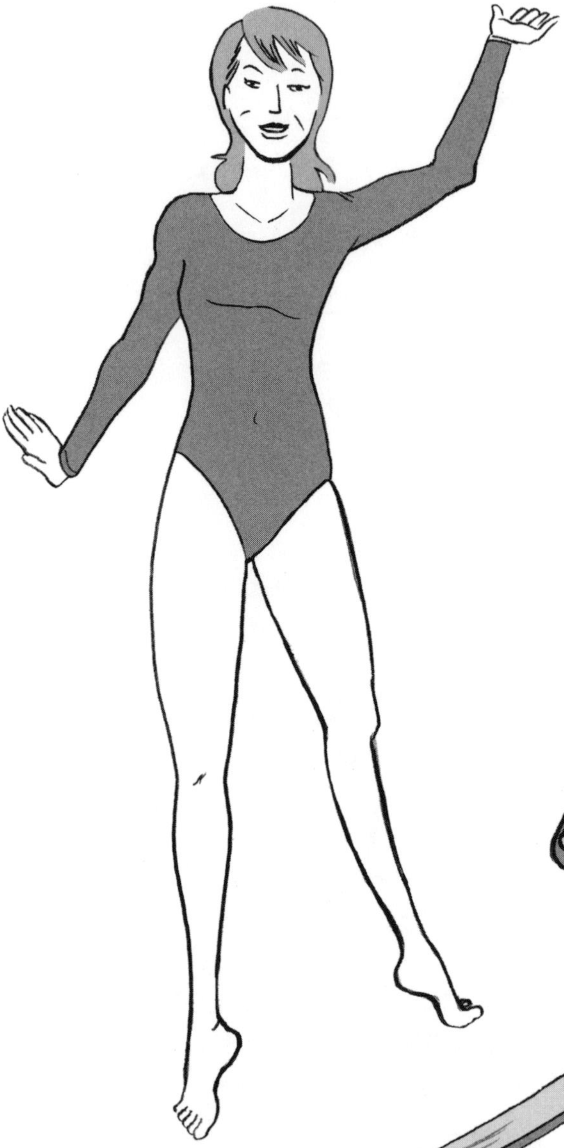

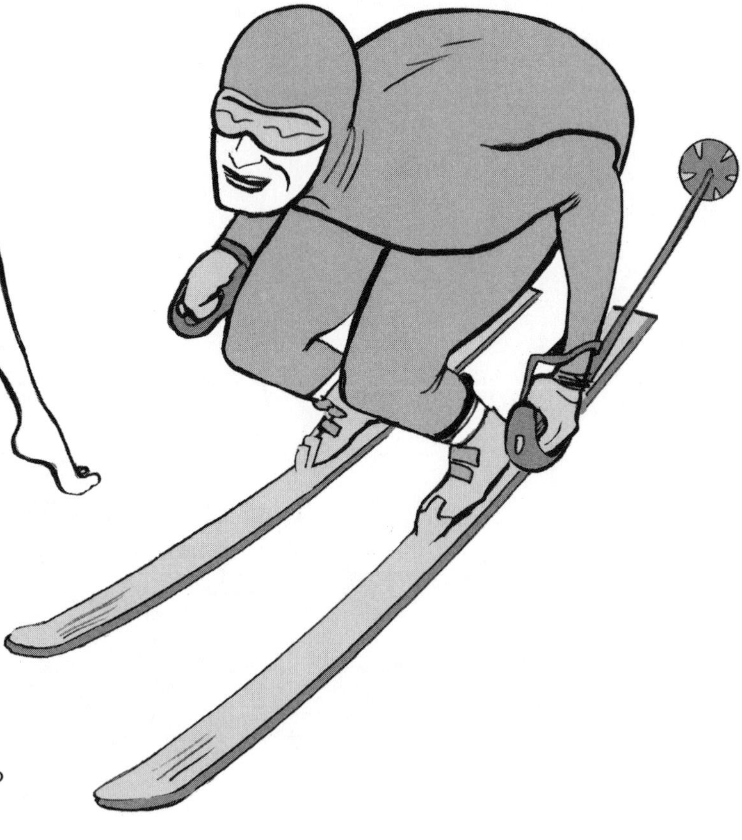

Many athletes with diabetes also give back to their communities by working as role models for kids with diabetes or helping organizations raise money for research for a cure.

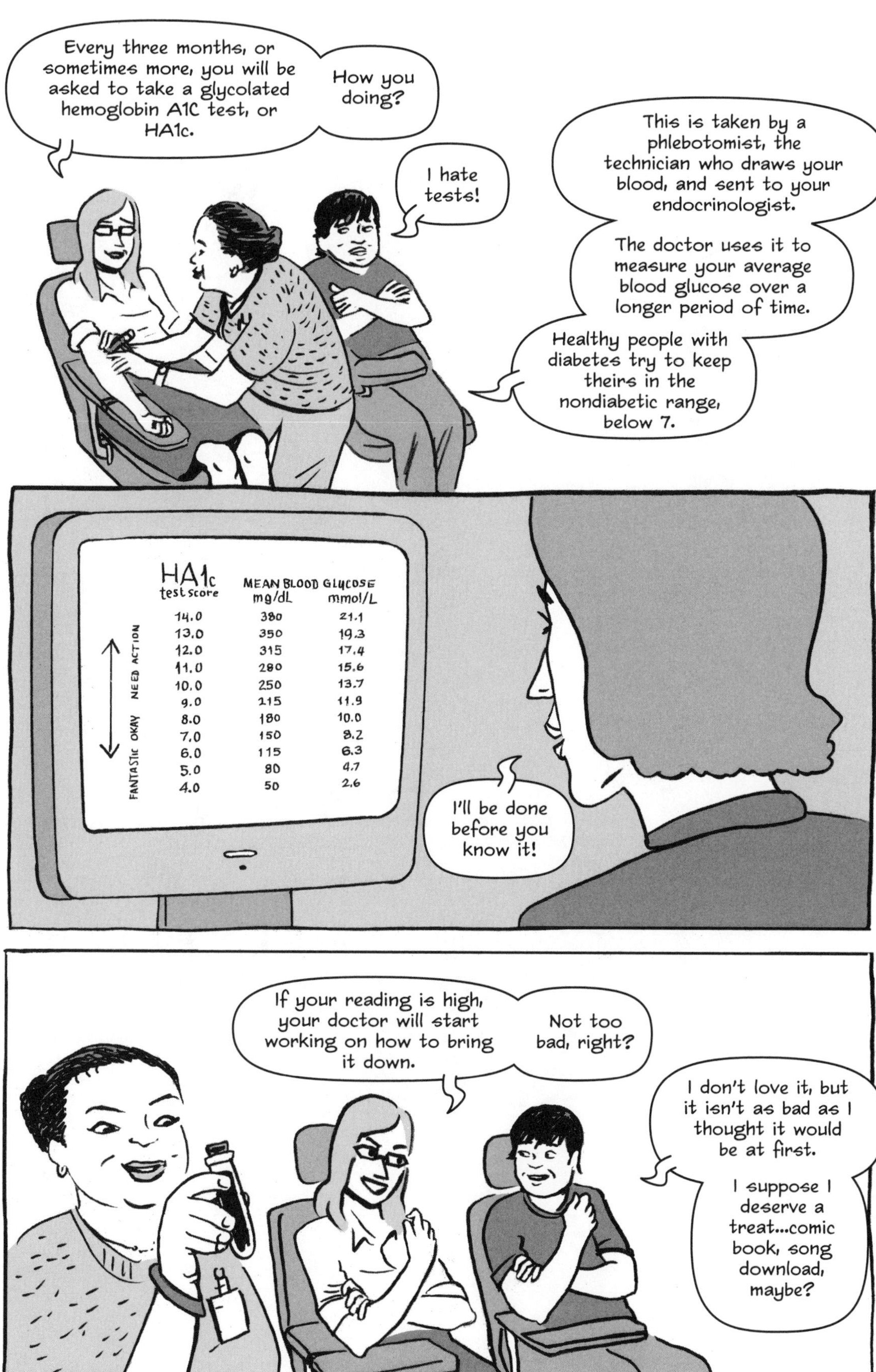
Every three months, or sometimes more, you will be asked to take a glycolated hemoglobin A1C test, or HA1c.
How you doing?
I hate tests!
This is taken by a phlebotomist, the technician who draws your blood, and sent to your endocrinologist.
The doctor uses it to measure your average blood glucose over a longer period of time.
Healthy people with diabetes try to keep theirs in the nondiabetic range, below 7.
HA1c test score
MEAN BLOOD GLUCOSE mg/dL mmol/L
14.0 380 21.1
13.0 350 19.3
12.0 315 17.4
11.0 280 15.6
10.0 250 13.7
9.0 215 11.9
8.0 180 10.0
7.0 150 8.2
6.0 115 6.3
5.0 80 4.7
4.0 50 2.6
NEED ACTION
OKAY
FANTASTIC
I'll be done before you know it!
If your reading is high, your doctor will start working on how to bring it down.
Not too bad, right?
I don't love it, but it isn't as bad as I thought it would be at first.
I suppose I deserve a treat...comic book, song download, maybe?

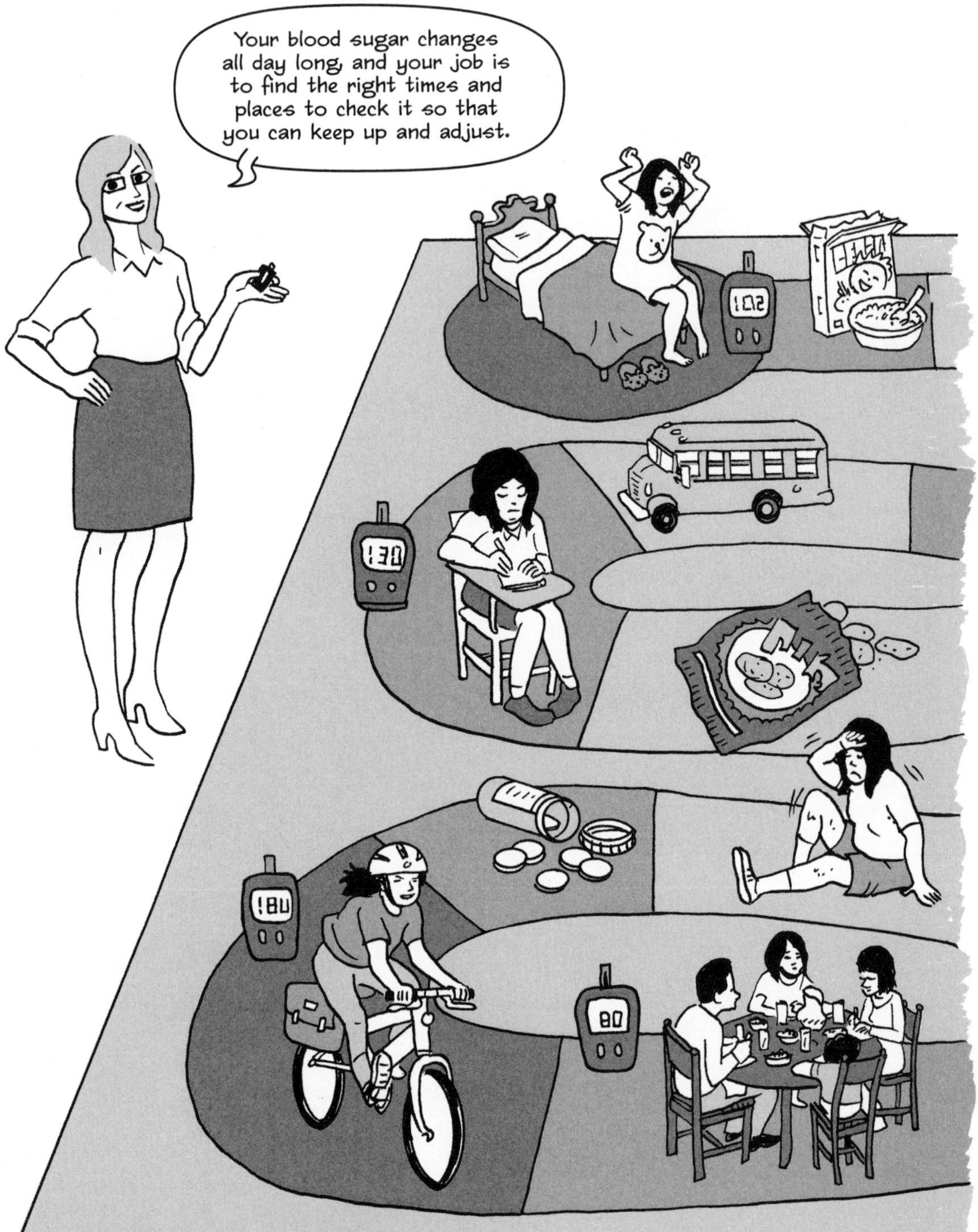
Your blood sugar changes all day long, and your job is to find the right times and places to check it so that you can keep up and adjust.

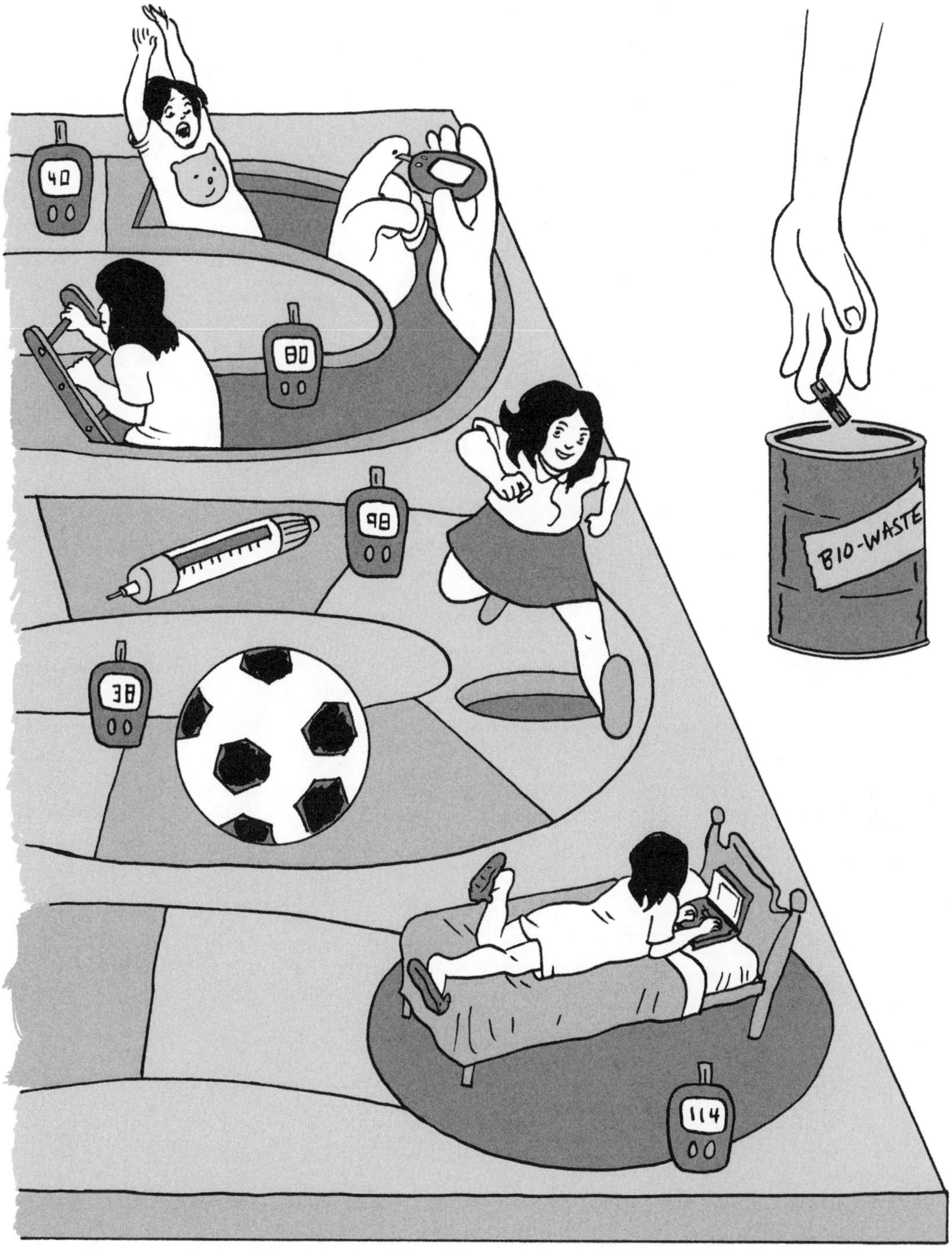
40
80
98
38
114
BIO-WASTE

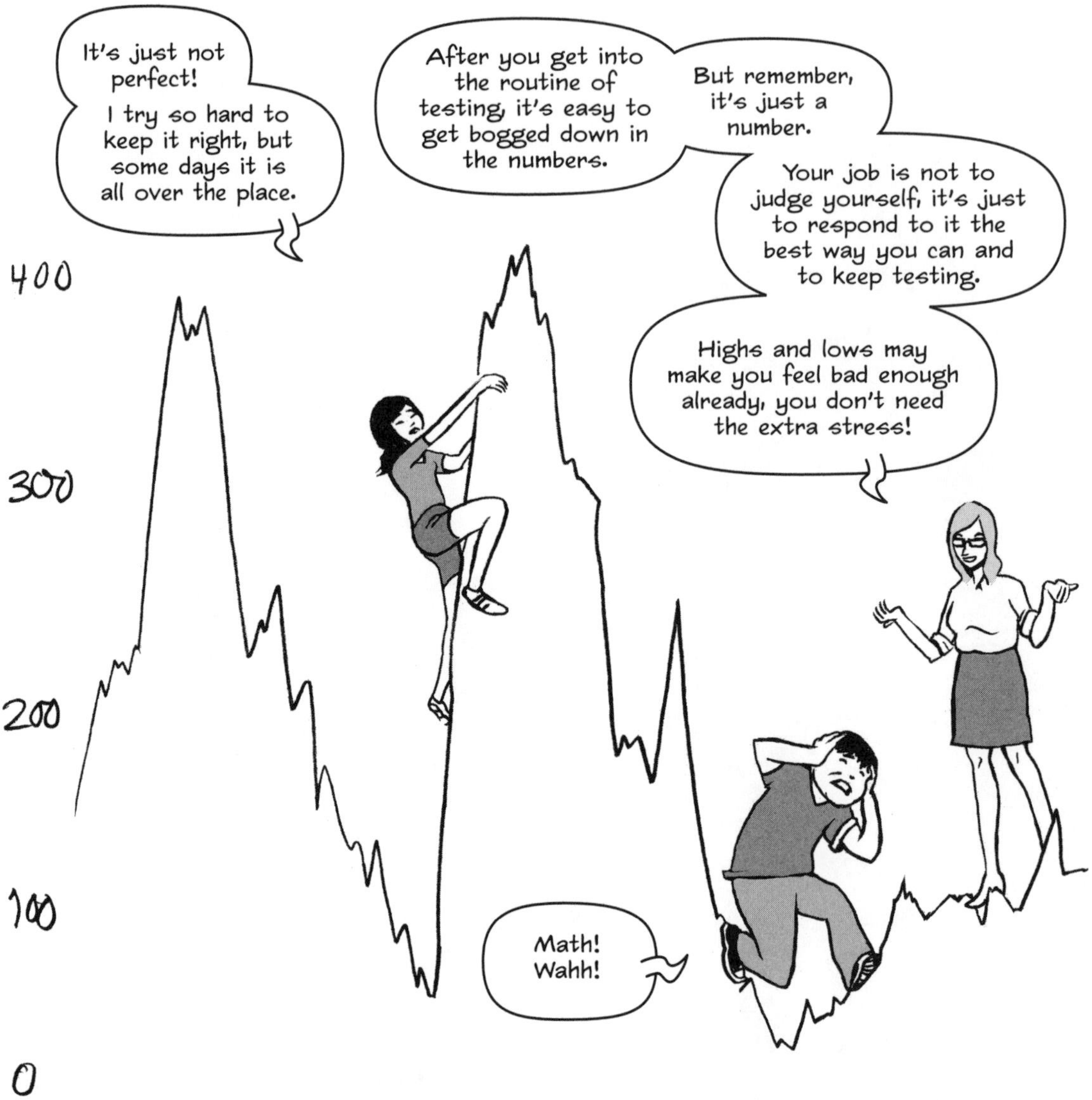
It's just not perfect!
I try so hard to keep it right, but some days it is all over the place.
After you get into the routine of testing, it's easy to get bogged down in the numbers.
But remember, it's just a number.
Your job is not to judge yourself, it's just to respond to it the best way you can and to keep testing.
Highs and lows may make you feel bad enough already, you don't need the extra stress!
400
300
200
100
0
Math! Wahh!

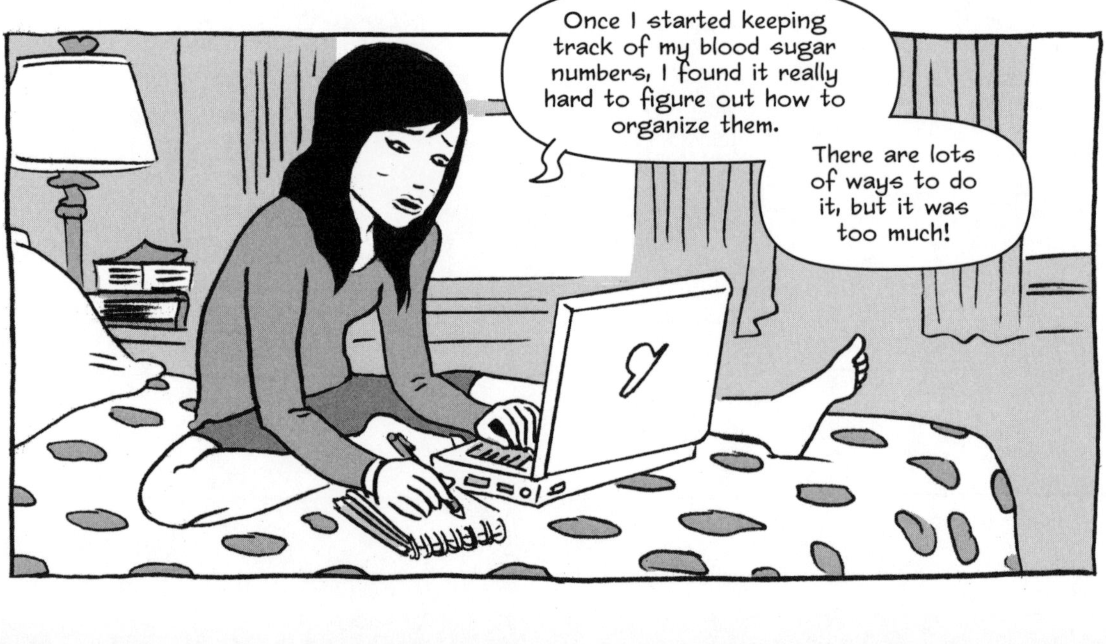
Once I started keeping track of my blood sugar numbers, I found it really hard to figure out how to organize them.
There are lots of ways to do it, but it was too much!

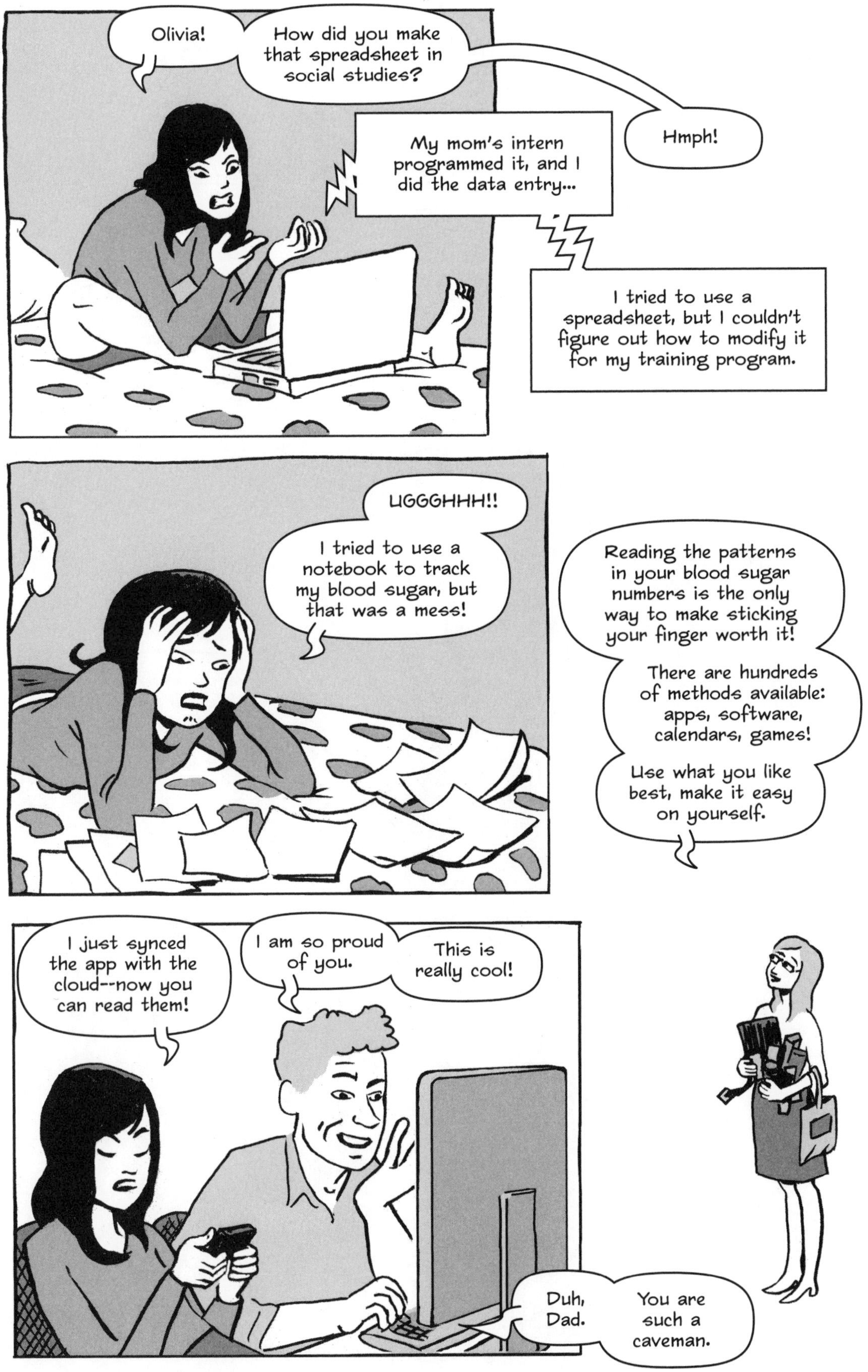
Olivia!
How did you make that spreadsheet in social studies?
Hmph!
My mom's intern programmed it, and I did the data entry...
I tried to use a spreadsheet, but I couldn't figure out how to modify it for my training program.
UGGGHHH!!
I tried to use a notebook to track my blood sugar, but that was a mess!
Reading the patterns in your blood sugar numbers is the only way to make sticking your finger worth it!
There are hundreds of methods available: apps, software, calendars, games!
Use what you like best, make it easy on yourself.
I just synced the app with the cloud--now you can read them!
I am so proud of you.
This is really cool!
Duh, Dad.
You are such a caveman.

EQUIPMENT #2: WHAT IS INSULIN, AND WHAT ARE ORAL MEDS?

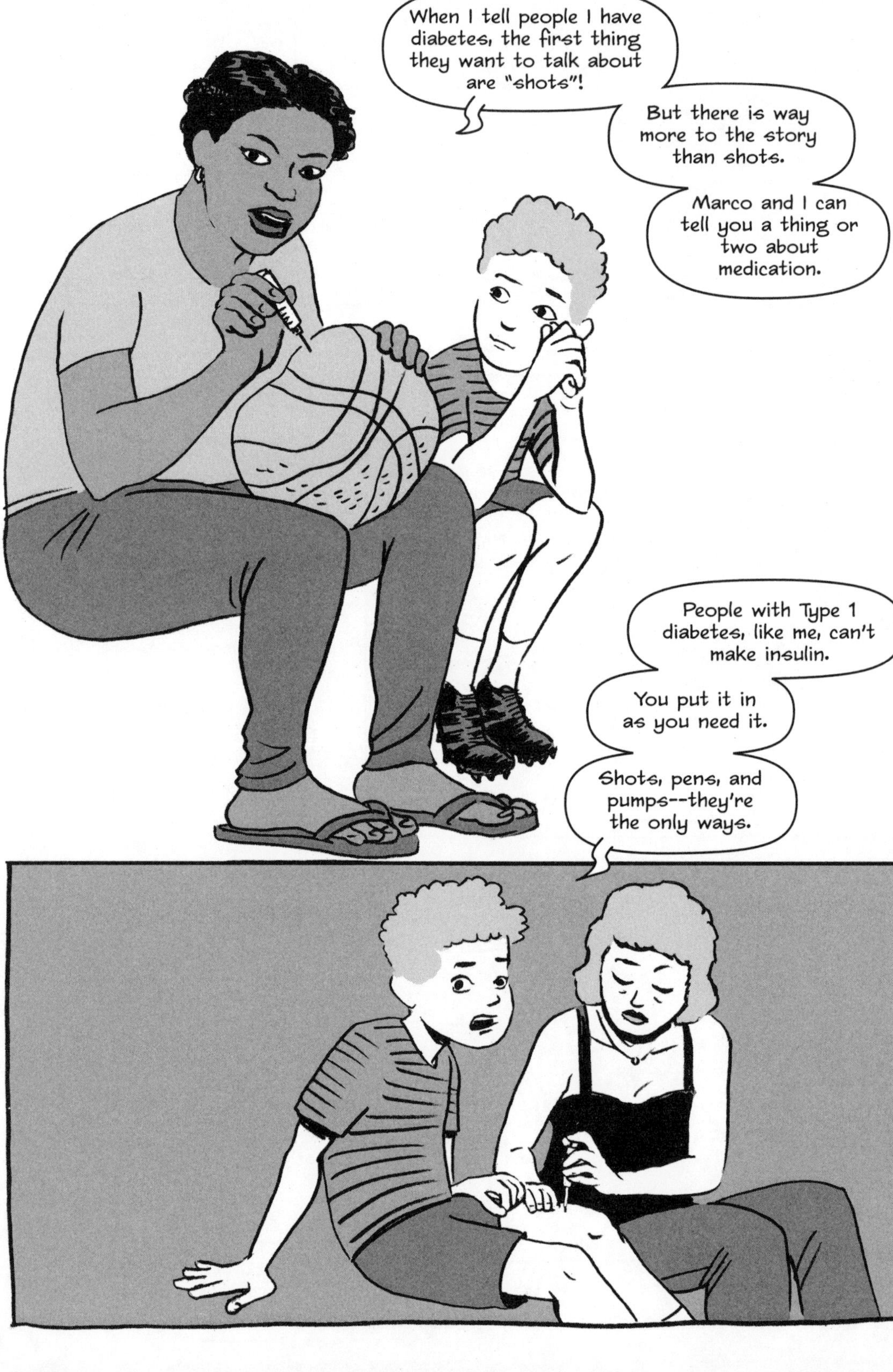
When I tell people I have diabetes, the first thing they want to talk about are "shots"!
But there is way more to the story than shots.
Marco and I can tell you a thing or two about medication.
People with Type 1 diabetes, like me, can't make insulin.
You put it in as you need it.
Shots, pens, and pumps--they're the only ways.

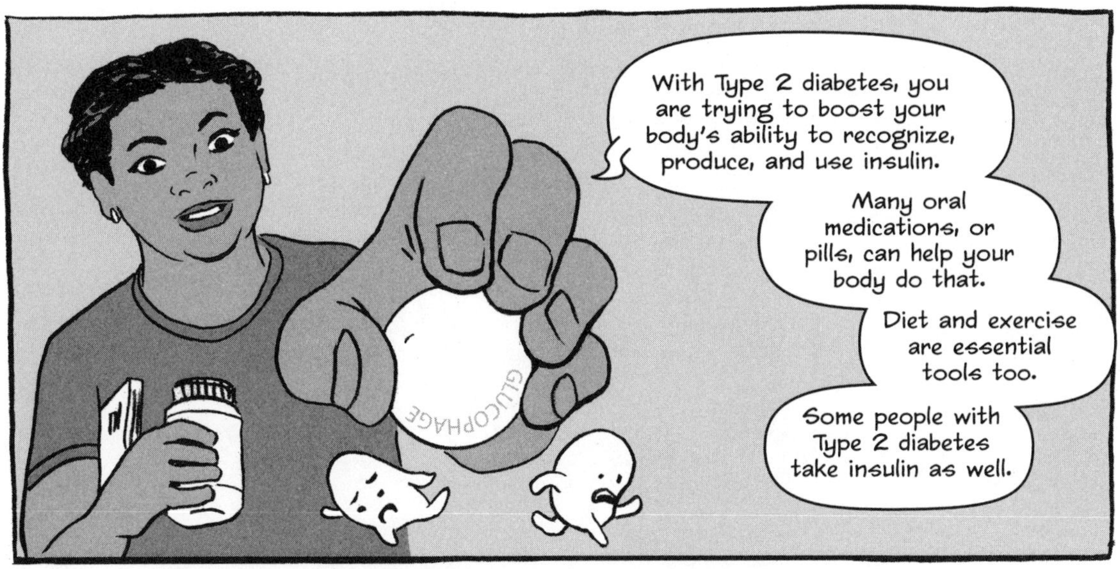
With Type 2 diabetes, you are trying to boost your body's ability to recognize, produce, and use insulin.
Many oral medications, or pills, can help your body do that.
Diet and exercise are essential tools too.
Some people with Type 2 diabetes take insulin as well.
GLUCOPHAGE

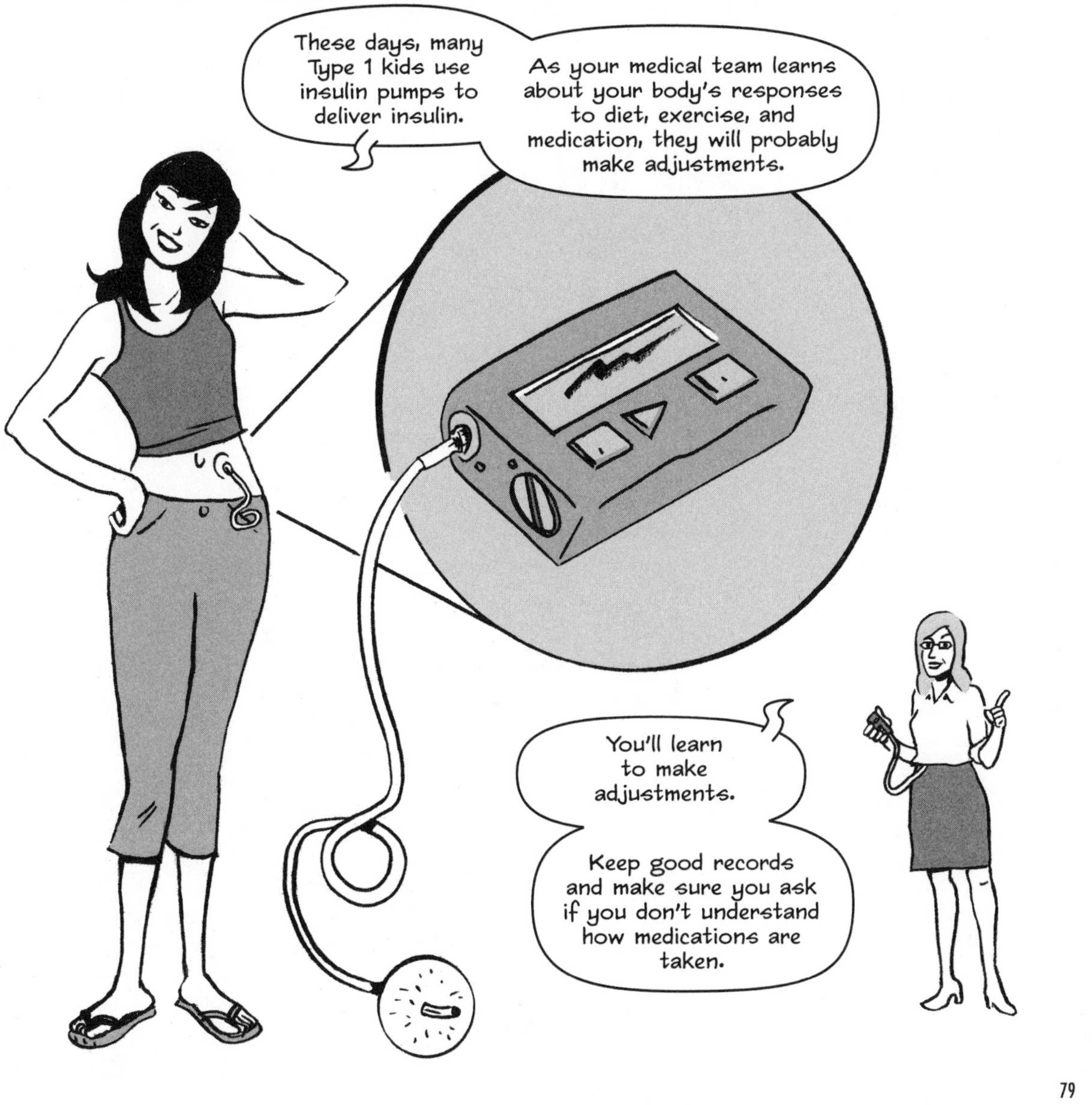
These days, many Type 1 kids use insulin pumps to deliver insulin.
As your medical team learns about your body's responses to diet, exercise, and medication, they will probably make adjustments.
You'll learn to make adjustments.
Keep good records and make sure you ask if you don't understand how medications are taken.

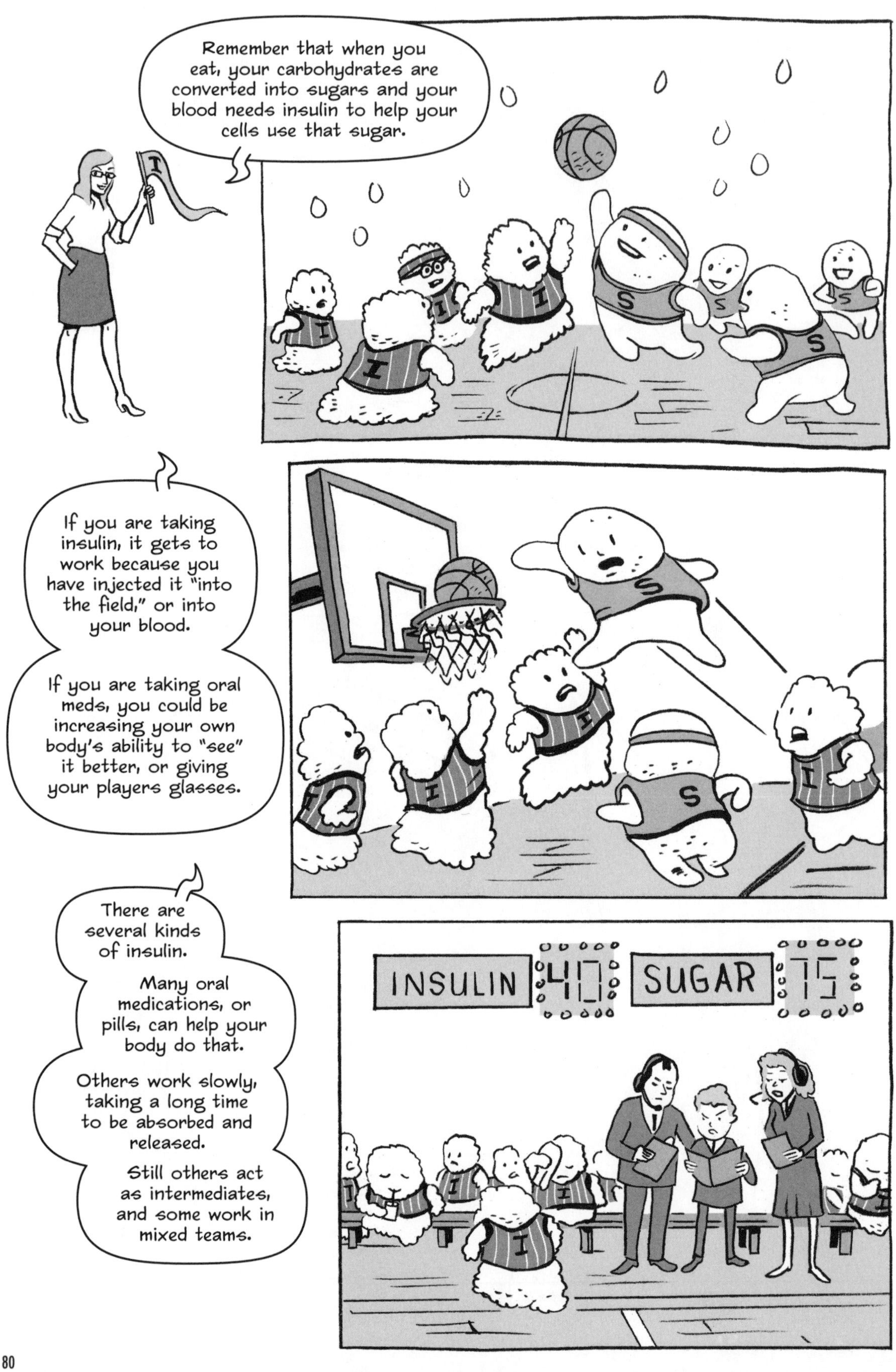

Remember that when you eat, your carbohydrates are converted into sugars and your blood needs insulin to help your cells use that sugar.
If you are taking insulin, it gets to work because you have injected it "into the field," or into your blood.
If you are taking oral meds, you could be increasing your own body's ability to "see" it better, or giving your players glasses.
There are several kinds of insulin.
Many oral medications, or pills, can help your body do that.
Others work slowly, taking a long time to be absorbed and released.
Still others act as intermediates, and some work in mixed teams.
INSULIN 40
SUGAR 15

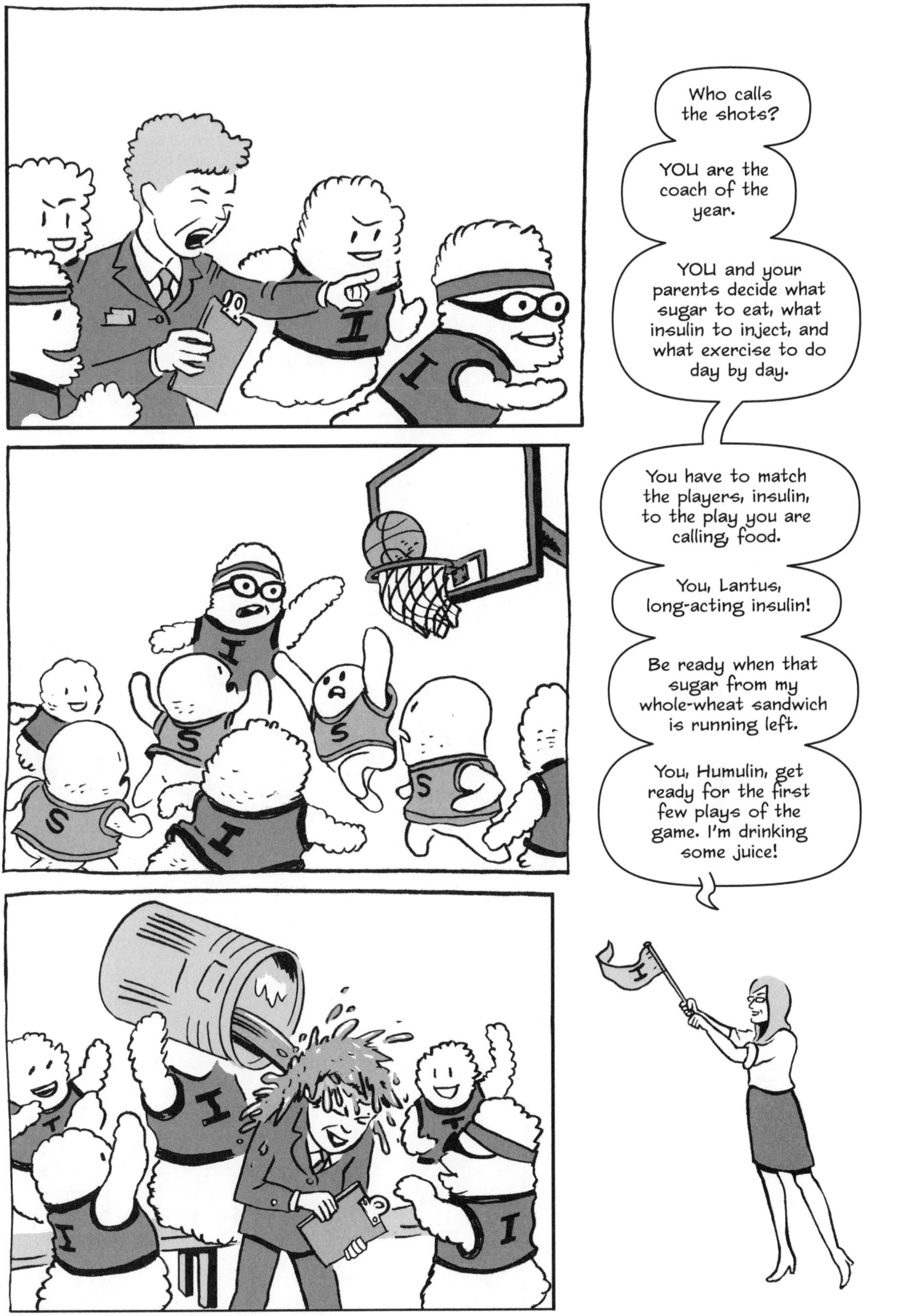

Who calls the shots?
YOU are the coach of the year.
YOU and your parents decide what sugar to eat, what insulin to inject, and what exercise to do day by day.
You have to match the players, insulin, to the play you are calling, food.
You, Lantus, long-acting insulin!
Be ready when that sugar from my whole-wheat sandwich is running left.
You, Humulin, get ready for the first few plays of the game. I'm drinking some juice!

THE PANCREAS PLAYBOOK

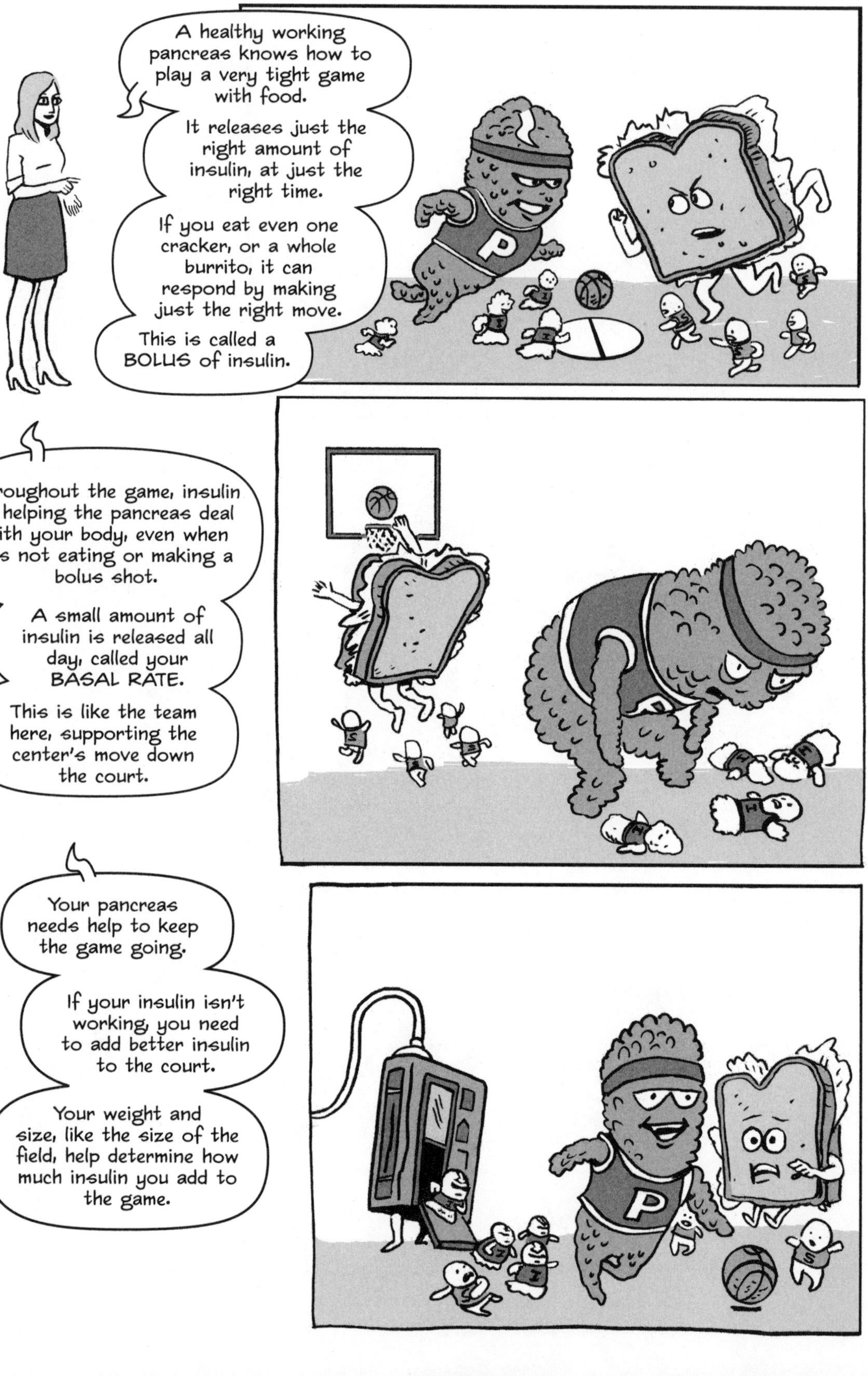

A healthy working pancreas knows how to play a very tight game with food.
It releases just the right amount of insulin, at just the right time.
If you eat even one cracker, or a whole burrito, it can respond by making just the right move.
This is called a BOLUS of insulin.
Throughout the game, insulin is helping the pancreas deal with your body, even when it's not eating or making a bolus shot.
A small amount of insulin is released all day, called your BASAL RATE.
This is like the team here, supporting the center's move down the court.
Your pancreas needs help to keep the game going.
If your insulin isn't working, you need to add better insulin to the court.
Your weight and size, like the size of the field, help determine how much insulin you add to the game.

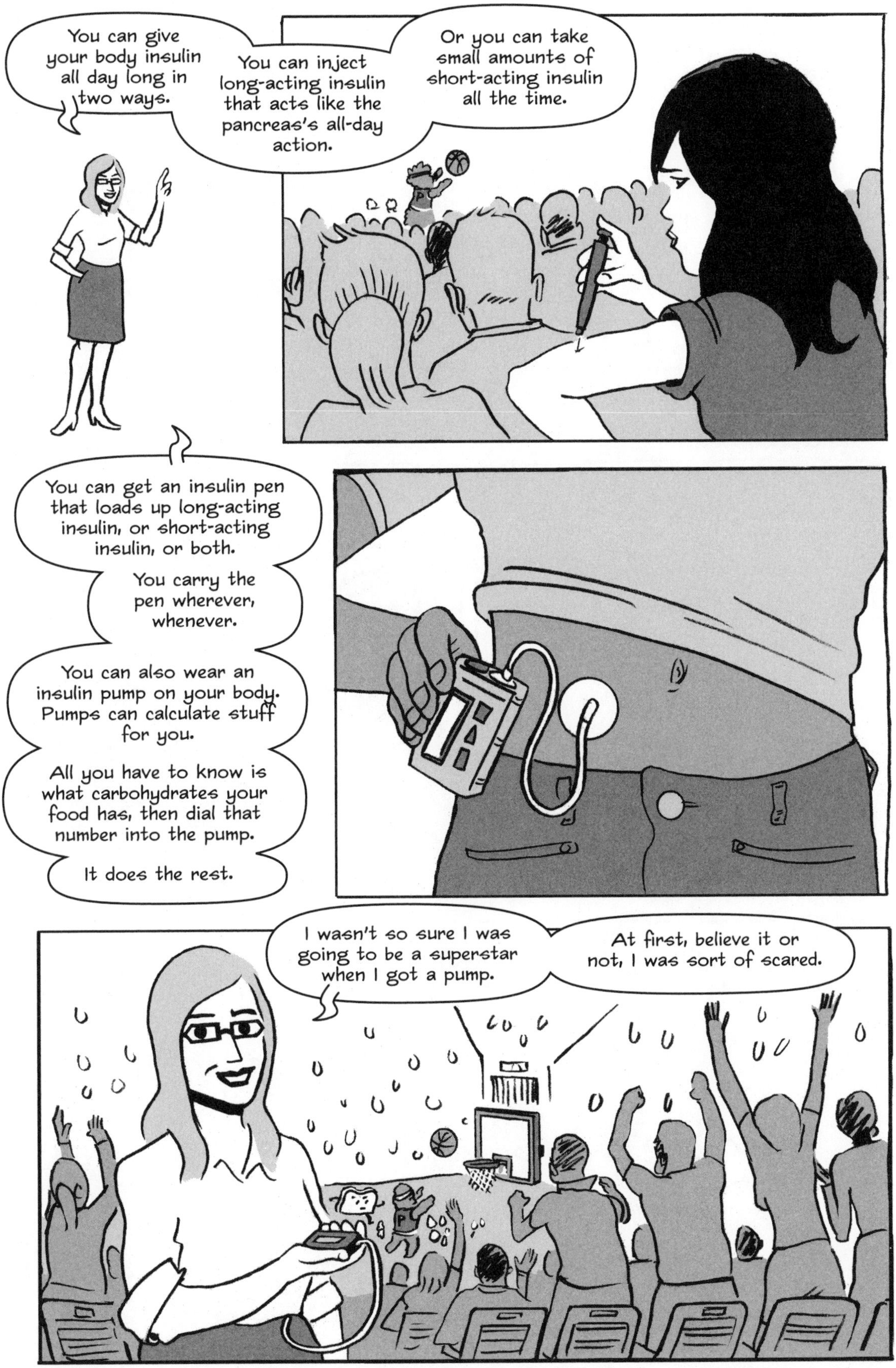
You can give your body insulin all day long in two ways.
You can inject long-acting insulin that acts like the pancreas's all-day action.
Or you can take small amounts of short-acting insulin all the time.
You can get an insulin pen that loads up long-acting insulin, or short-acting insulin, or both.
You carry the pen wherever, whenever.
You can also wear an insulin pump on your body. Pumps can calculate stuff for you.
All you have to know is what carbohydrates your food has, then dial that number into the pump.
It does the rest.
I wasn't so sure I was going to be a superstar when I got a pump.
At first, believe it or not, I was sort of scared.

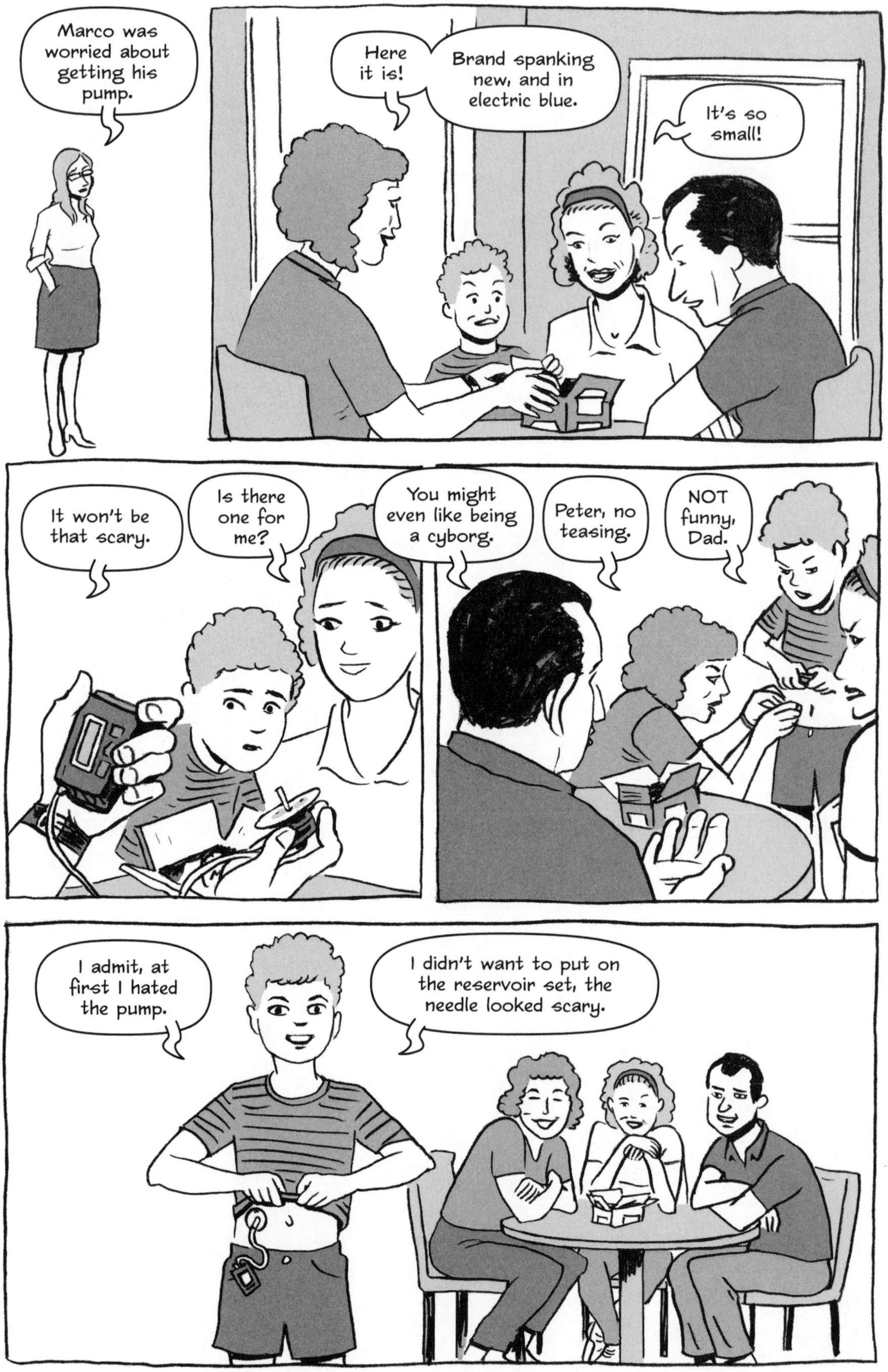
Marco was worried about getting his pump.
Here it is!
Brand spanking new, and in electric blue.
It's so small!
It won't be that scary.
Is there one for me?
You might even like being a cyborg.
Peter, no teasing.
NOT funny, Dad.
I admit, at first I hated the pump.
I didn't want to put on the reservoir set, the needle looked scary.

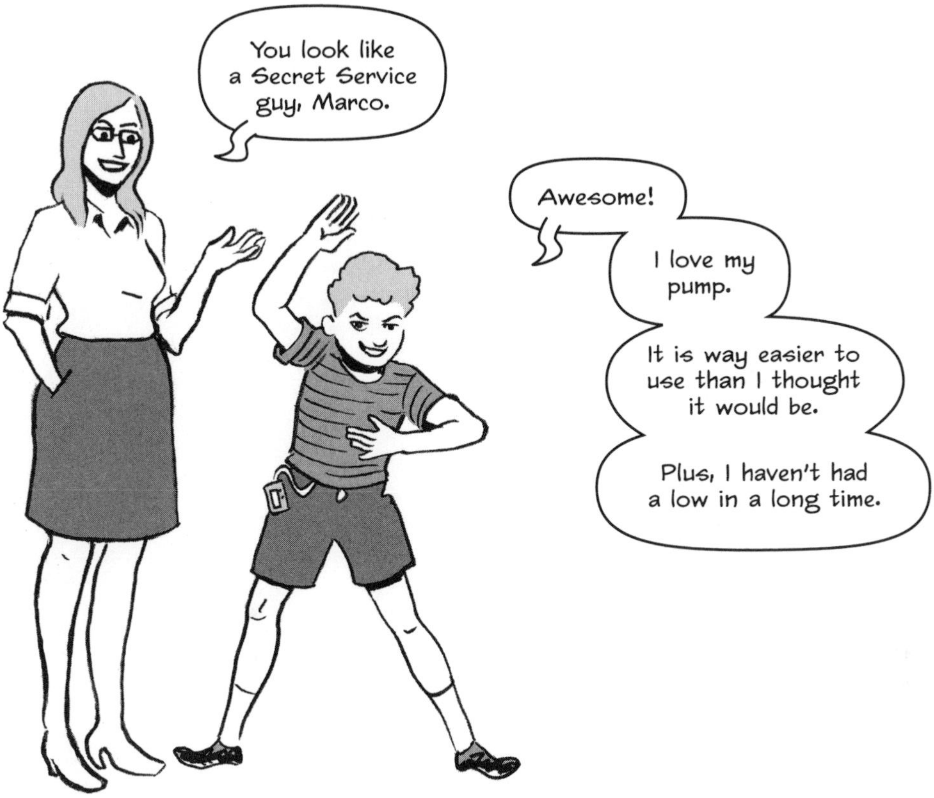
You look like a Secret Service guy, Marco.
Awesome!
I love my pump.
It is way easier to use than I thought it would be.
Plus, I haven't had a low in a long time.

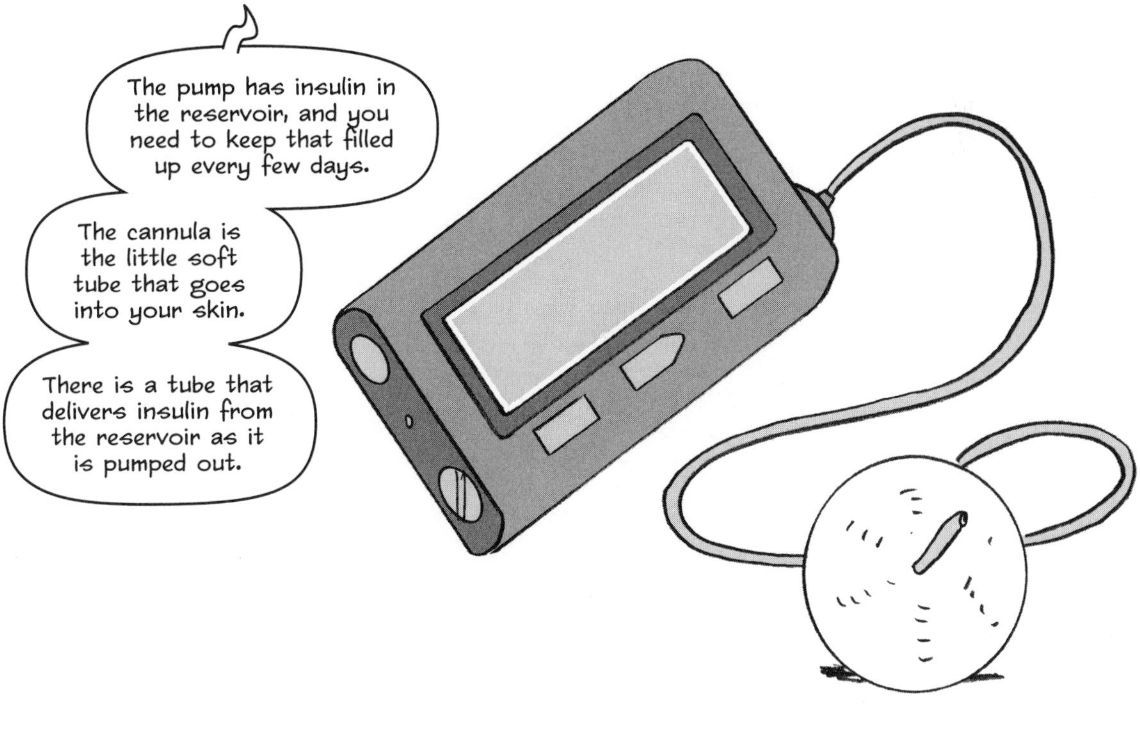
The pump has insulin in the reservoir, and you need to keep that filled up every few days.
The cannula is the little soft tube that goes into your skin.
There is a tube that delivers insulin from the reservoir as it is pumped out.

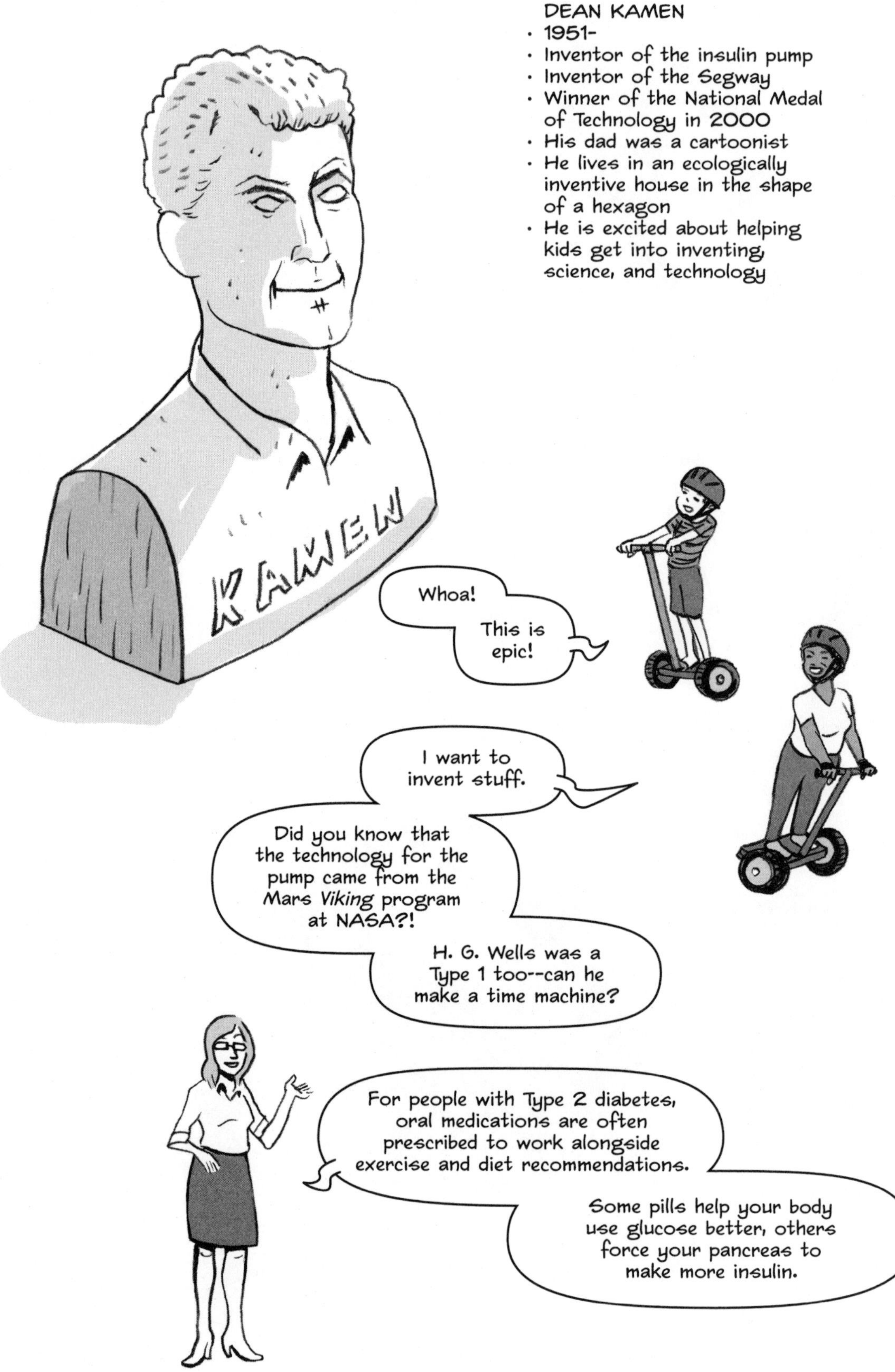
DEAN KAMEN
• 1951-
• Inventor of the insulin pump
• Inventor of the Segway
• Winner of the National Medal of Technology in 2000
• His dad was a cartoonist
• He lives in an ecologically inventive house in the shape of a hexagon
• He is excited about helping kids get into inventing, science, and technology
KAMEN
Whoa!
This is epic!
I want to invent stuff.
Did you know that the technology for the pump came from the Mars *Viking* program at NASA?!
H. G. Wells was a Type 1 too--can he make a time machine?
For people with Type 2 diabetes, oral medications are often prescribed to work alongside exercise and diet recommendations.
Some pills help your body use glucose better, others force your pancreas to make more insulin.

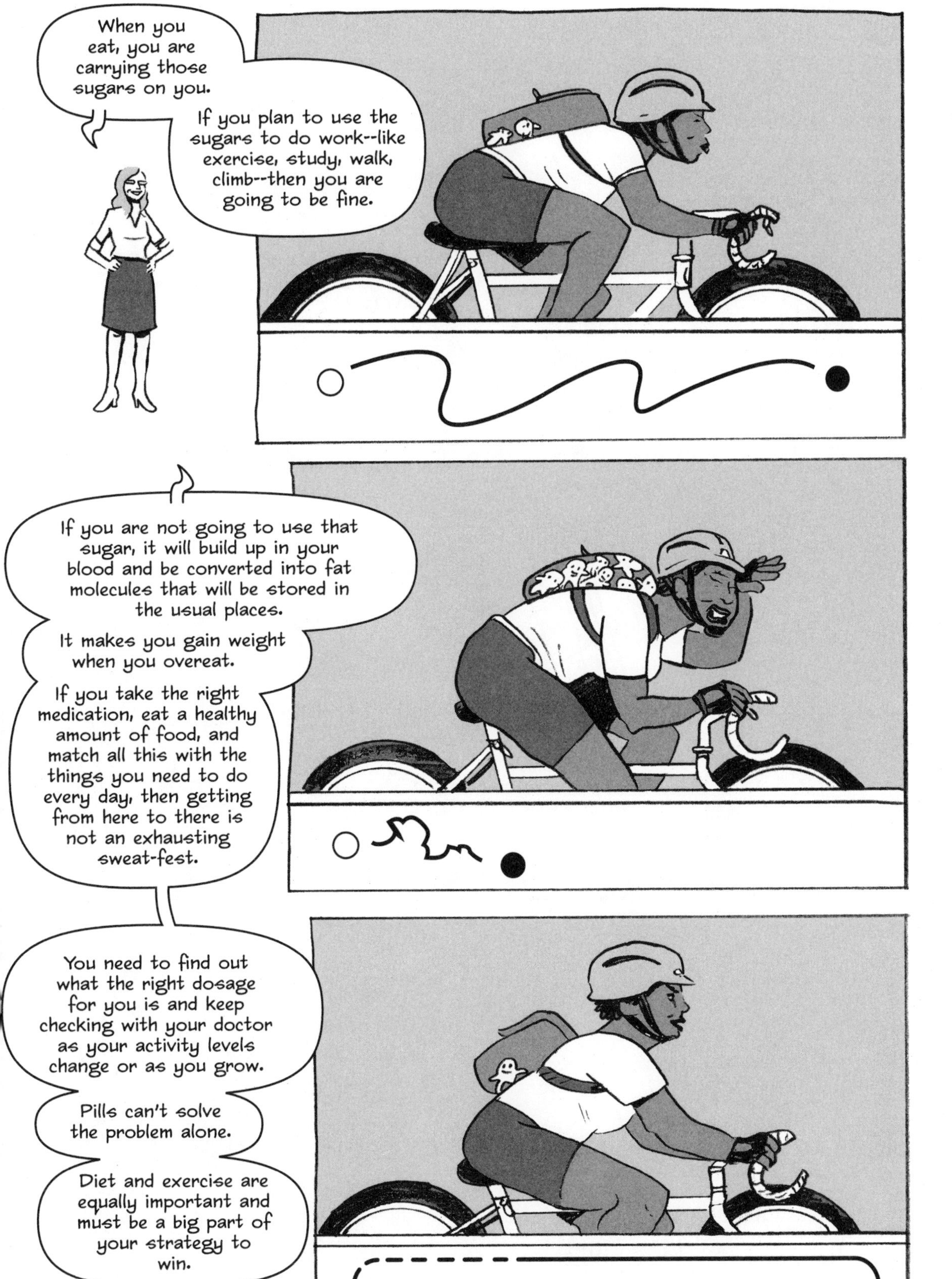
When you eat, you are carrying those sugars on you.
If you plan to use the sugars to do work--like exercise, study, walk, climb--then you are going to be fine.
If you are not going to use that sugar, it will build up in your blood and be converted into fat molecules that will be stored in the usual places.
It makes you gain weight when you overeat.
If you take the right medication, eat a healthy amount of food, and match all this with the things you need to do every day, then getting from here to there is not an exhausting sweat-fest.
You need to find out what the right dosage for you is and keep checking with your doctor as your activity levels change or as you grow.
Pills can't solve the problem alone.
Diet and exercise are equally important and must be a big part of your strategy to win.

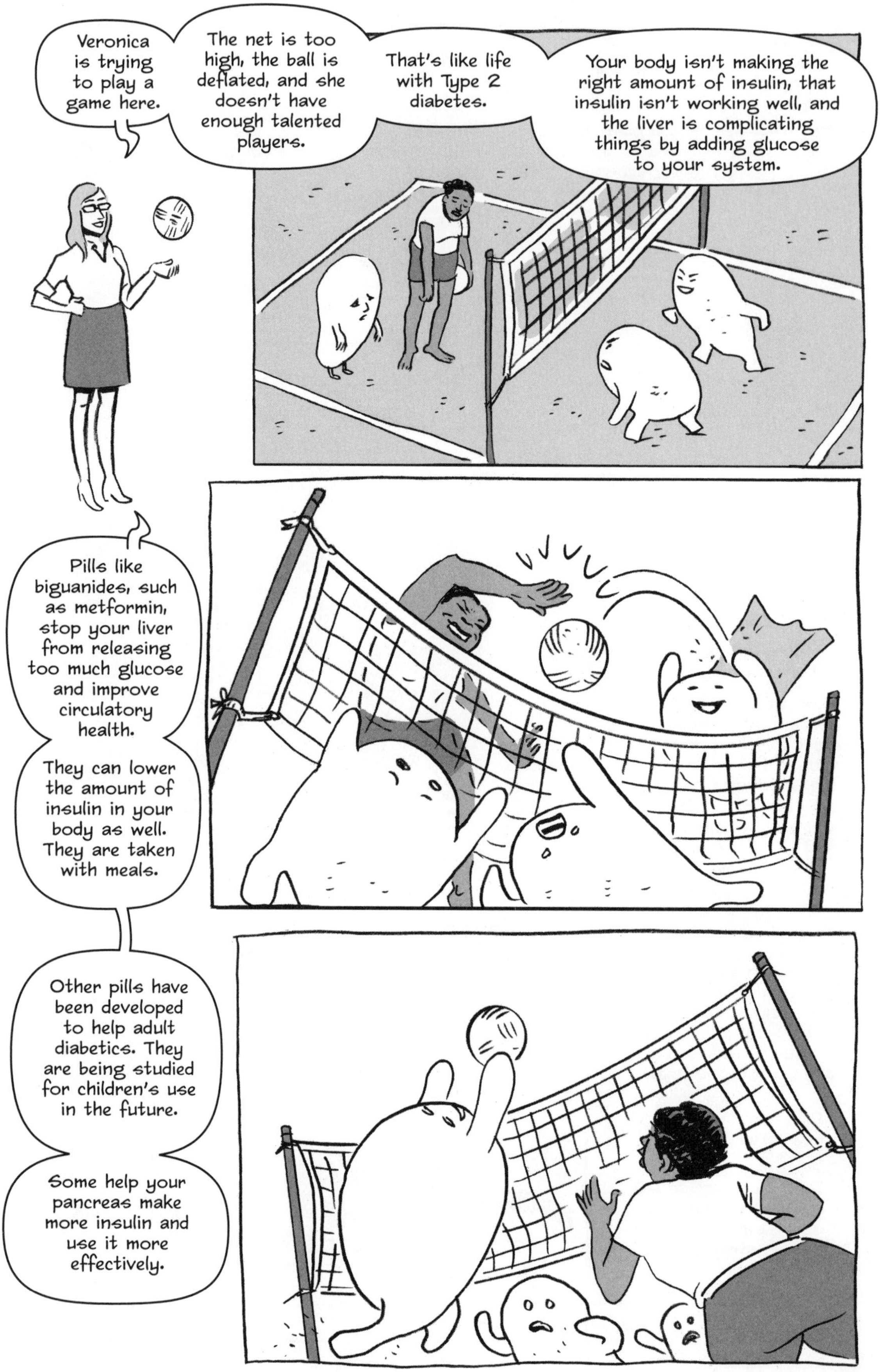

Veronica is trying to play a game here.
The net is too high, the ball is deflated, and she doesn't have enough talented players.
That's like life with Type 2 diabetes.
Your body isn't making the right amount of insulin, that insulin isn't working well, and the liver is complicating things by adding glucose to your system.
Pills like biguanides, such as metformin, stop your liver from releasing too much glucose and improve circulatory health.
They can lower the amount of insulin in your body as well. They are taken with meals.
Other pills have been developed to help adult diabetics. They are being studied for children's use in the future.
Some help your pancreas make more insulin and use it more effectively.

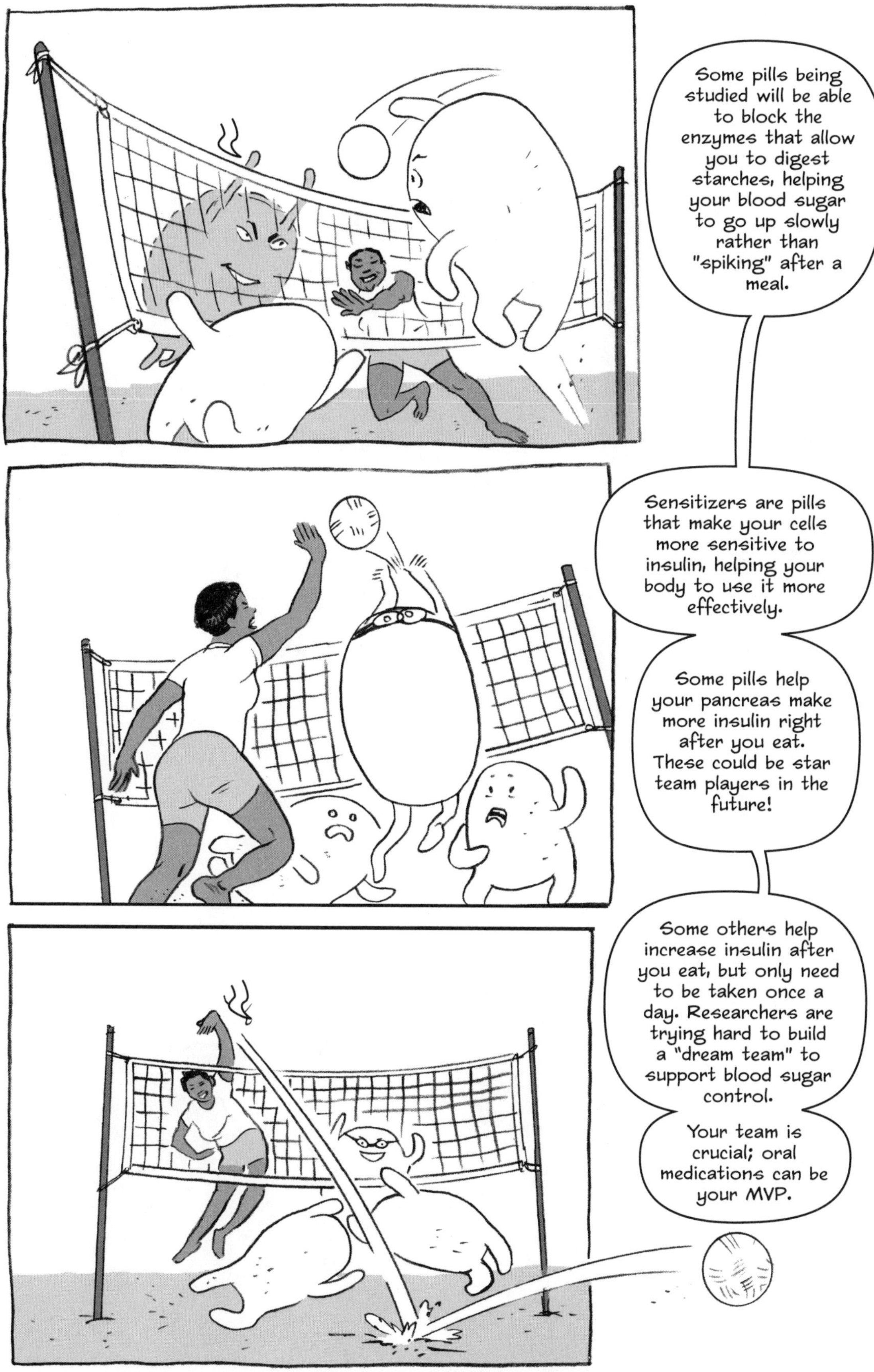

Some pills being studied will be able to block the enzymes that allow you to digest starches, helping your blood sugar to go up slowly rather than "spiking" after a meal.
Sensitizers are pills that make your cells more sensitive to insulin, helping your body to use it more effectively.
Some pills help your pancreas make more insulin right after you eat. These could be star team players in the future!
Some others help increase insulin after you eat, but only need to be taken once a day. Researchers are trying hard to build a "dream team" to support blood sugar control.
Your team is crucial; oral medications can be your MVP.

PART FOUR: FUEL

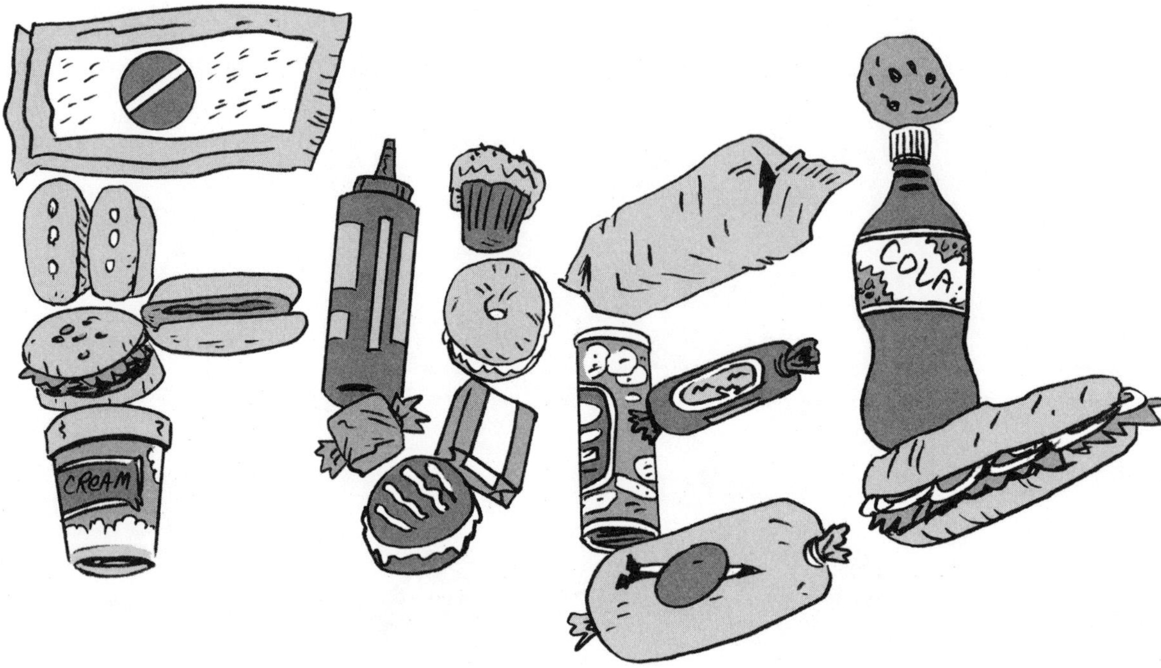
CREAM
COLA

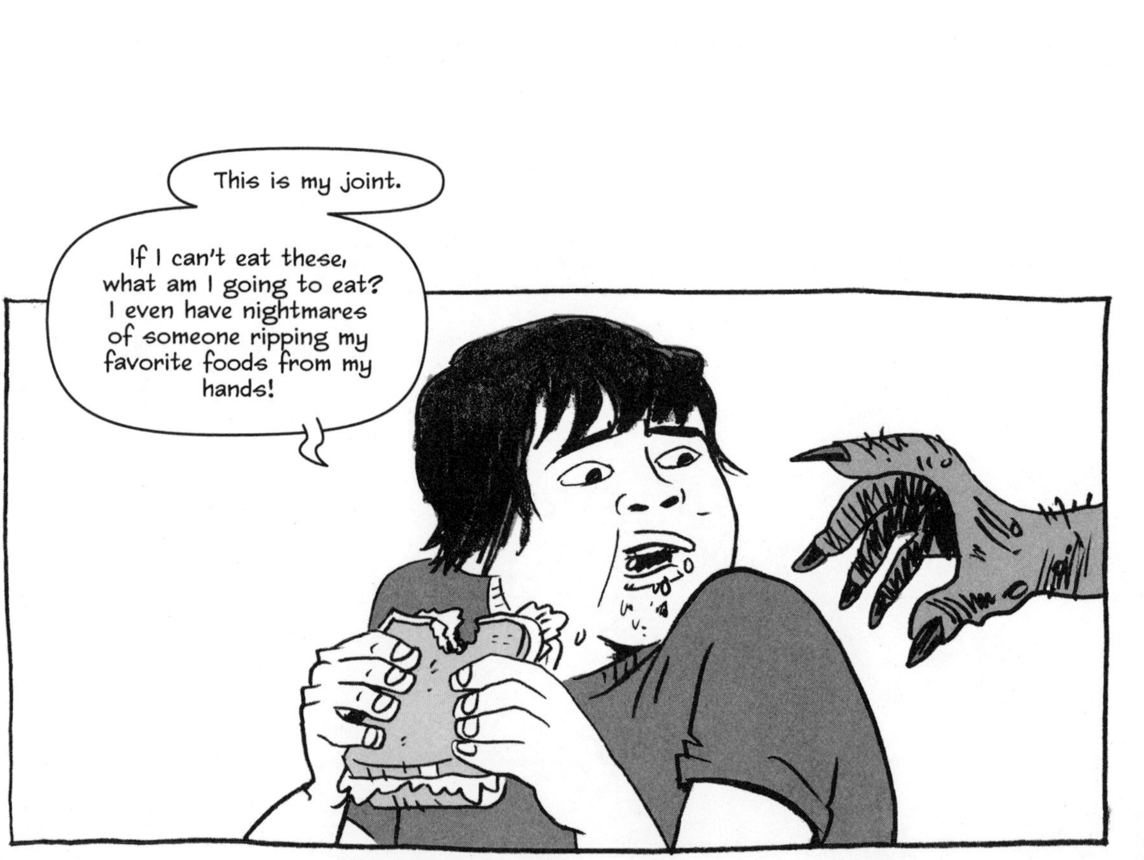
This is my joint.
If I can't eat these, what am I going to eat? I even have nightmares of someone ripping my favorite foods from my hands!

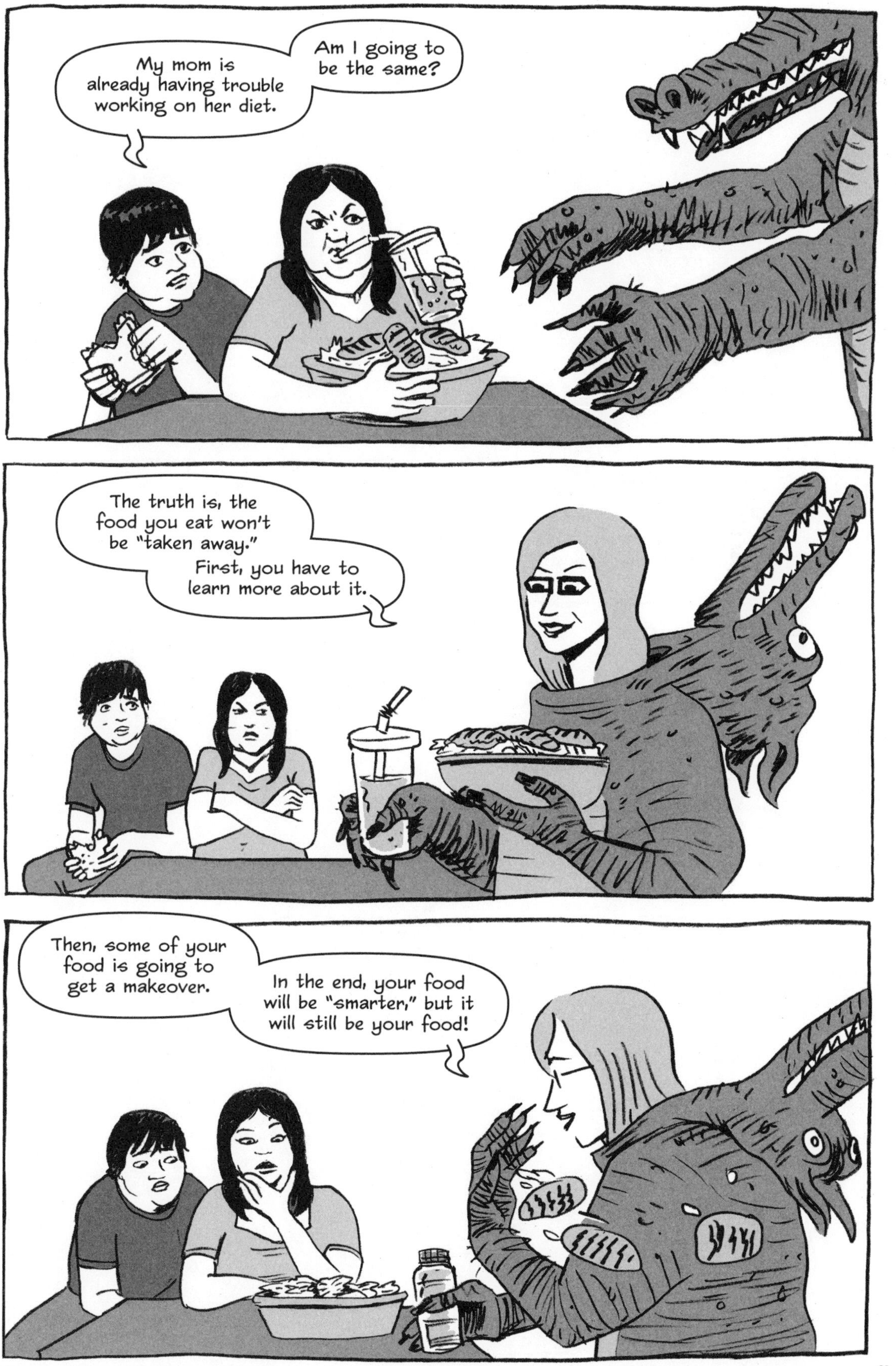
My mom is already having trouble working on her diet.
Am I going to be the same?
The truth is, the food you eat won't be "taken away."
First, you have to learn more about it.
Then, some of your food is going to get a makeover.
In the end, your food will be "smarter," but it will still be your food!

WHAT IS A CARBOHYDRATE?

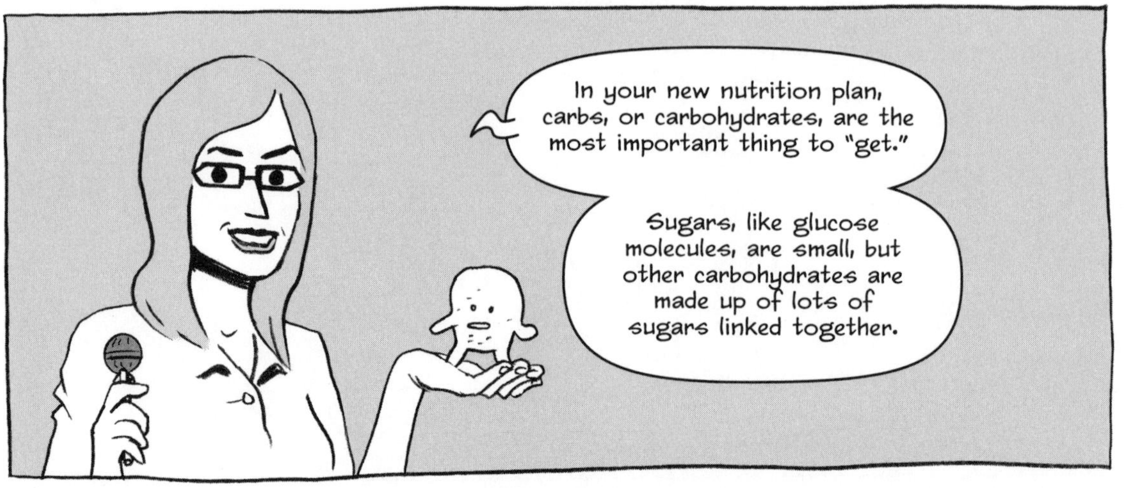
In your new nutrition plan, carbs, or carbohydrates, are the most important thing to "get."
Sugars, like glucose molecules, are small, but other carbohydrates are made up of lots of sugars linked together.

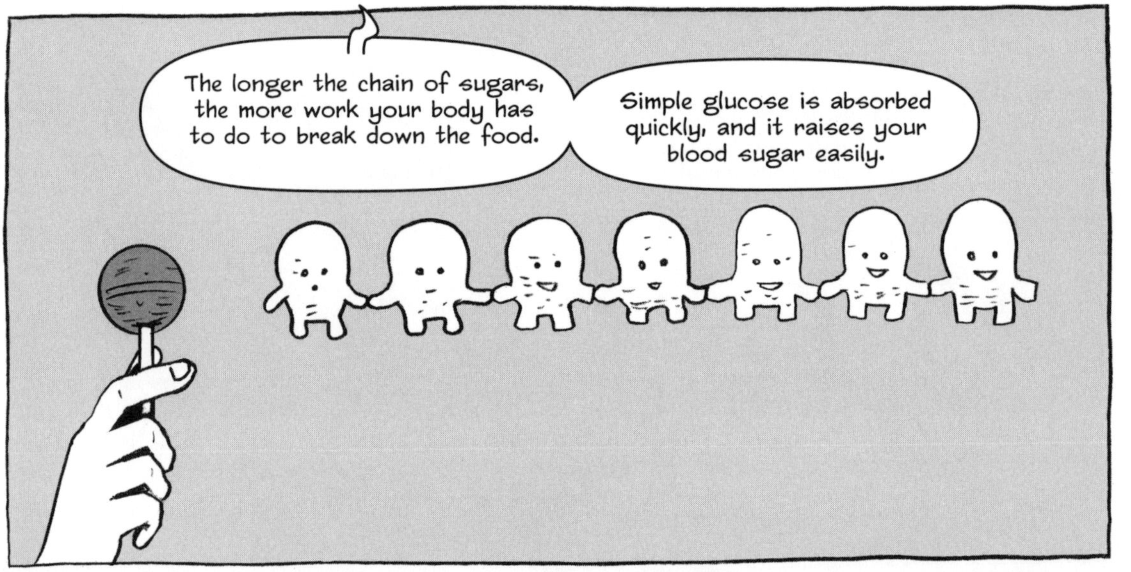
The longer the chain of sugars, the more work your body has to do to break down the food.
Simple glucose is absorbed quickly, and it raises your blood sugar easily.

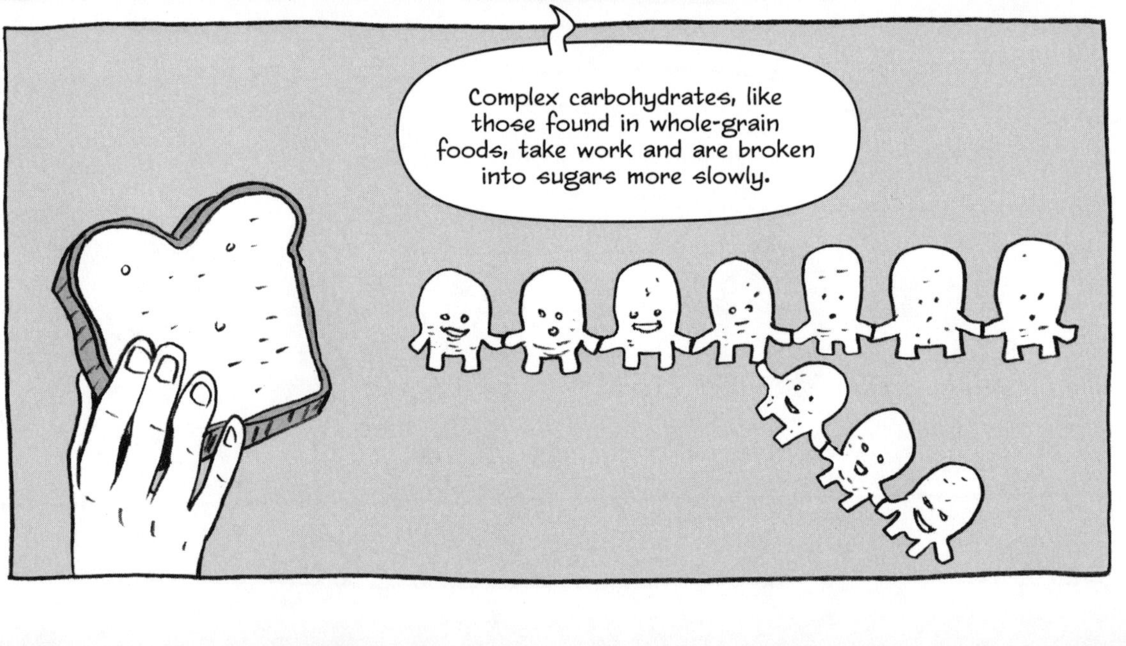
Complex carbohydrates, like those found in whole-grain foods, take work and are broken into sugars more slowly.

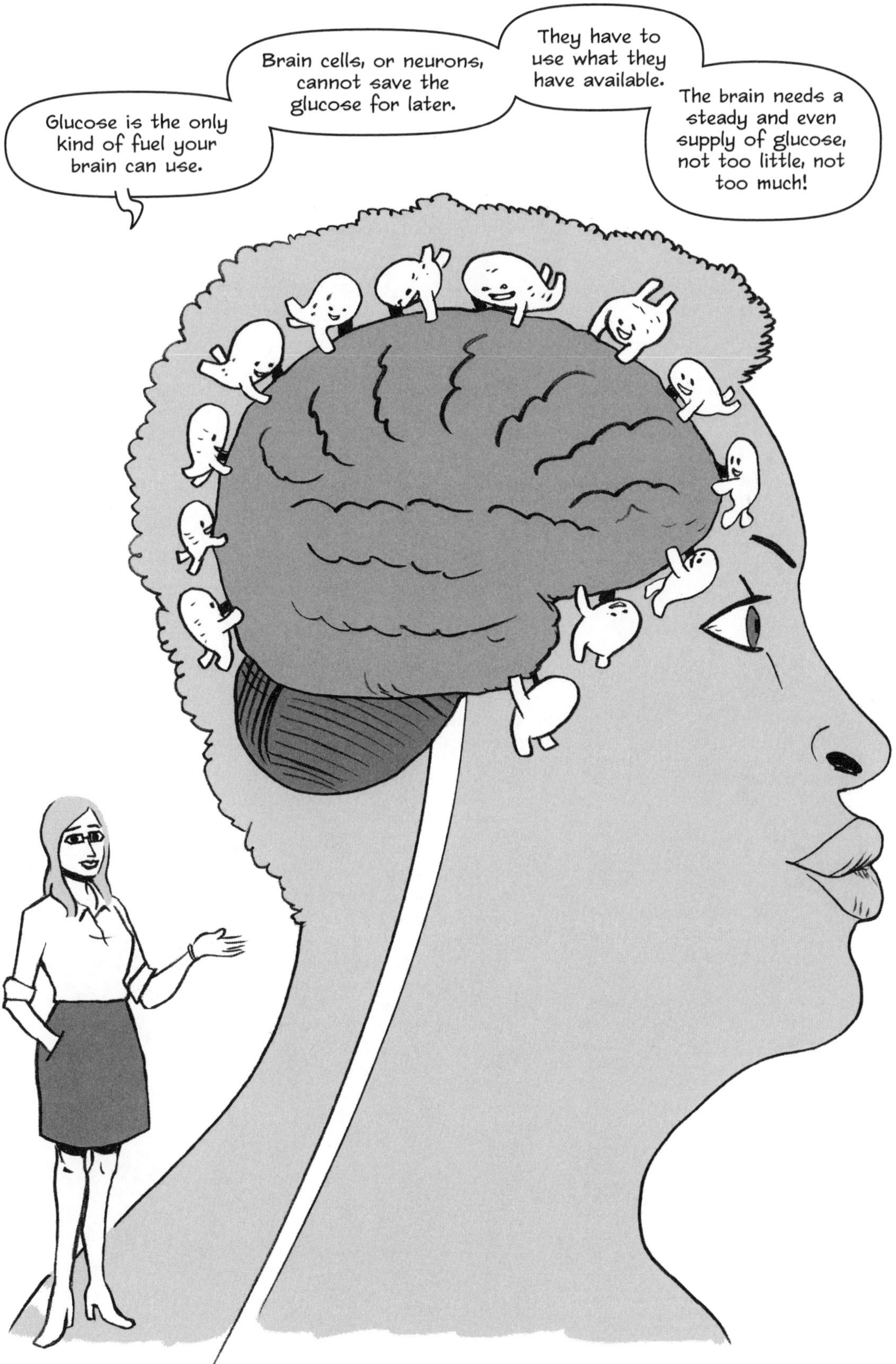
Glucose is the only kind of fuel your brain can use.
Brain cells, or neurons, cannot save the glucose for later.
They have to use what they have available.
The brain needs a steady and even supply of glucose, not too little, not too much!

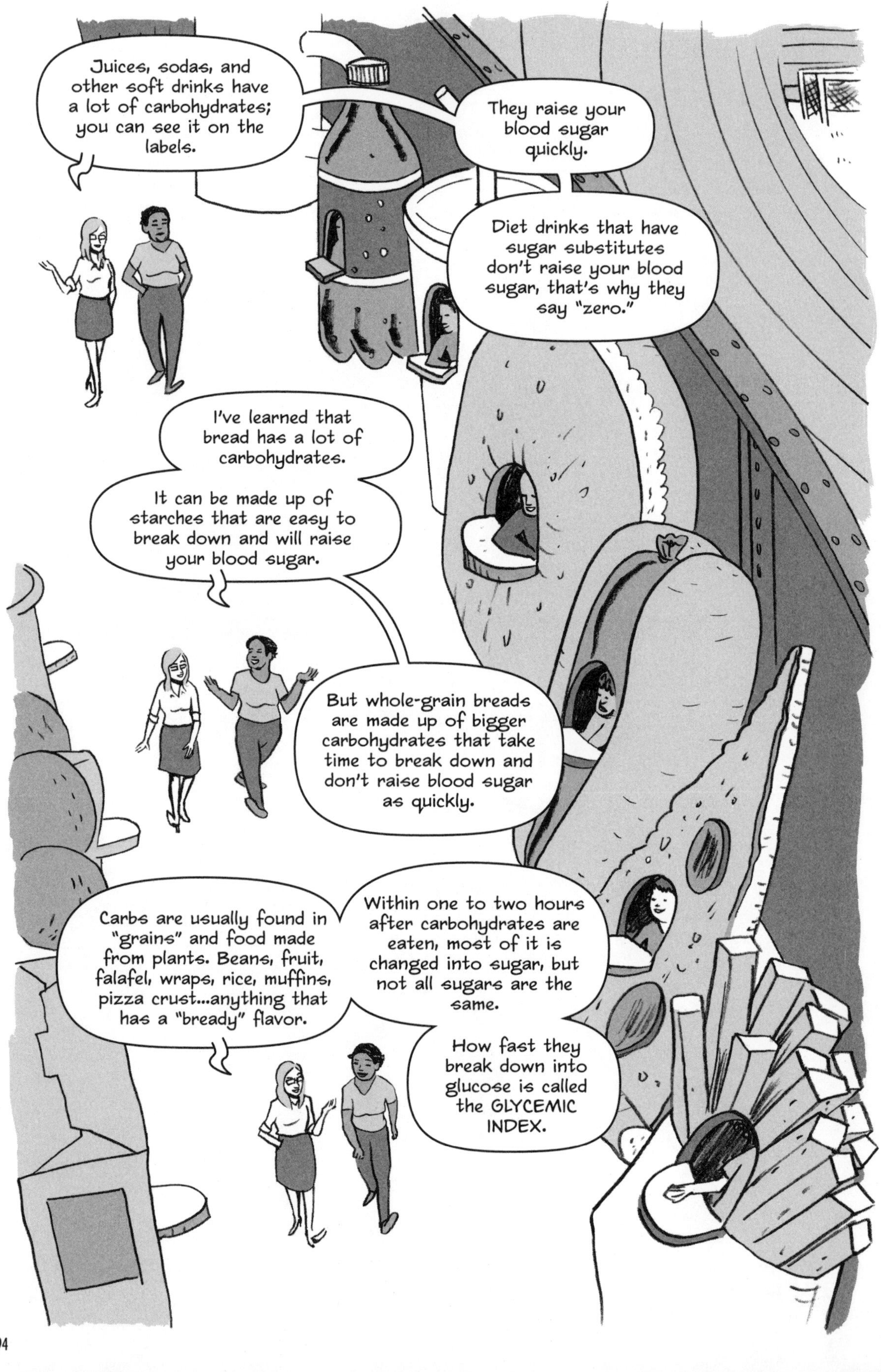
Juices, sodas, and other soft drinks have a lot of carbohydrates; you can see it on the labels.
They raise your blood sugar quickly.
Diet drinks that have sugar substitutes don't raise your blood sugar, that's why they say "zero."
I've learned that bread has a lot of carbohydrates.
It can be made up of starches that are easy to break down and will raise your blood sugar.
But whole-grain breads are made up of bigger carbohydrates that take time to break down and don't raise blood sugar as quickly.
Carbs are usually found in "grains" and food made from plants. Beans, fruit, falafel, wraps, rice, muffins, pizza crust...anything that has a "bready" flavor.
Within one to two hours after carbohydrates are eaten, most of it is changed into sugar, but not all sugars are the same.
How fast they break down into glucose is called the GLYCEMIC INDEX.

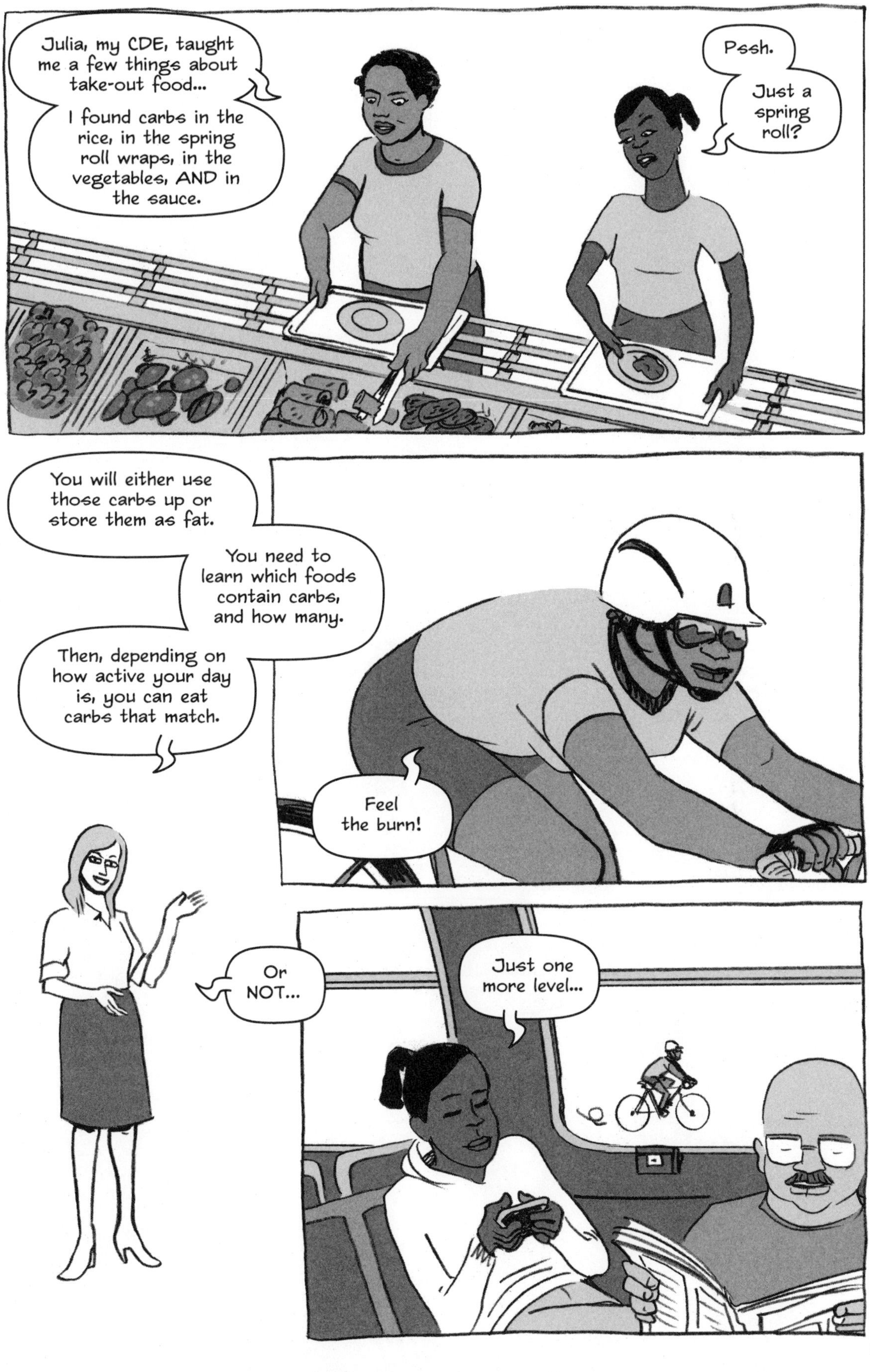
Julia, my CDE, taught me a few things about take-out food...
I found carbs in the rice, in the spring roll wraps, in the vegetables, AND in the sauce.
Pssh.
Just a spring roll?
You will either use those carbs up or store them as fat.
You need to learn which foods contain carbs, and how many.
Then, depending on how active your day is, you can eat carbs that match.
Feel the burn!
Or NOT...
Just one more level...

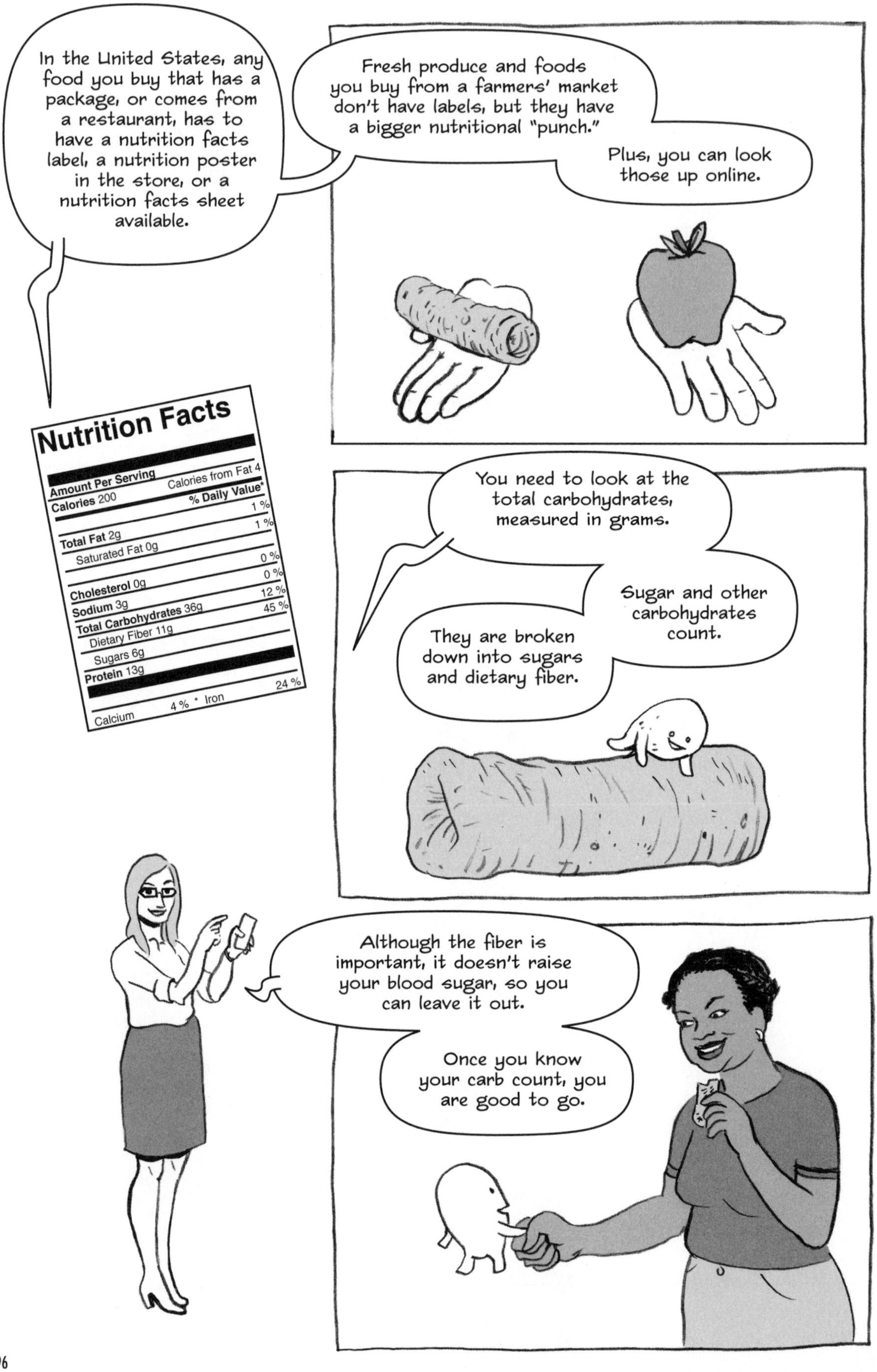
In the United States, any food you buy that has a package, or comes from a restaurant, has to have a nutrition facts label, a nutrition poster in the store, or a nutrition facts sheet available.
Nutrition Facts
Amount Per Serving
Calories 200 Calories from Fat 4
% Daily Value*
Total Fat 2g 1 %
Saturated Fat 0g 1 %
Cholesterol 0g 0 %
Sodium 3g 0 %
Total Carbohydrates 36g 12 %
Dietary Fiber 11g 45 %
Sugars 6g
Protein 13g
Calcium 4 % * Iron 24 %
Fresh produce and foods you buy from a farmers' market don't have labels, but they have a bigger nutritional "punch."
Plus, you can look those up online.
You need to look at the total carbohydrates, measured in grams.
Sugar and other carbohydrates count.
They are broken down into sugars and dietary fiber.
Although the fiber is important, it doesn't raise your blood sugar, so you can leave it out.
Once you know your carb count, you are good to go.

WHAT ARE FATS?

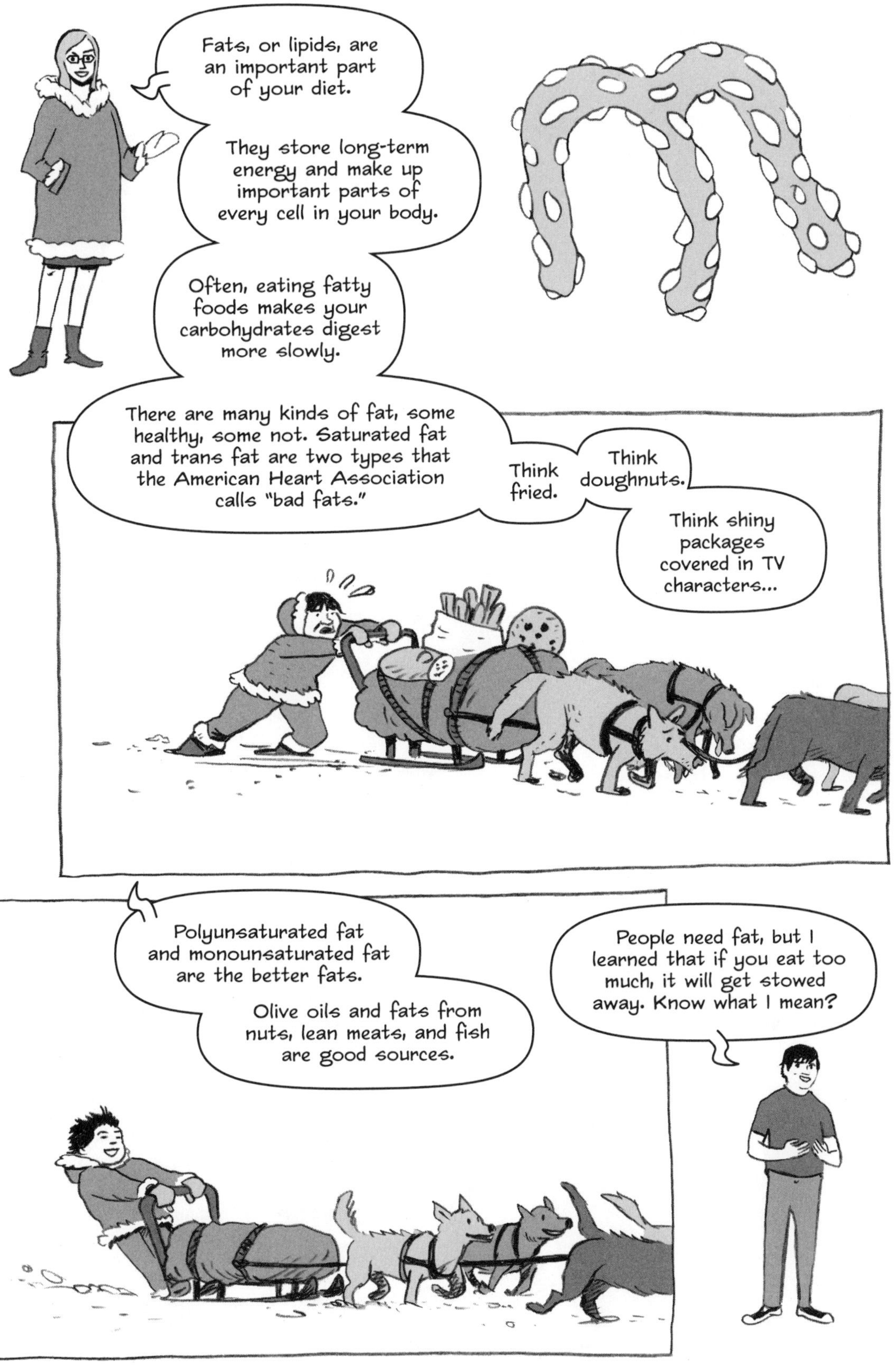

Fats, or lipids, are an important part of your diet.
They store long-term energy and make up important parts of every cell in your body.
Often, eating fatty foods makes your carbohydrates digest more slowly.
There are many kinds of fat, some healthy, some not. Saturated fat and trans fat are two types that the American Heart Association calls "bad fats."
Think fried.
Think doughnuts.
Think shiny packages covered in TV characters...
Polyunsaturated fat and monounsaturated fat are the better fats.
Olive oils and fats from nuts, lean meats, and fish are good sources.
People need fat, but I learned that if you eat too much, it will get stowed away. Know what I mean?

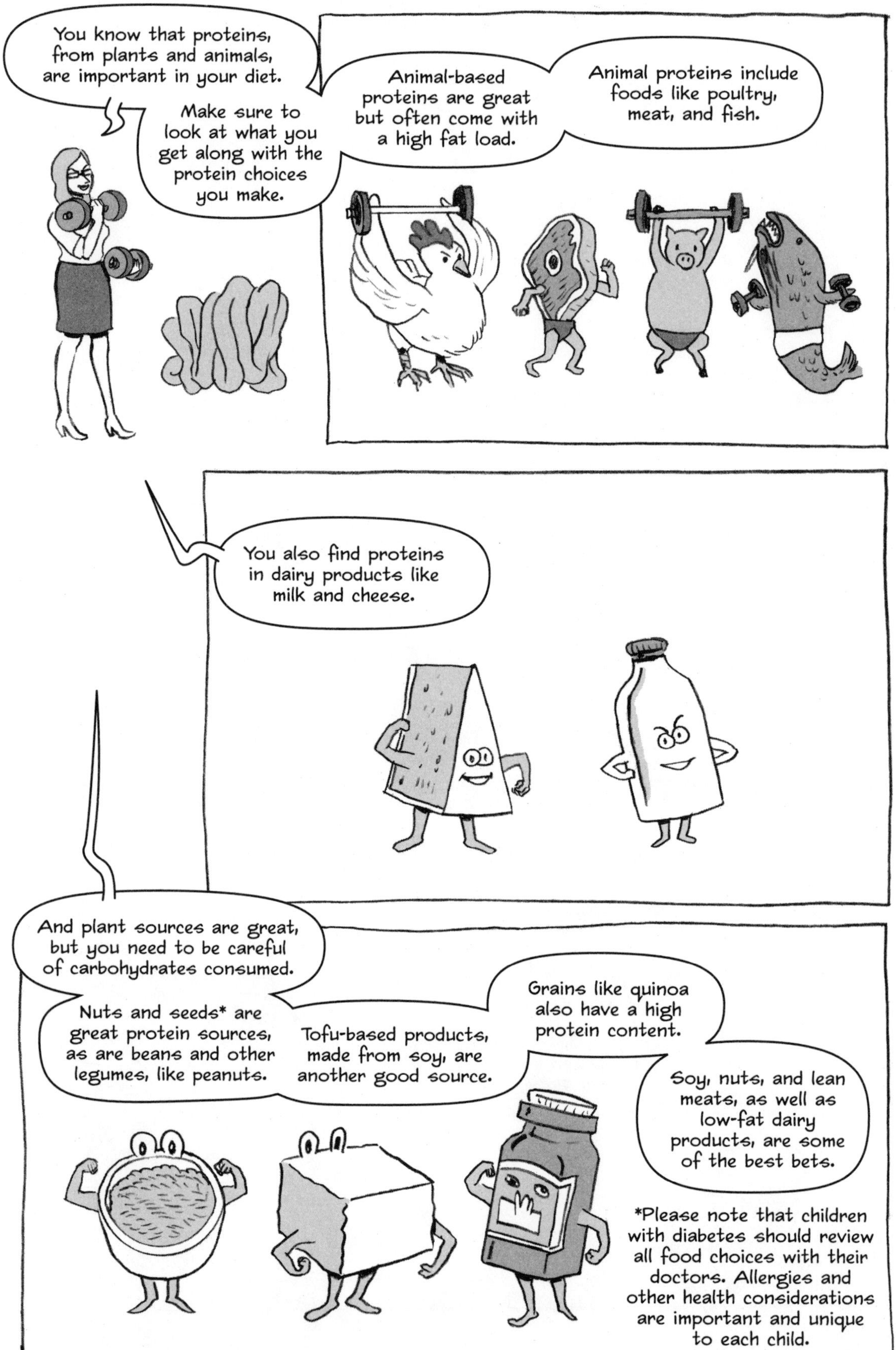
You know that proteins, from plants and animals, are important in your diet.
Make sure to look at what you get along with the protein choices you make.
Animal-based proteins are great but often come with a high fat load.
Animal proteins include foods like poultry, meat, and fish.
You also find proteins in dairy products like milk and cheese.
And plant sources are great, but you need to be careful of carbohydrates consumed.
Nuts and seeds* are great protein sources, as are beans and other legumes, like peanuts.
Tofu-based products, made from soy, are another good source.
Grains like quinoa also have a high protein content.
Soy, nuts, and lean meats, as well as low-fat dairy products, are some of the best bets.
*Please note that children with diabetes should review all food choices with their doctors. Allergies and other health considerations are important and unique to each child.

CARB COUNTING

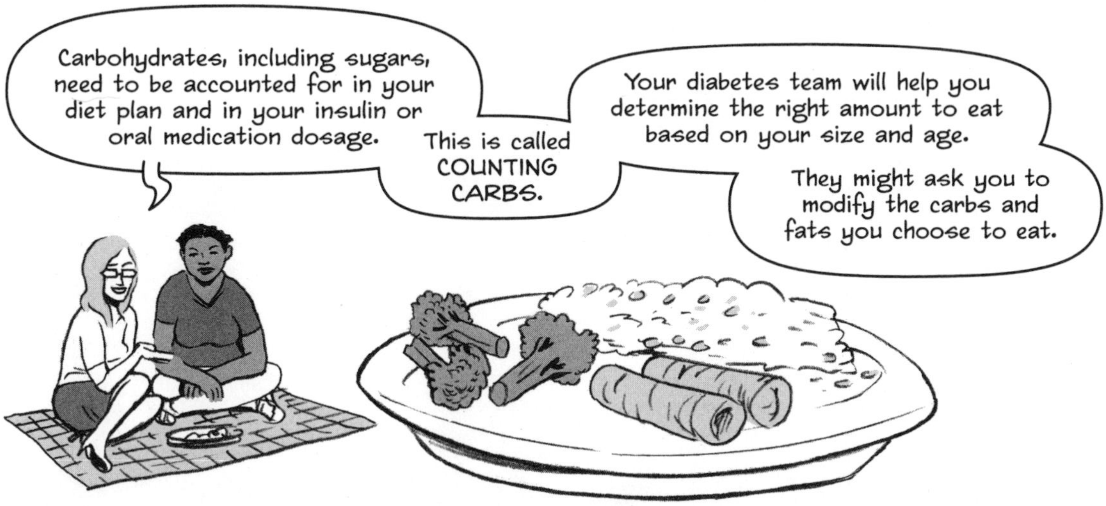

Carbohydrates, including sugars, need to be accounted for in your diet plan and in your insulin or oral medication dosage.
This is called COUNTING CARBS.
Your diabetes team will help you determine the right amount to eat based on your size and age.
They might ask you to modify the carbs and fats you choose to eat.

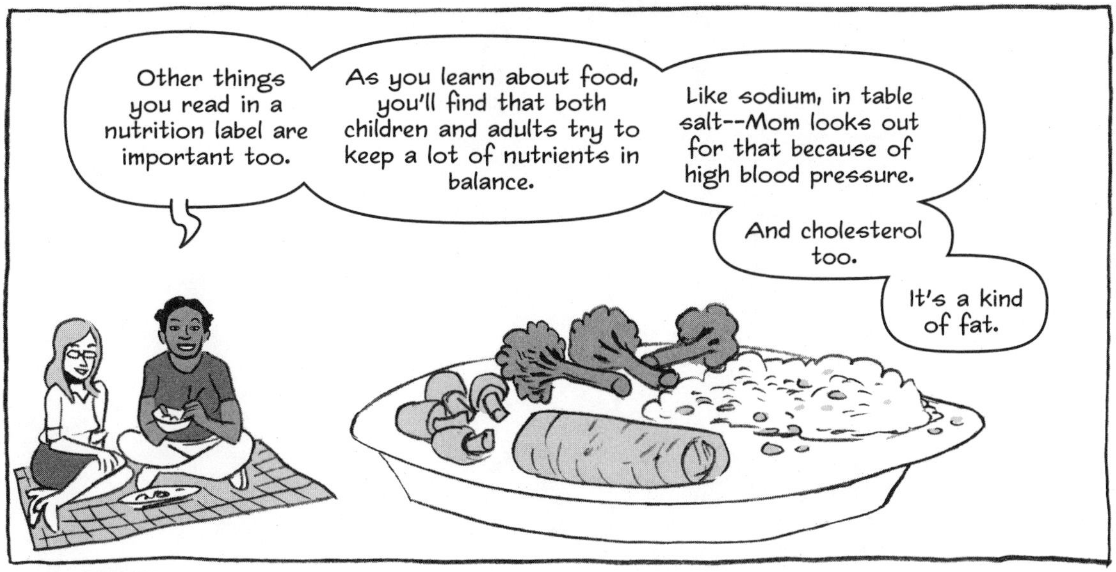

Other things you read in a nutrition label are important too.
As you learn about food, you'll find that both children and adults try to keep a lot of nutrients in balance.
Like sodium, in table salt--Mom looks out for that because of high blood pressure.
And cholesterol too.
It's a kind of fat.

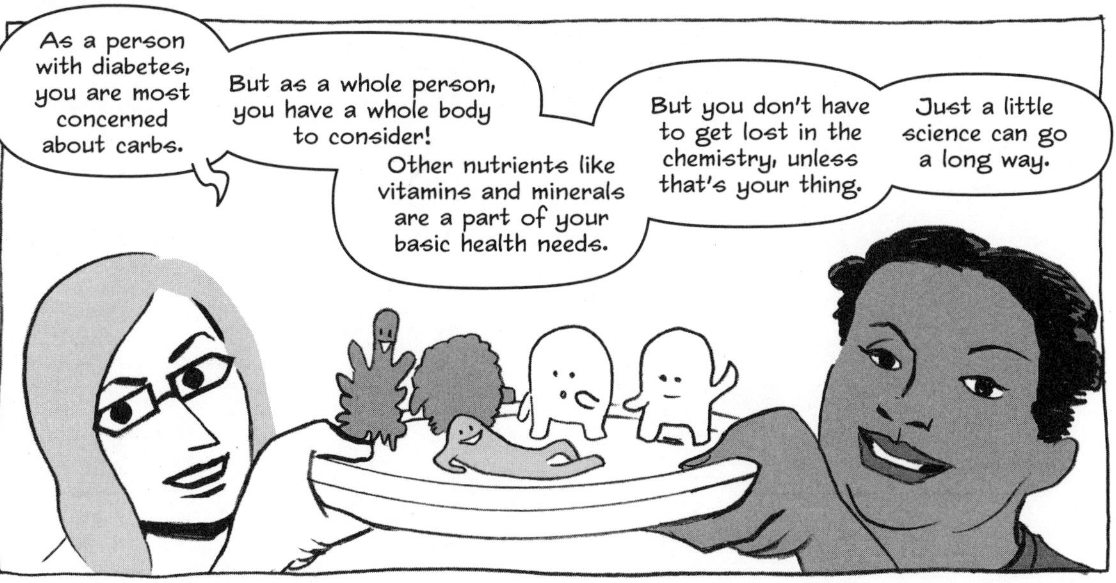

As a person with diabetes, you are most concerned about carbs.
But as a whole person, you have a whole body to consider!
Other nutrients like vitamins and minerals are a part of your basic health needs.
But you don't have to get lost in the chemistry, unless that's your thing.
Just a little science can go a long way.

BEWARE! DON'T JUDGE A TEAM BY THE COLOR OF ITS UNIFORM!

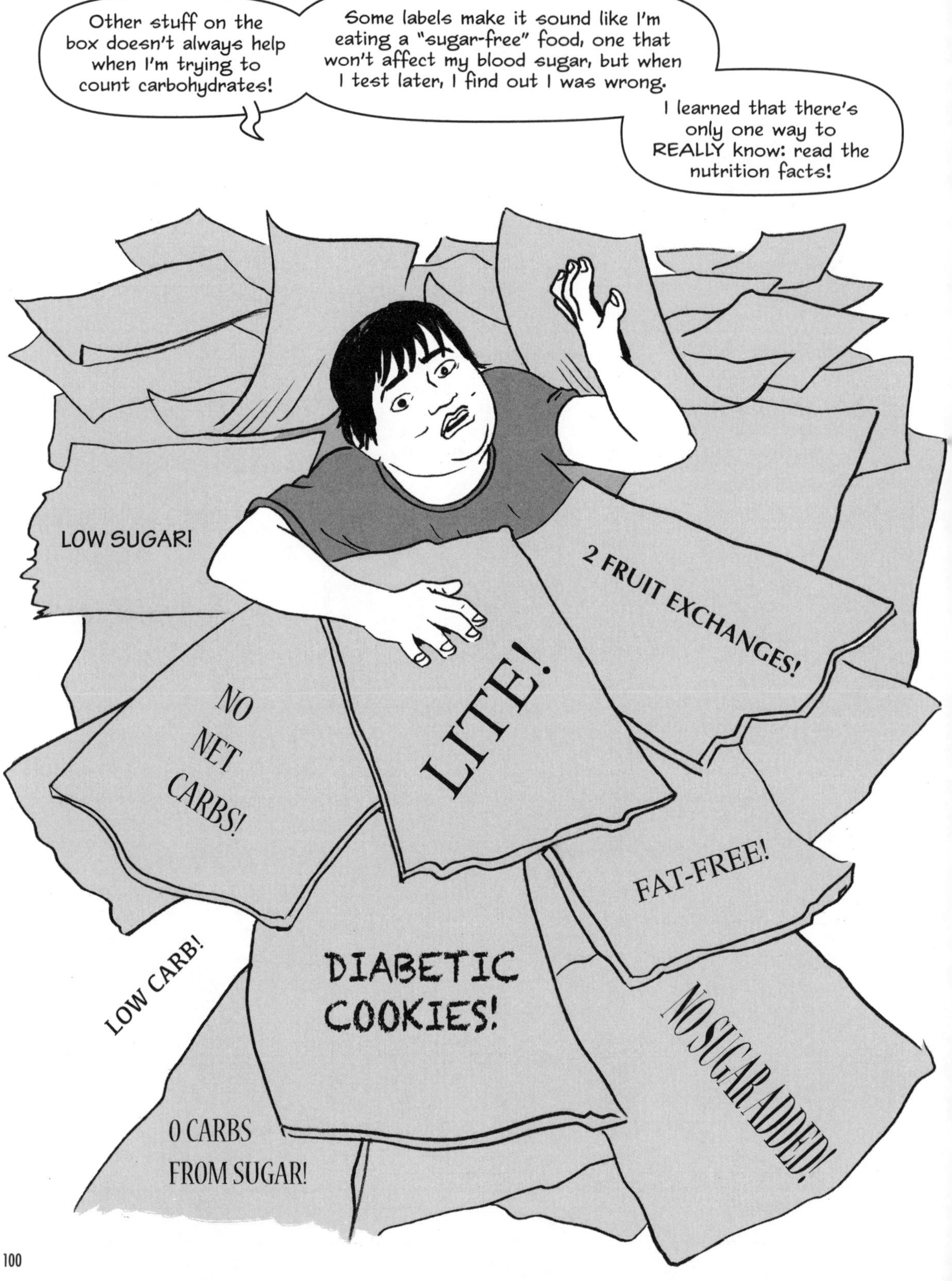

Other stuff on the box doesn't always help when I'm trying to count carbohydrates!
Some labels make it sound like I'm eating a "sugar-free" food, one that won't affect my blood sugar, but when I test later, I find out I was wrong.
I learned that there's only one way to REALLY know: read the nutrition facts!
LOW SUGAR!
2 FRUIT EXCHANGES!
NO NET CARBS!
LITE!
FAT-FREE!
LOW CARB!
DIABETIC COOKIES!
NO SUGAR ADDED!
0 CARBS FROM SUGAR!

NEW WAYS TO FUEL UP

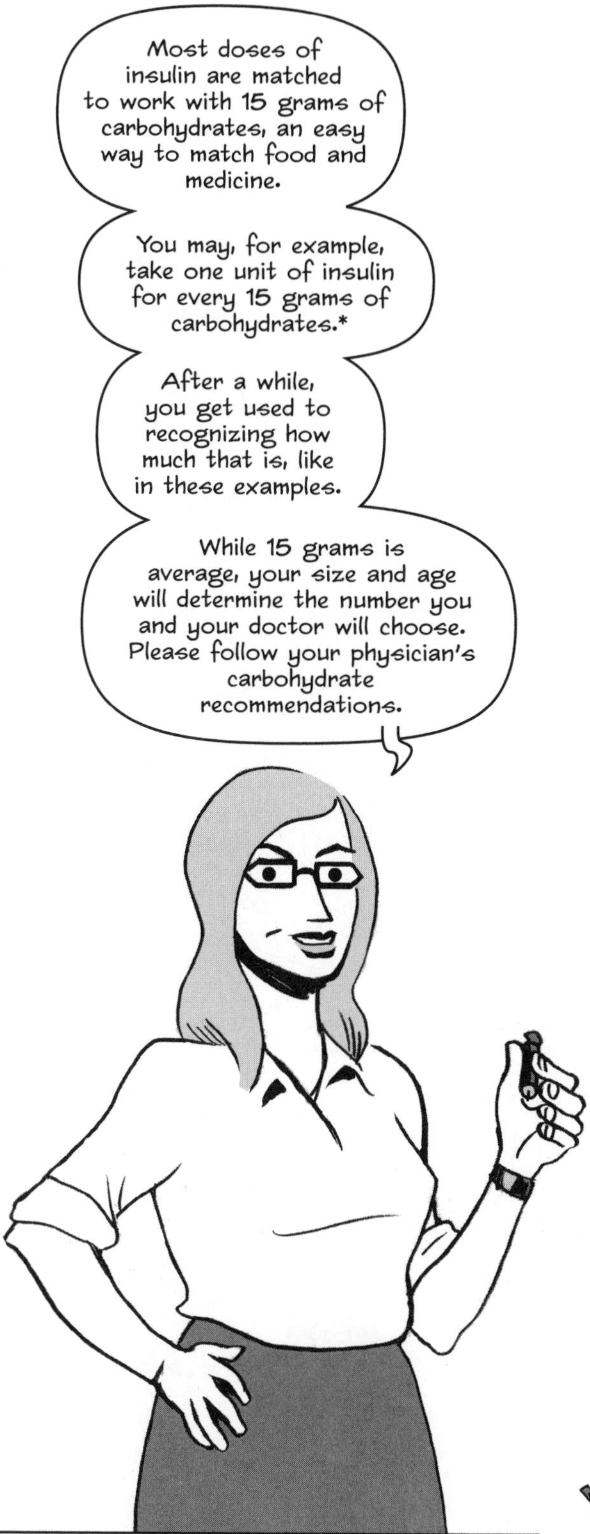

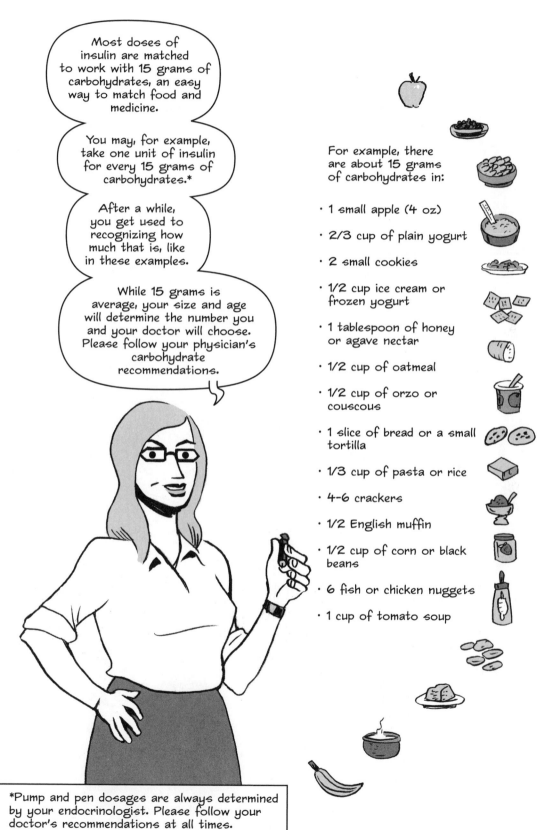

Most doses of insulin are matched to work with 15 grams of carbohydrates, an easy way to match food and medicine.
You may, for example, take one unit of insulin for every 15 grams of carbohydrates.*
After a while, you get used to recognizing how much that is, like in these examples.
While 15 grams is average, your size and age will determine the number you and your doctor will choose. Please follow your physician's carbohydrate recommendations.

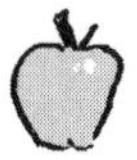

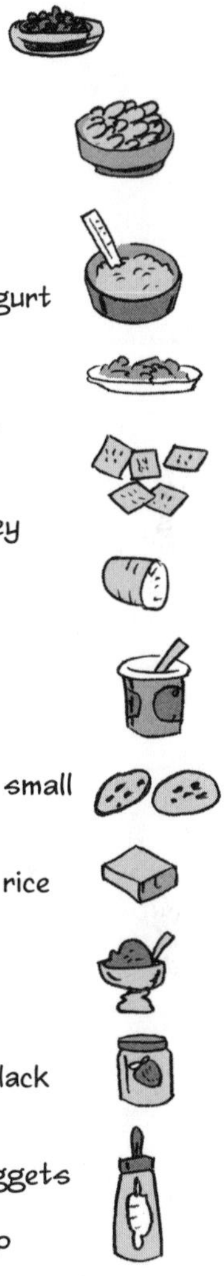

For example, there are about 15 grams of carbohydrates in:

- 1 small apple (4 oz)
- 2/3 cup of plain yogurt
- 2 small cookies
- 1/2 cup ice cream or frozen yogurt
- 1 tablespoon of honey or agave nectar
- 1/2 cup of oatmeal
- 1/2 cup of orzo or couscous
- 1 slice of bread or a small tortilla
- 1/3 cup of pasta or rice
- 4-6 crackers
- 1/2 English muffin
- 1/2 cup of corn or black beans
- 6 fish or chicken nuggets
- 1 cup of tomato soup

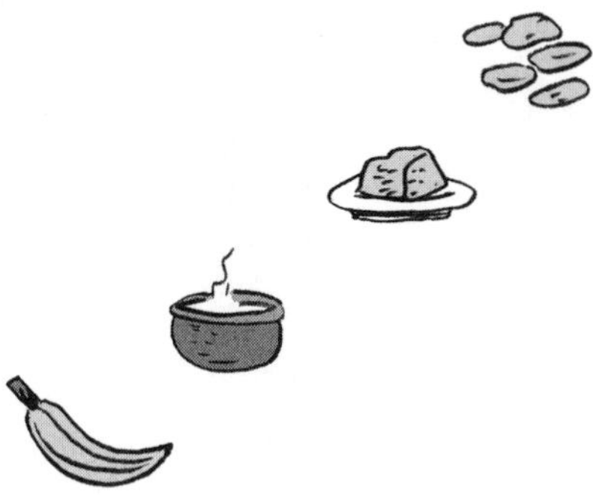

*Pump and pen dosages are always determined by your endocrinologist. Please follow your doctor's recommendations at all times.

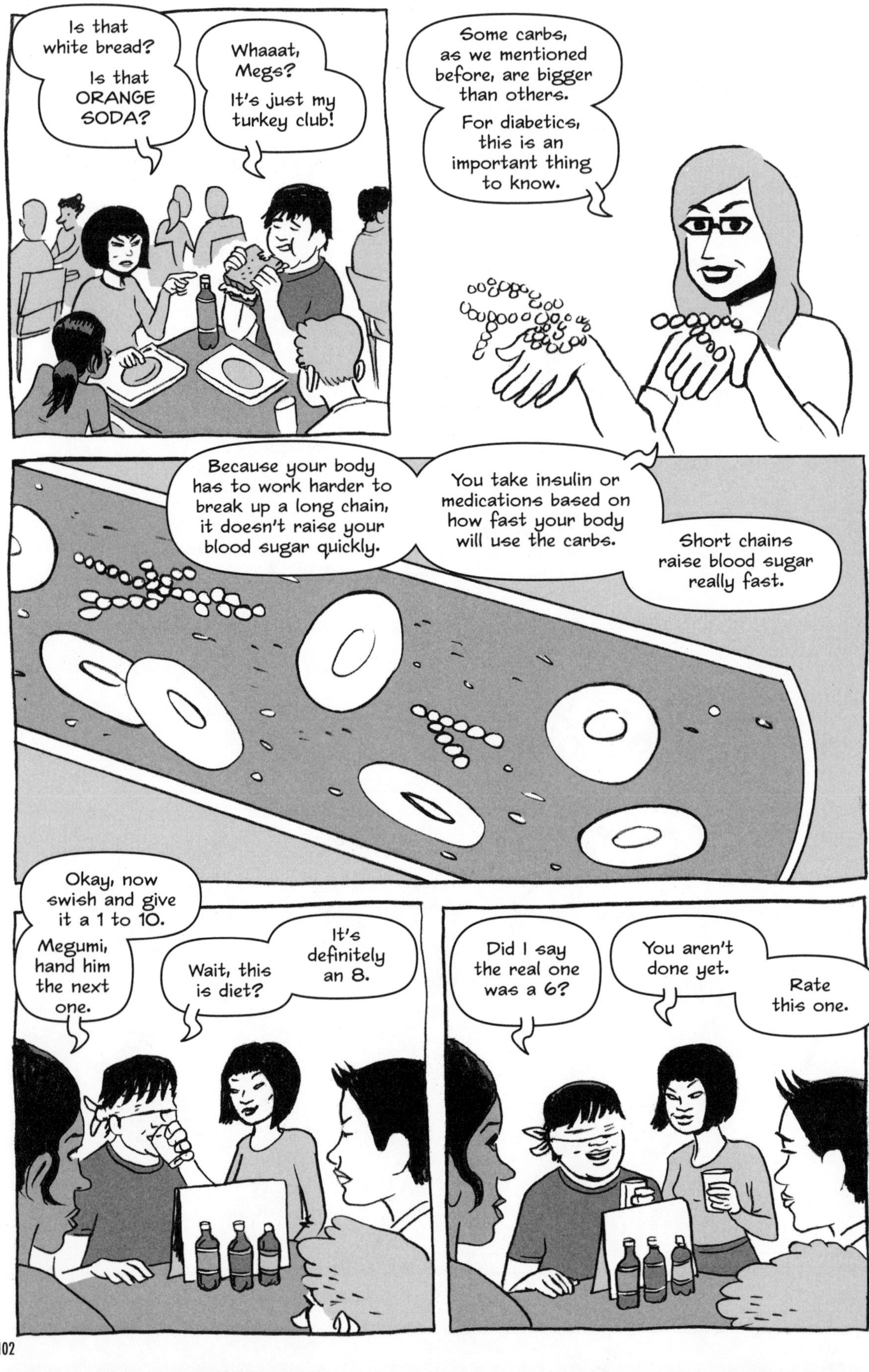
Is that white bread?
Is that ORANGE SODA?
Whaaat, Megs?
It's just my turkey club!
Some carbs, as we mentioned before, are bigger than others.
For diabetics, this is an important thing to know.
Because your body has to work harder to break up a long chain, it doesn't raise your blood sugar quickly.
You take insulin or medications based on how fast your body will use the carbs.
Short chains raise blood sugar really fast.
Okay, now swish and give it a 1 to 10.
Megumi, hand him the next one.
Wait, this is diet?
It's definitely an 8.
Did I say the real one was a 6?
You aren't done yet.
Rate this one.

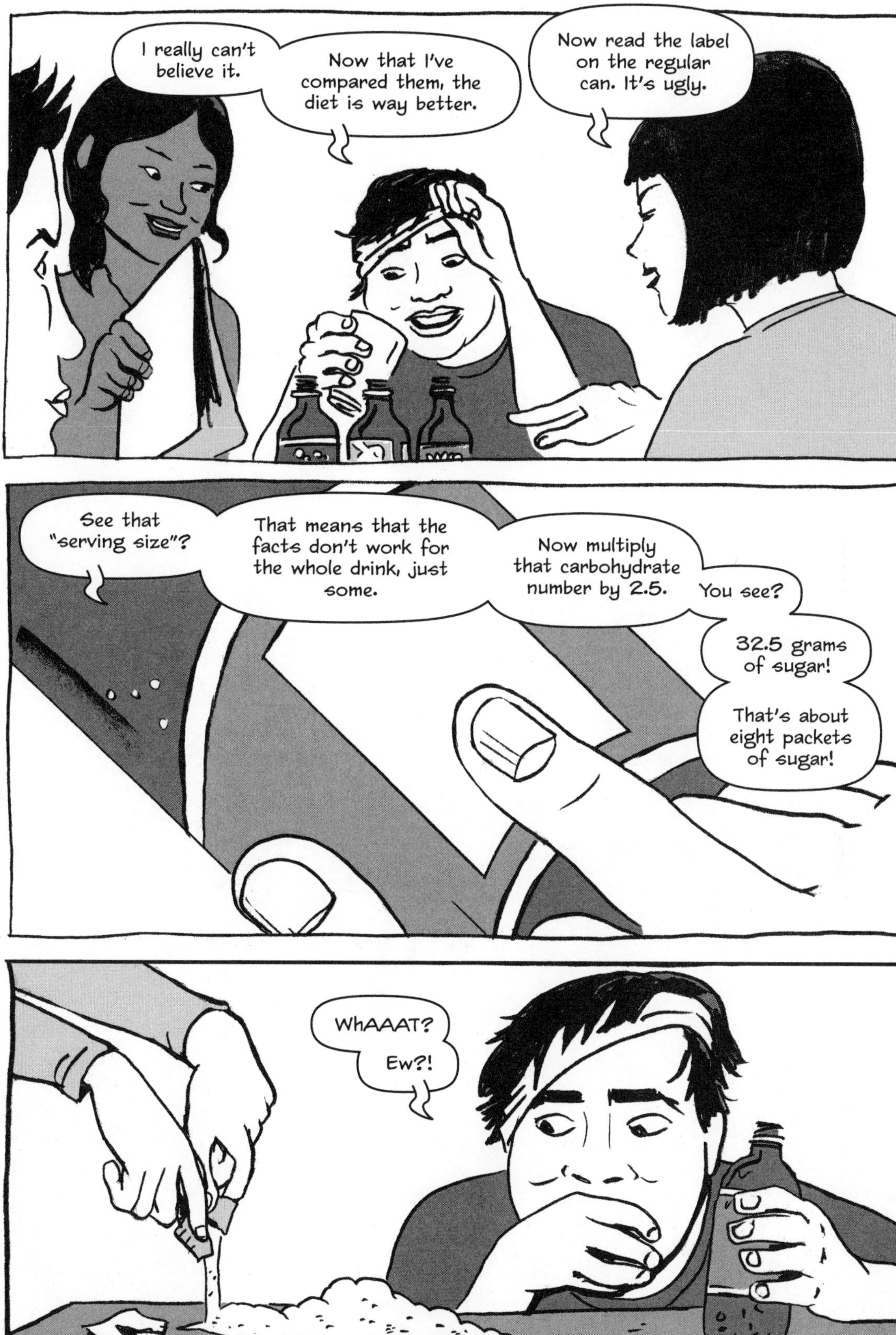
I really can't believe it.
Now that I've compared them, the diet is way better.
Now read the label on the regular can. It's ugly.
See that "serving size"?
That means that the facts don't work for the whole drink, just some.
Now multiply that carbohydrate number by 2.5.
You see?
32.5 grams of sugar!
That's about eight packets of sugar!
WhAAAT?
Ew?!

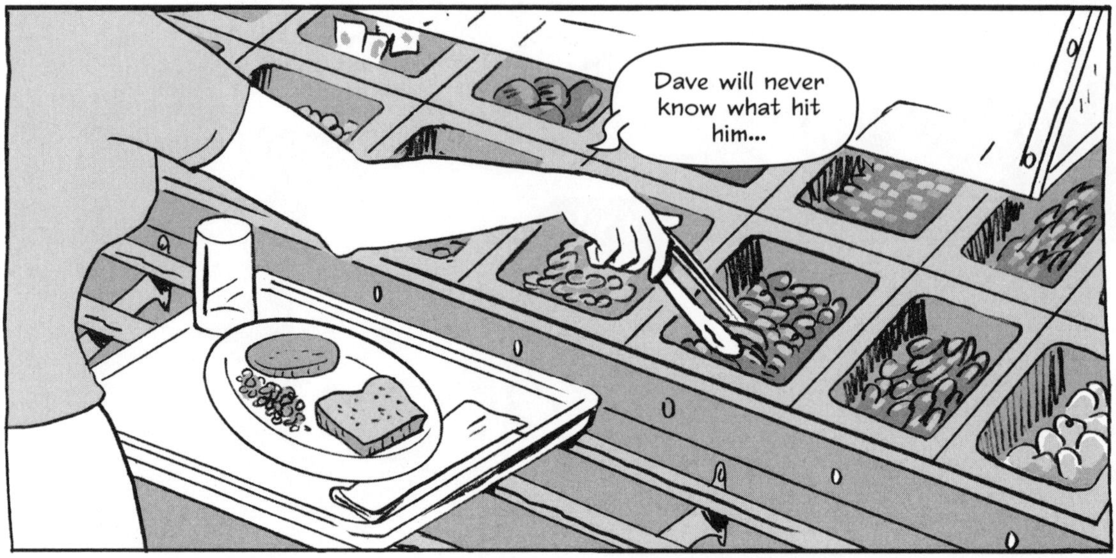
Dave will never know what hit him...

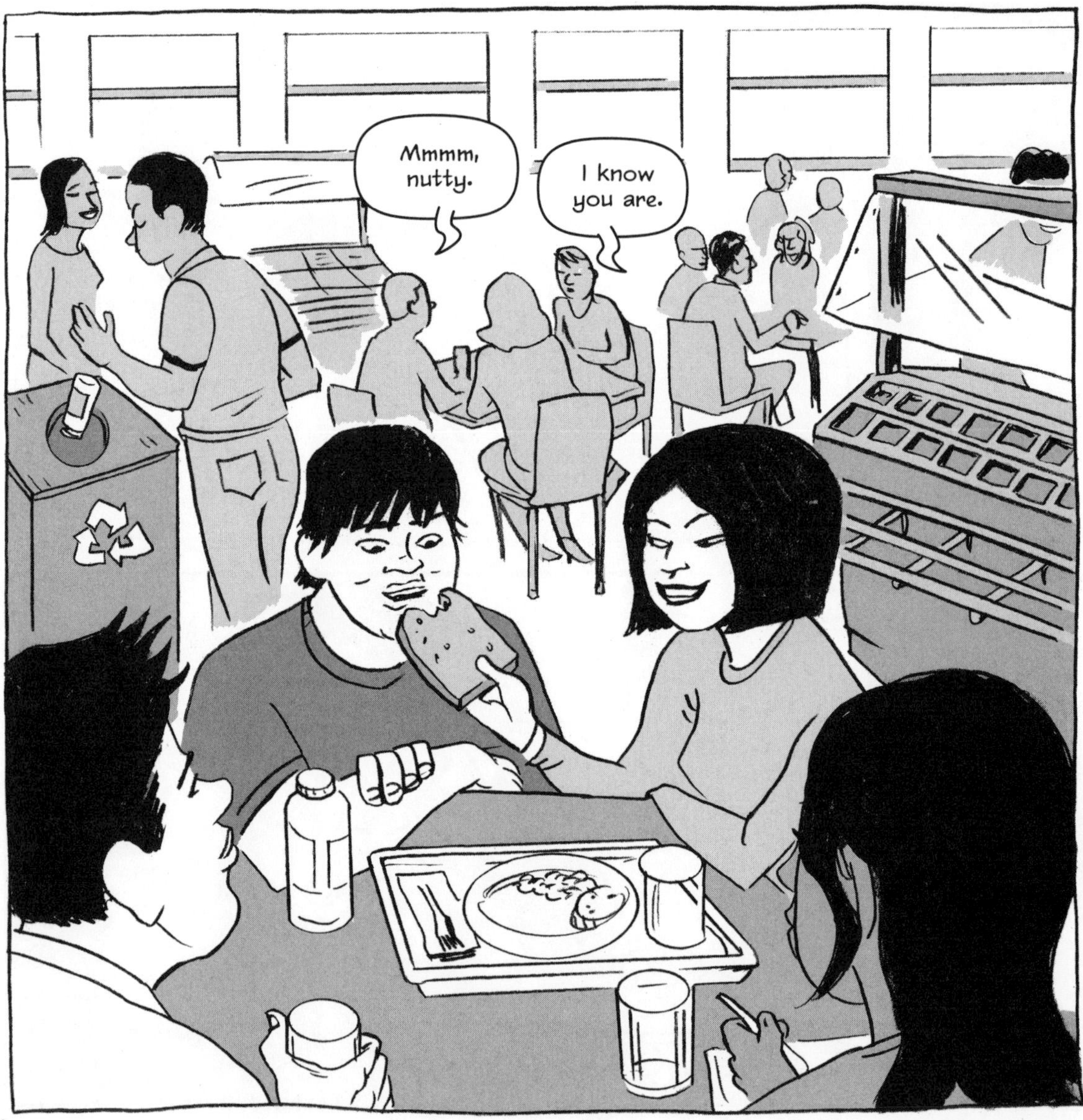
Mmmm, nutty.
I know you are.

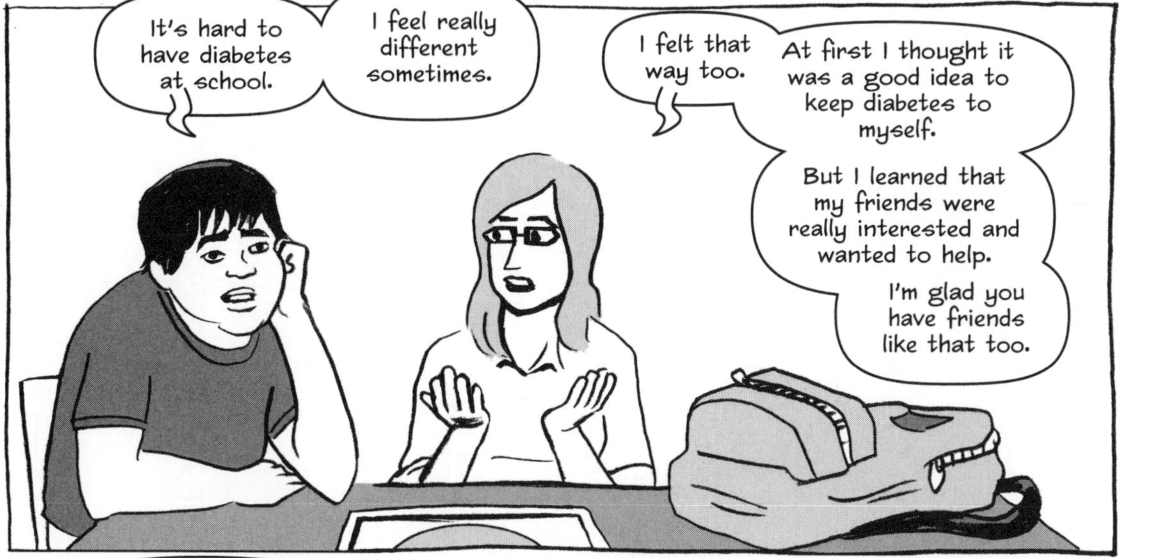
It's hard to have diabetes at school.
I feel really different sometimes.
I felt that way too.
At first I thought it was a good idea to keep diabetes to myself.
But I learned that my friends were really interested and wanted to help.
I'm glad you have friends like that too.

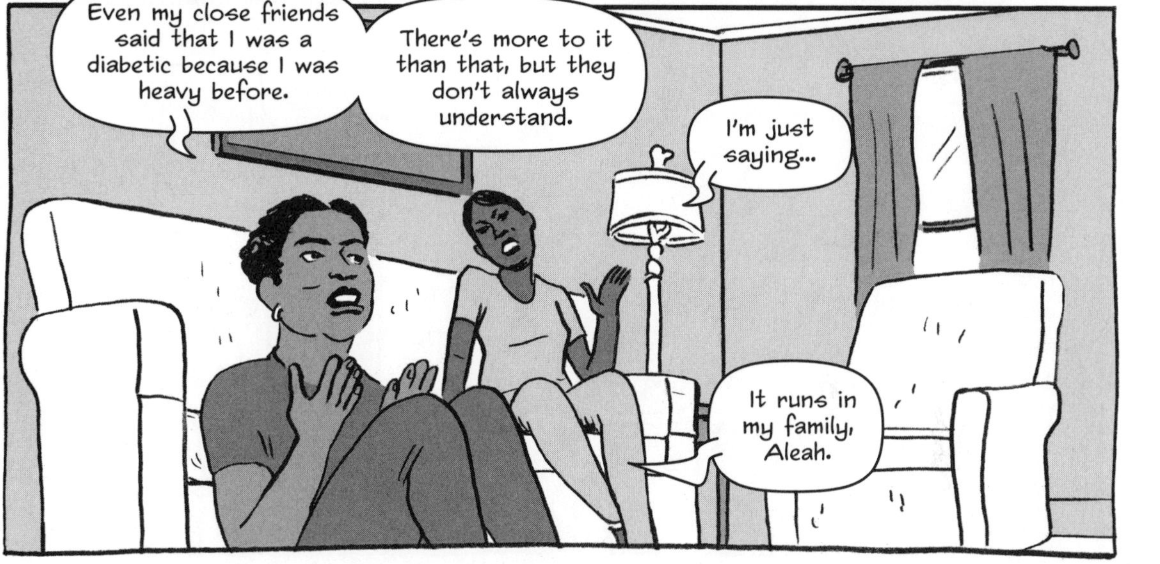
Even my close friends said that I was a diabetic because I was heavy before.
There's more to it than that, but they don't always understand.
I'm just saying...
It runs in my family, Aleah.

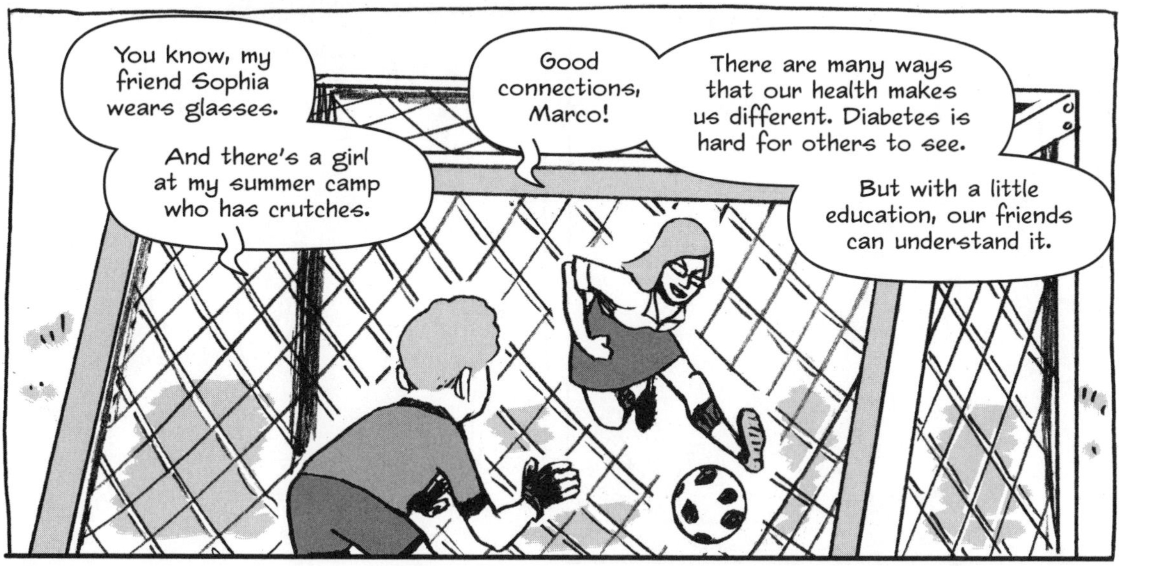
You know, my friend Sophia wears glasses.
And there's a girl at my summer camp who has crutches.
Good connections, Marco!
There are many ways that our health makes us different. Diabetes is hard for others to see.
But with a little education, our friends can understand it.

FOOD MAKEOVER #1: THE BURRITO COMEBACK KID

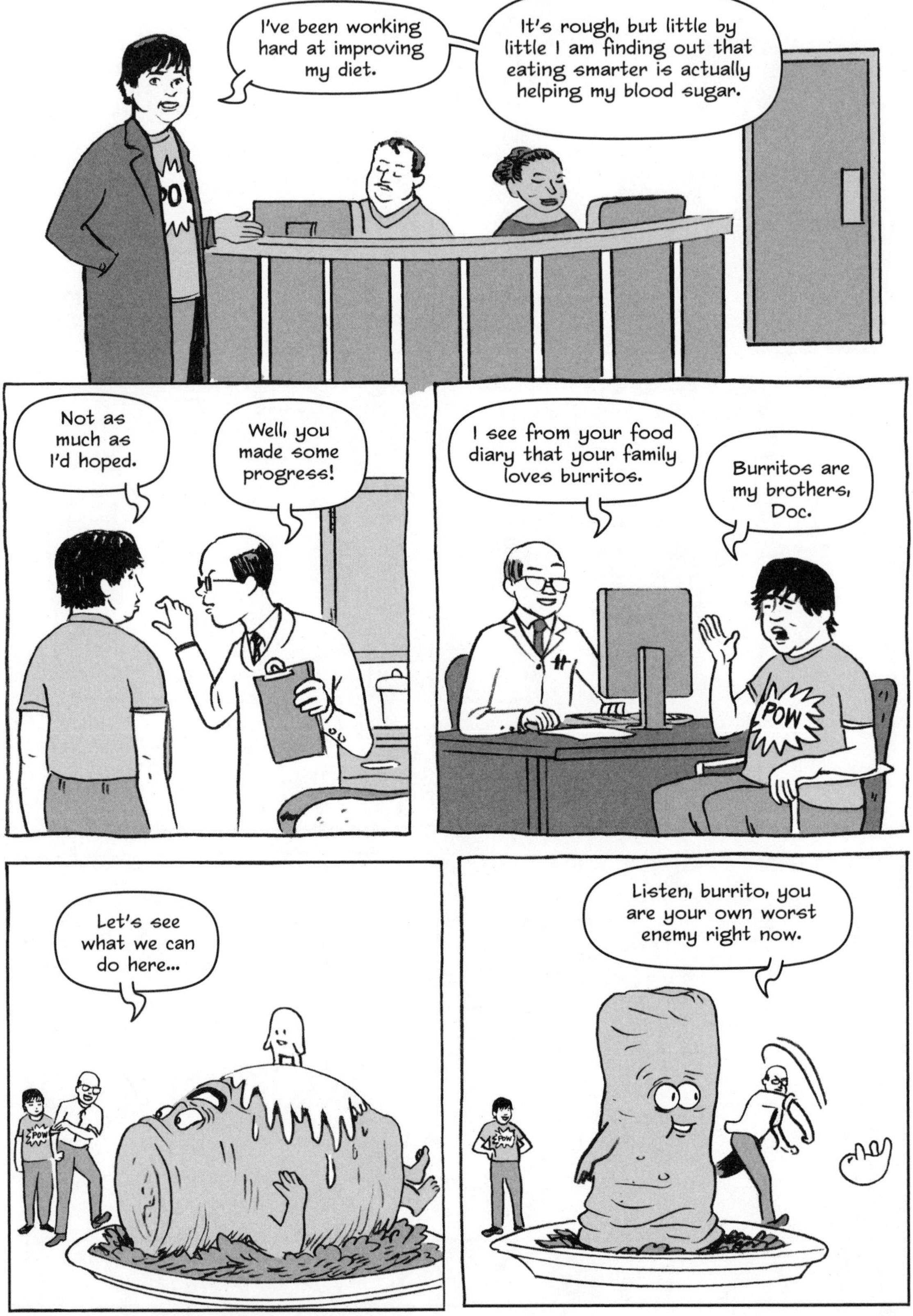
I've been working hard at improving my diet.
It's rough, but little by little I am finding out that eating smarter is actually helping my blood sugar.
POW
Not as much as I'd hoped.
Well, you made some progress!
I see from your food diary that your family loves burritos.
Burritos are my brothers, Doc.
POW
Let's see what we can do here...
POW
Listen, burrito, you are your own worst enemy right now.
POW

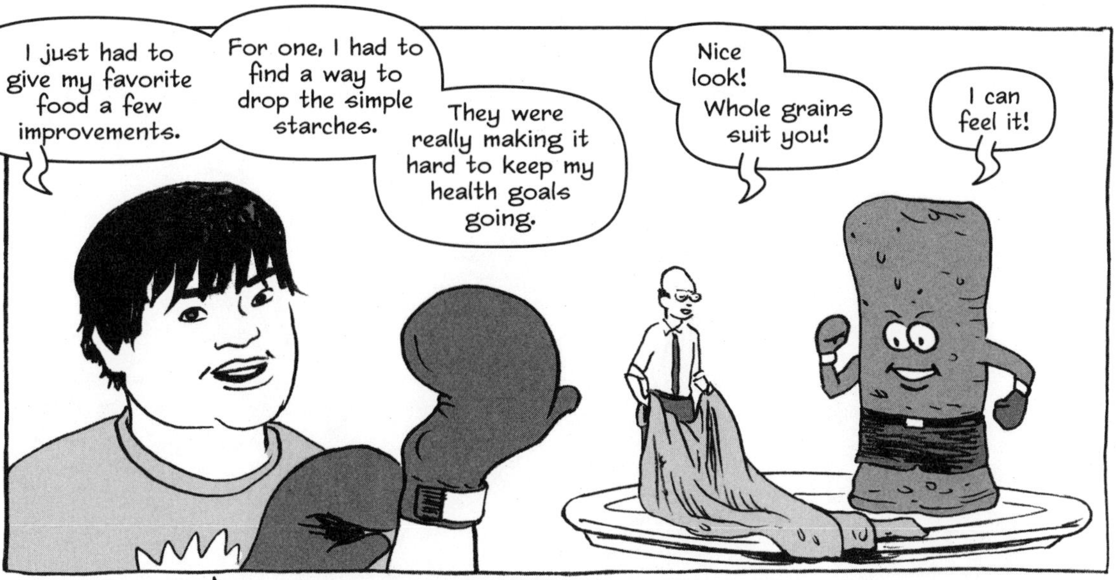
I just had to give my favorite food a few improvements.
For one, I had to find a way to drop the simple starches.
They were really making it hard to keep my health goals going.
Nice look! Whole grains suit you!
I can feel it!

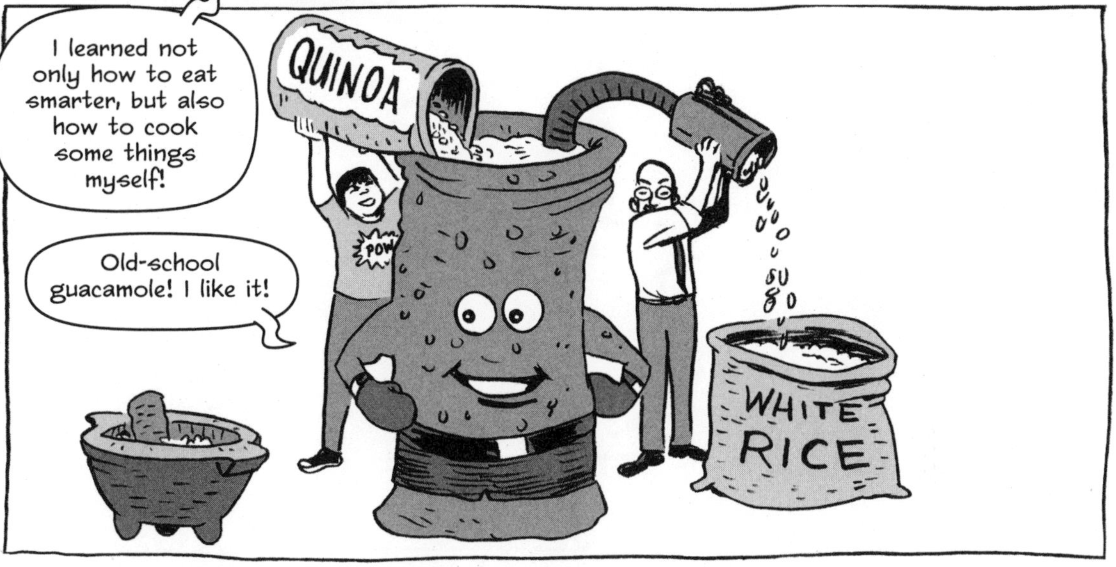
I learned not only how to eat smarter, but also how to cook some things myself!
Old-school guacamole! I like it!
QUINOA
POW
WHITE RICE

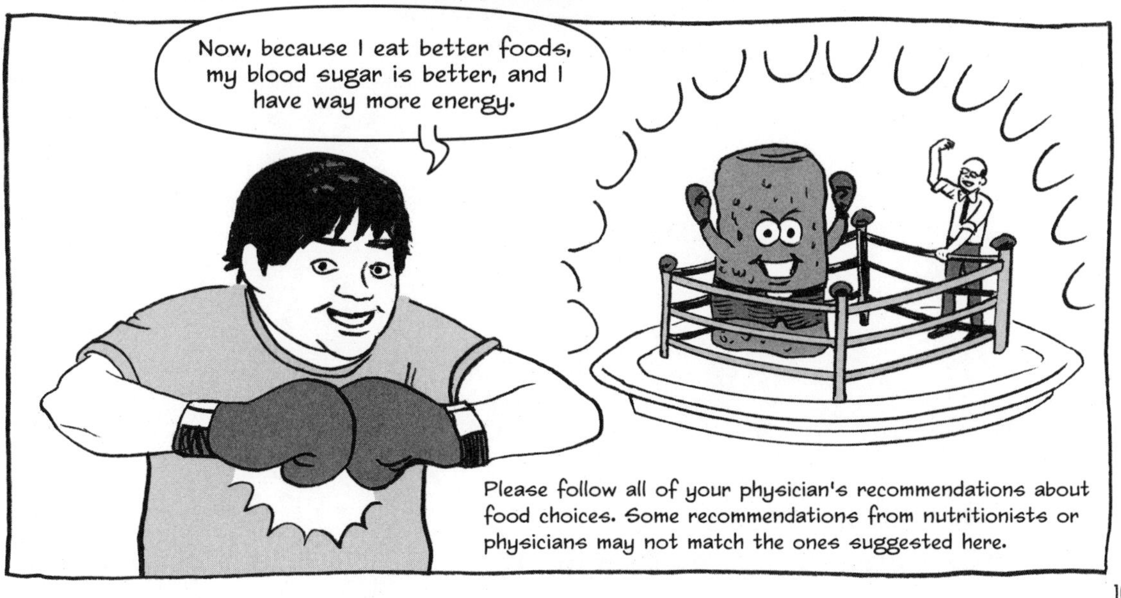
Now, because I eat better foods, my blood sugar is better, and I have way more energy.
Please follow all of your physician's recommendations about food choices. Some recommendations from nutritionists or physicians may not match the ones suggested here.

FOOD MAKEOVER #2: REAL PIZZA, REAL TASTY

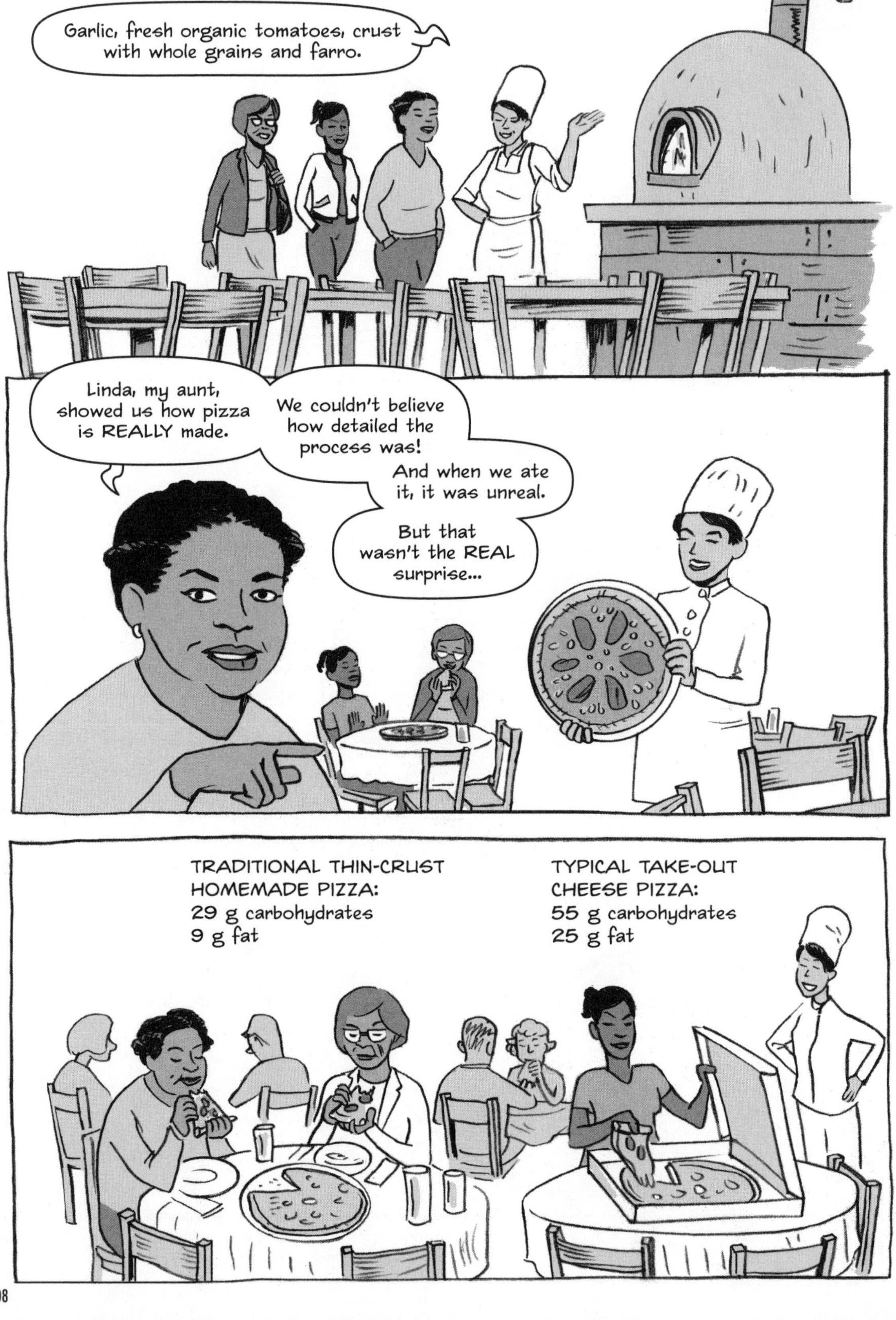

Garlic, fresh organic tomatoes, crust with whole grains and farro.
Linda, my aunt, showed us how pizza is REALLY made.
We couldn't believe how detailed the process was!
And when we ate it, it was unreal.
But that wasn't the REAL surprise...
TRADITIONAL THIN-CRUST HOMEMADE PIZZA:
29 g carbohydrates
9 g fat
TYPICAL TAKE-OUT CHEESE PIZZA:
55 g carbohydrates
25 g fat

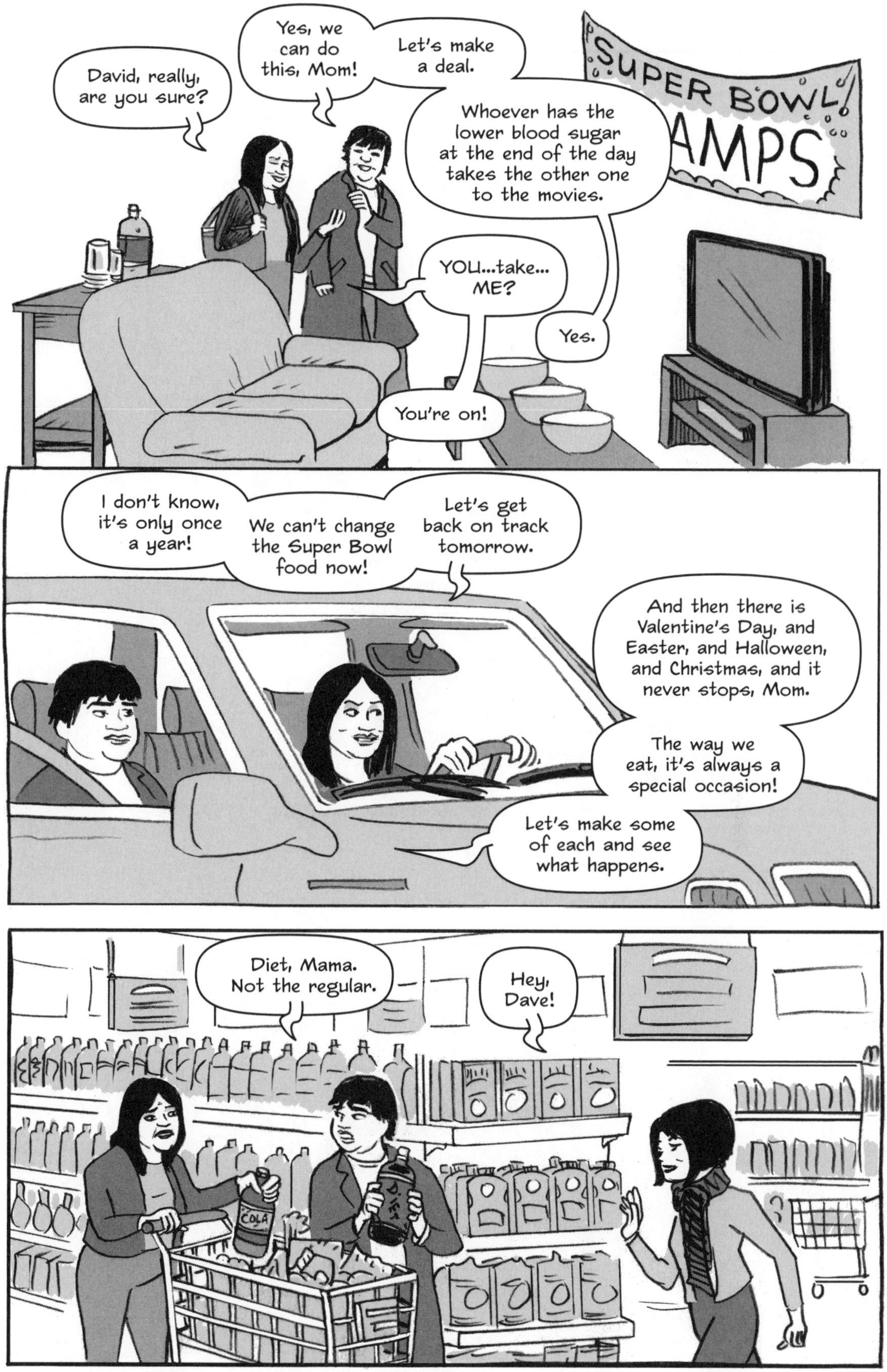
SUPER BOWL
AMPS
David, really, are you sure?
Yes, we can do this, Mom!
Let's make a deal.
Whoever has the lower blood sugar at the end of the day takes the other one to the movies.
YOU...take... ME?
Yes.
You're on!
I don't know, it's only once a year!
We can't change the Super Bowl food now!
Let's get back on track tomorrow.
And then there is Valentine's Day, and Easter, and Halloween, and Christmas, and it never stops, Mom.
The way we eat, it's always a special occasion!
Let's make some of each and see what happens.
Diet, Mama. Not the regular.
Hey, Dave!
COLA

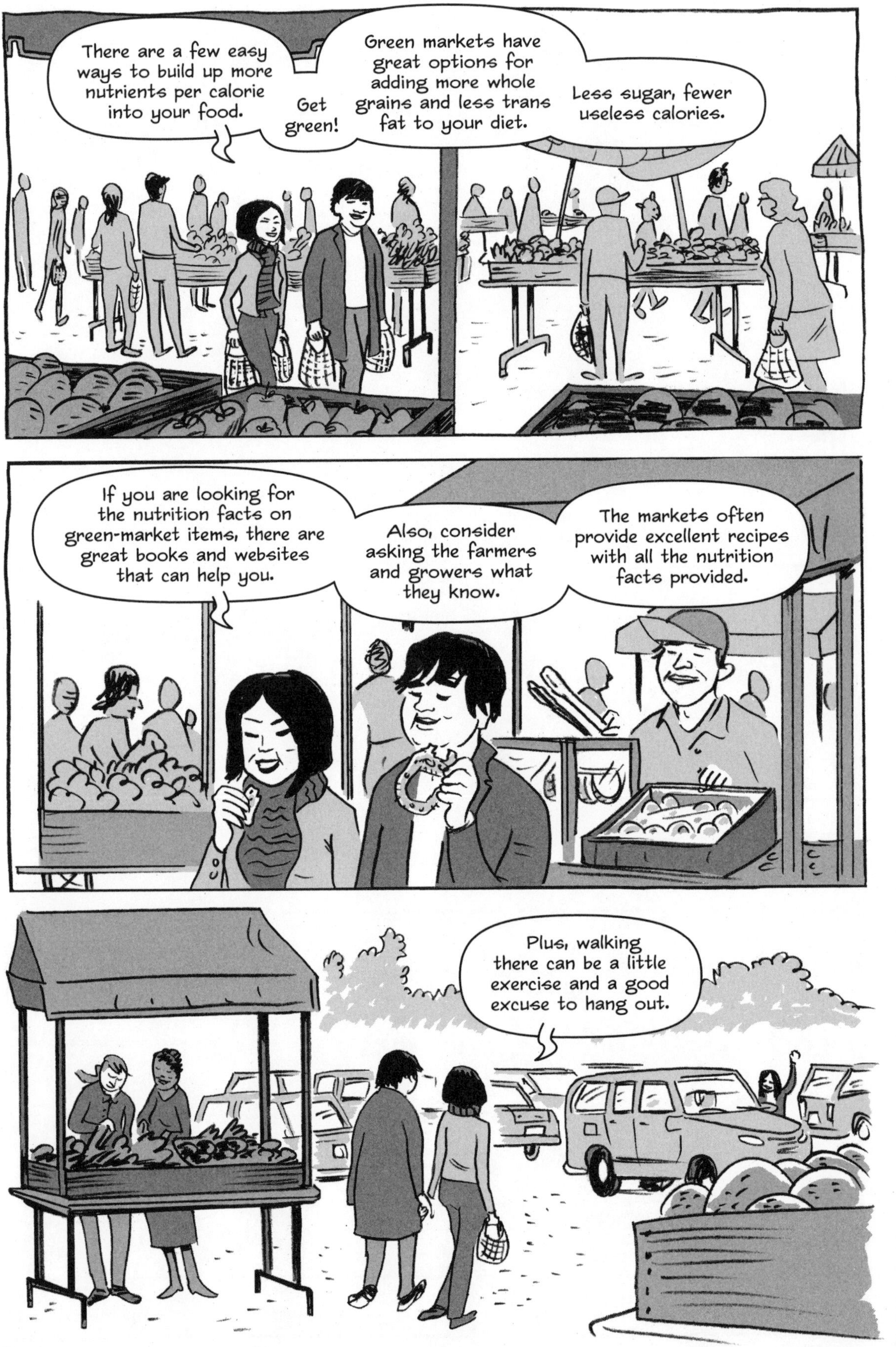
There are a few easy ways to build up more nutrients per calorie into your food.
Get green!
Green markets have great options for adding more whole grains and less trans fat to your diet.
Less sugar, fewer useless calories.
If you are looking for the nutrition facts on green-market items, there are great books and websites that can help you.
Also, consider asking the farmers and growers what they know.
The markets often provide excellent recipes with all the nutrition facts provided.
Plus, walking there can be a little exercise and a good excuse to hang out.

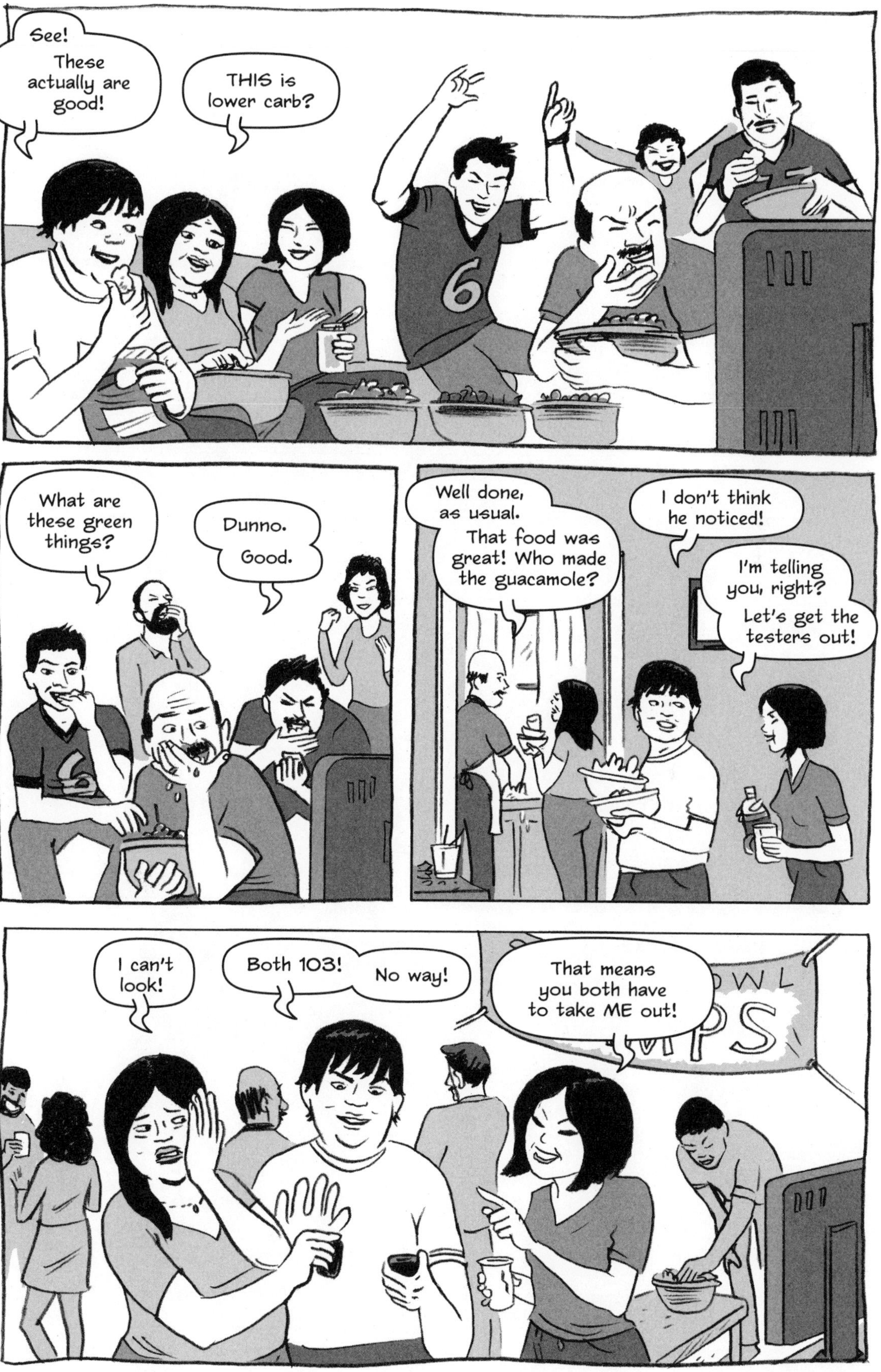
See!
These actually are good!
THIS is lower carb?
What are these green things?
Dunno.
Good.
Well done, as usual.
That food was great! Who made the guacamole?
I don't think he noticed!
I'm telling you, right?
Let's get the testers out!
I can't look!
Both 103!
No way!
That means you both have to take ME out!
OWL
PS

Oven-Baked Sweet Potato Home Fries

1. Cut 3 medium-size sweet potatoes into ½-inch-thick strips. Toss with 1 tbsp. olive oil. Put on a nonstick cookie sheet with cooking spray or oil.

2. Bake at 400 degrees for 15 to 20 minutes, until strips are golden brown on the bottom.

3. Turn and bake for 15 to 20 minutes more, until strips are golden brown all over.

4. Add coarse salt and parsley to taste. Makes 2 servings.

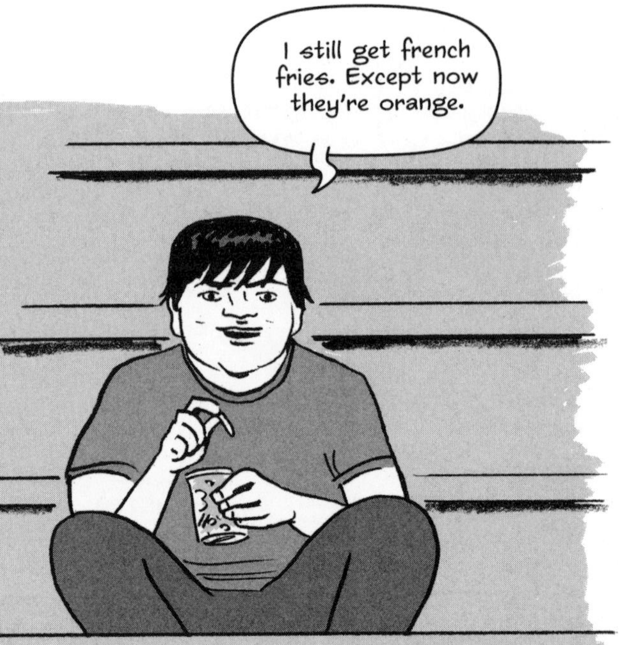
I still get french fries. Except now they're orange.

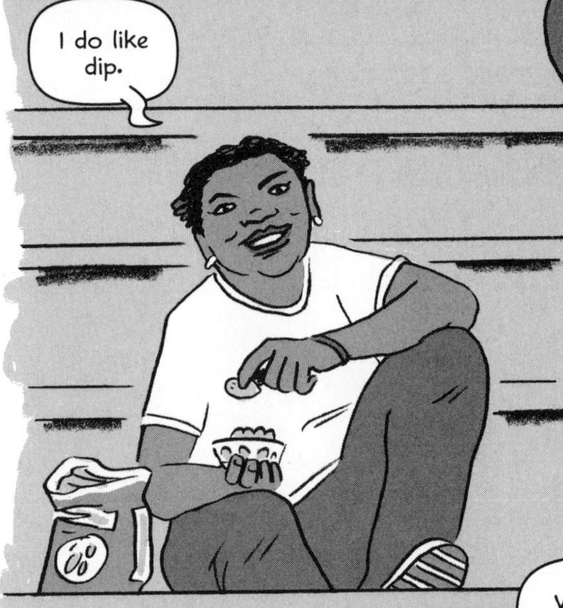
I do like dip.

Curry Dip

1. Sauté 1/2 cup of chopped scallions in 1 tbsp. butter.

2. Add 1 tsp. curry powder and mix well. Remove from the heat.

3. Mix the curried scallions with 1 cup of 2 percent fat yogurt.

4. Add 1/4 cup of chopped golden raisins. Chill well before serving.

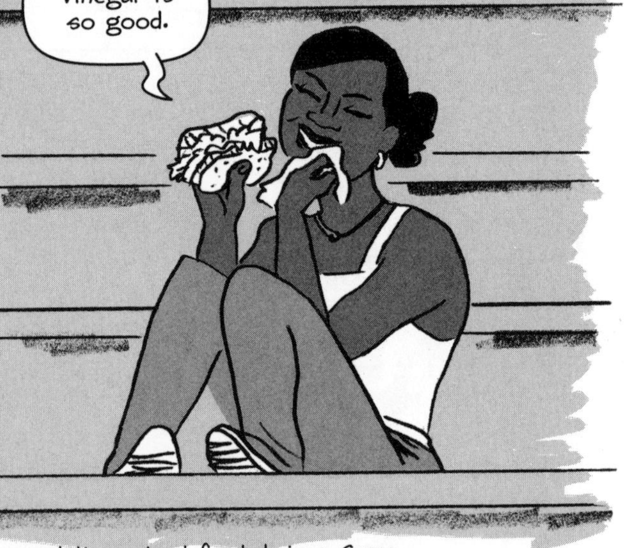
Vinegar is so good.

Veggie Panini Sandwiches

1. Grill about 1 cup of your favorite veggies, roughly chopped, in olive oil.

2. On thick, whole wheat panini bread, spread a balsamic-vinegar-and-mustard mix (1 tsp. each) on each side. Before grilling, add 2 thin slices or sprinkle with 1/4 cup grated sharp cheese such as Asiago or Parmesan.

3. Press in a panini grill or grill like a cheese sandwich.

Please follow all of your physician's recommendations about food choices. Some recommendations from nutritionists or physicians may not match the ones suggested here.

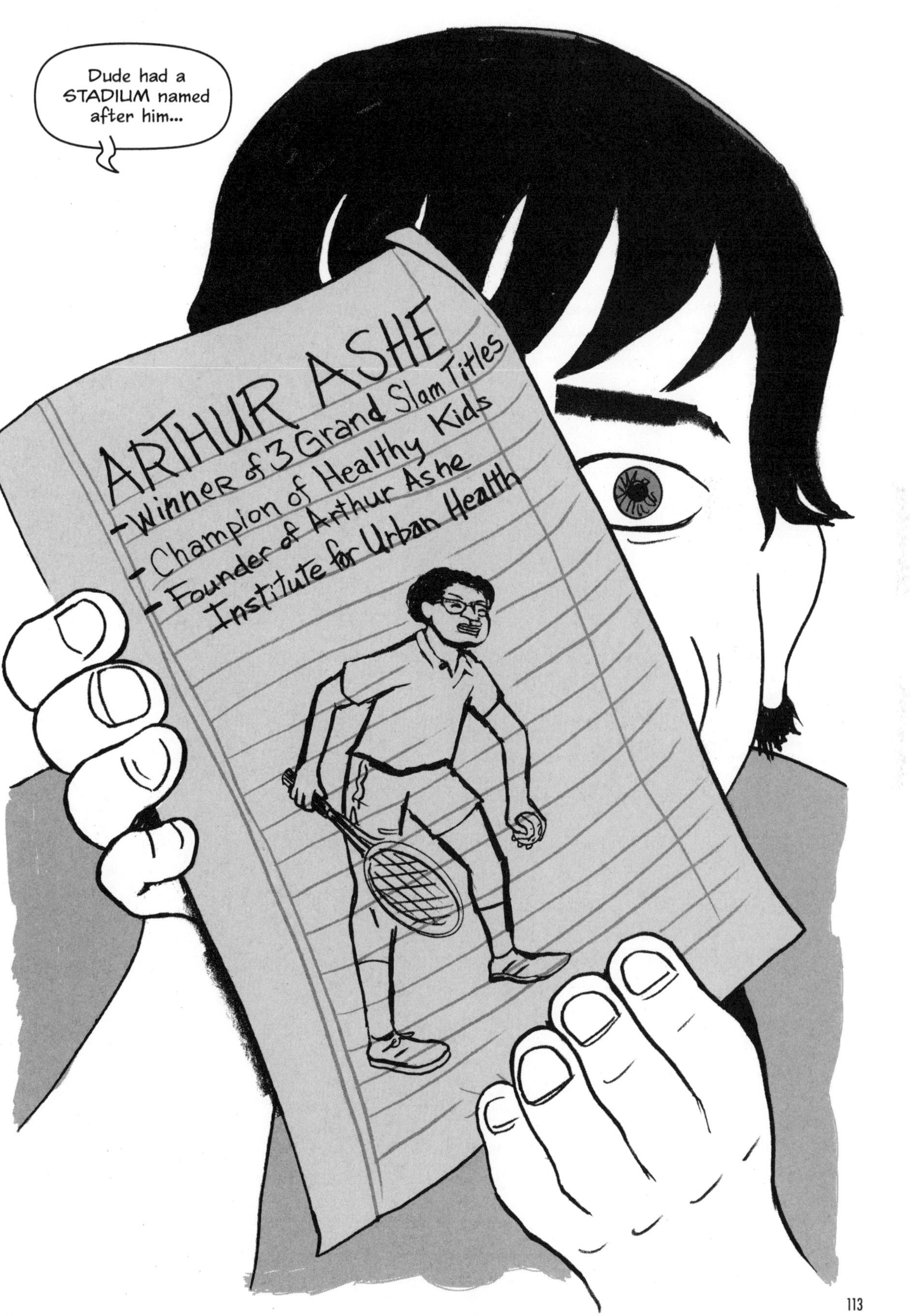

Dude had a STADIUM named after him...
ARTHUR ASHE
-Winner of 3 Grand Slam Titles
-Champion of Healthy Kids
-Founder of Arthur Ashe Institute for Urban Health

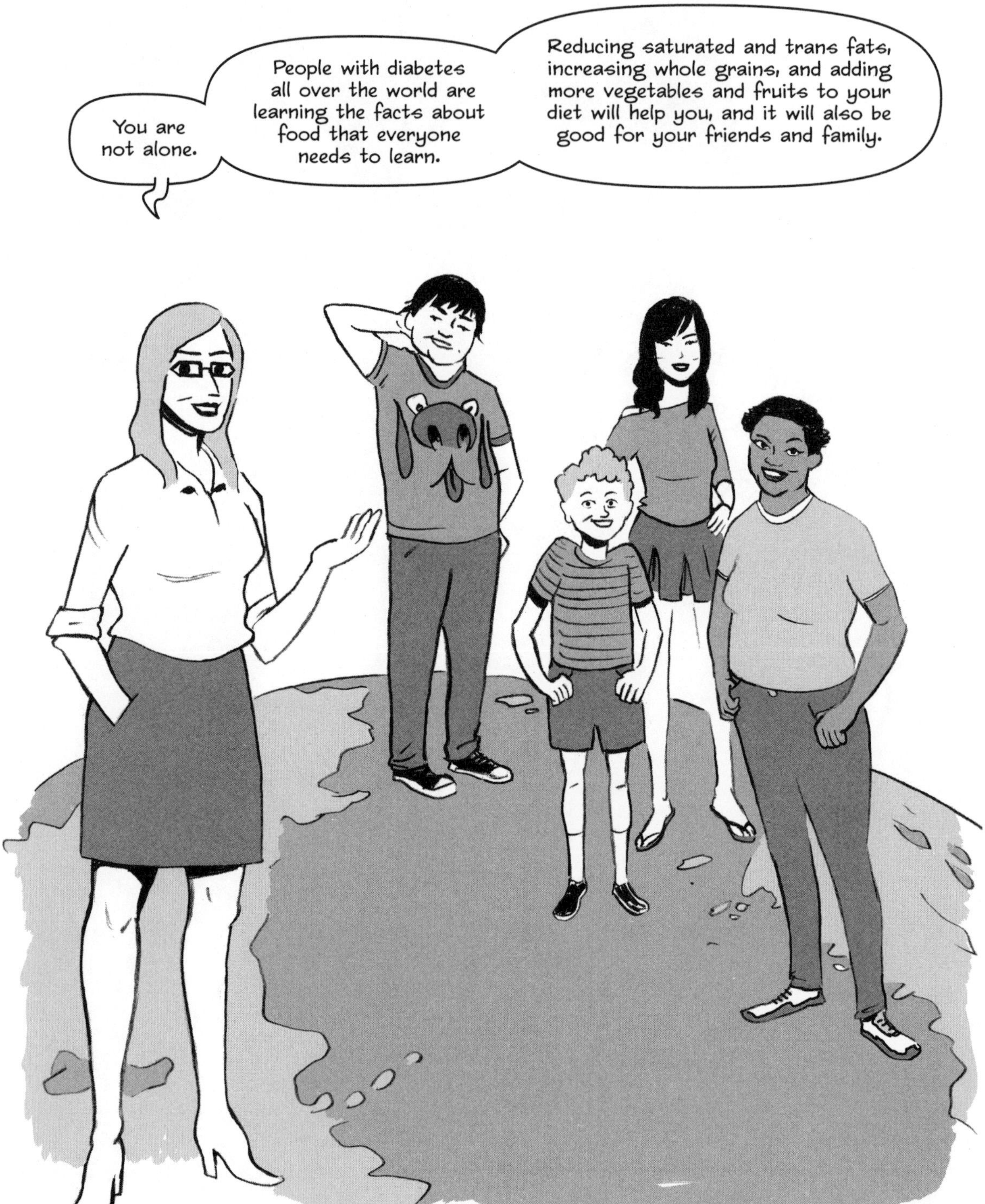
You are not alone.
People with diabetes all over the world are learning the facts about food that everyone needs to learn.
Reducing saturated and trans fats, increasing whole grains, and adding more vegetables and fruits to your diet will help you, and it will also be good for your friends and family.

TIME-OUT: DEALING WITH EMERGENCIES AND FOOD

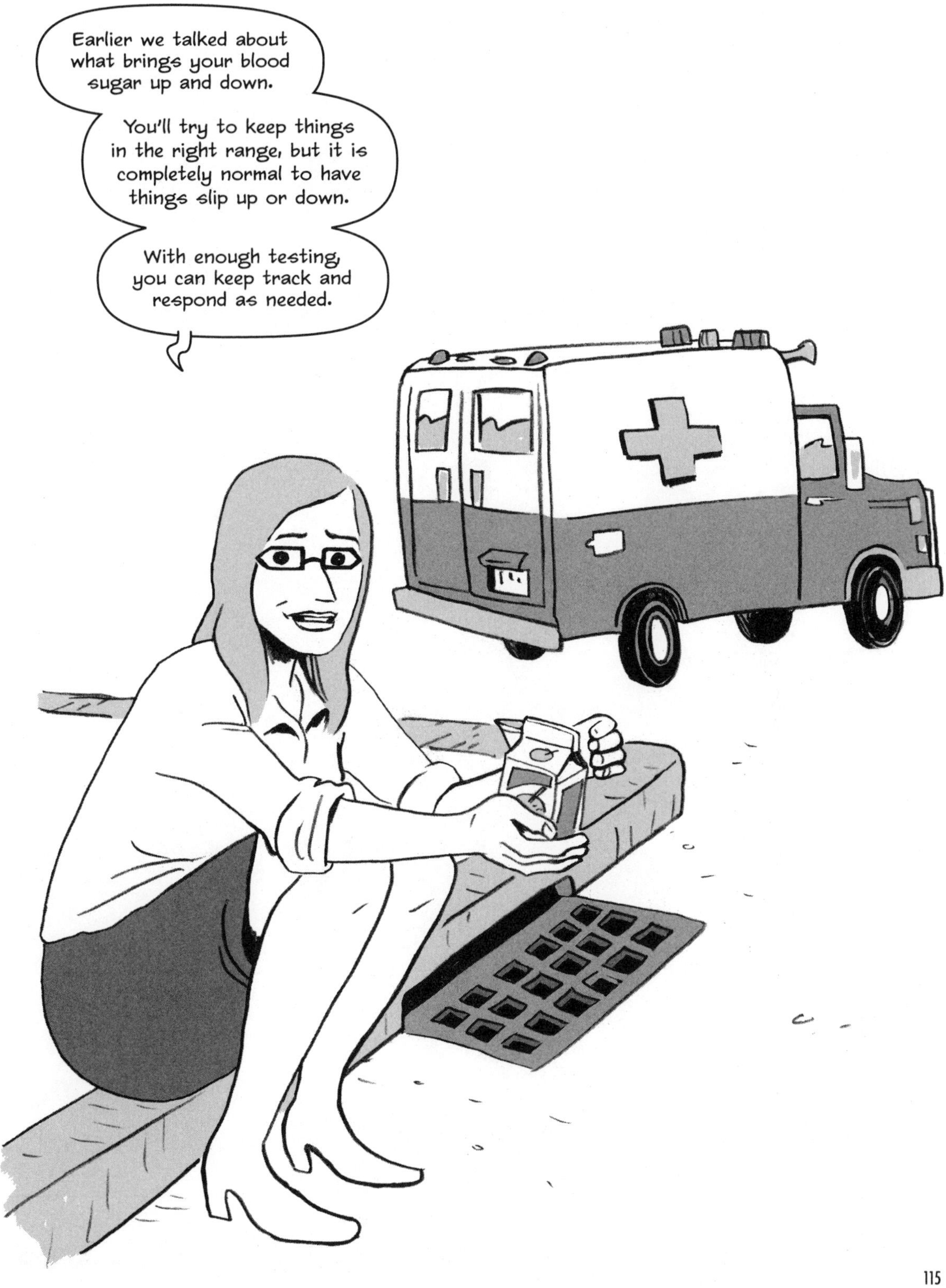
Earlier we talked about what brings your blood sugar up and down.
You'll try to keep things in the right range, but it is completely normal to have things slip up or down.
With enough testing, you can keep track and respond as needed.

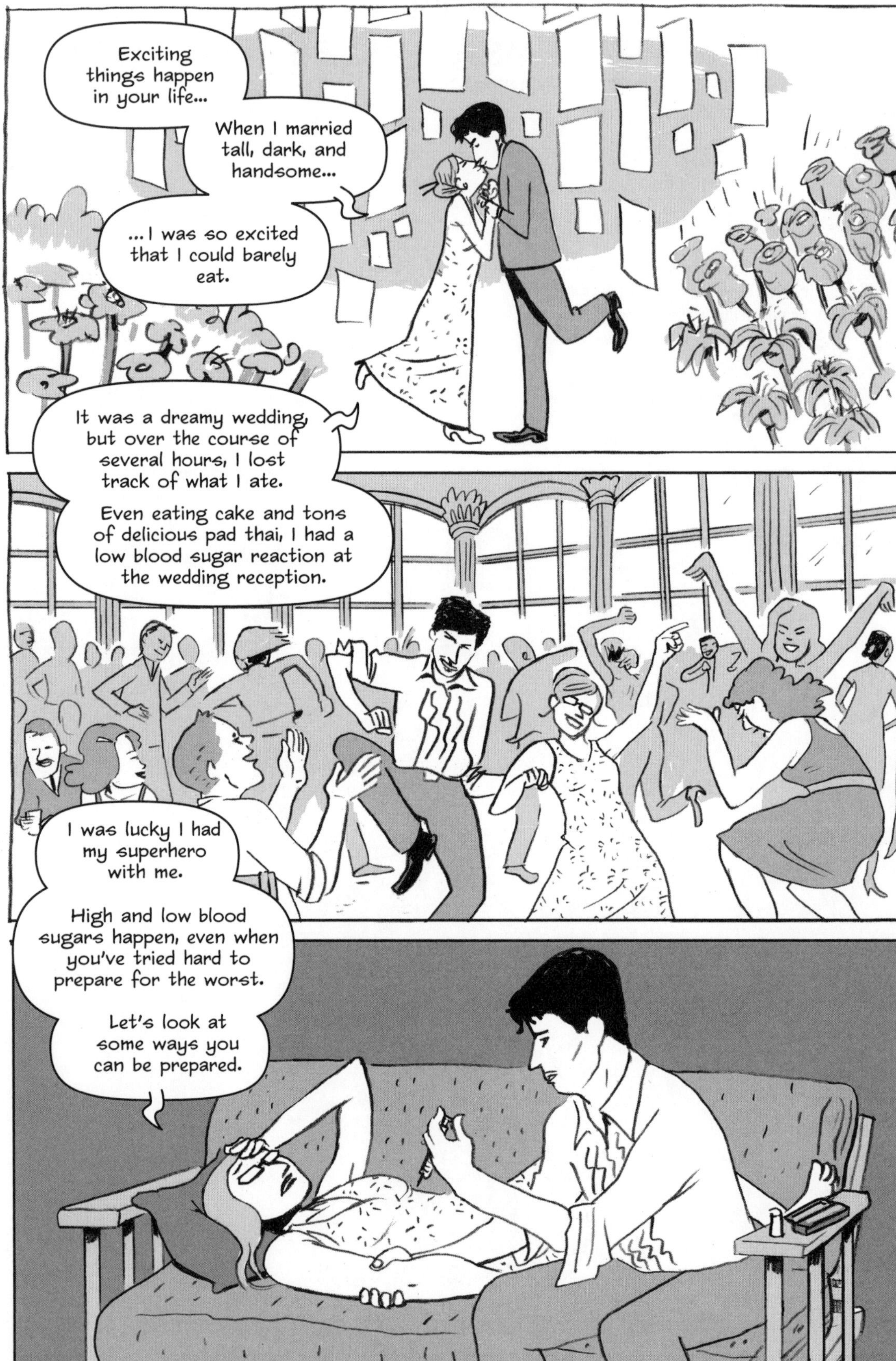
Exciting things happen in your life...
When I married tall, dark, and handsome...
...I was so excited that I could barely eat.
It was a dreamy wedding, but over the course of several hours, I lost track of what I ate.
Even eating cake and tons of delicious pad thai, I had a low blood sugar reaction at the wedding reception.
I was lucky I had my superhero with me.
High and low blood sugars happen, even when you've tried hard to prepare for the worst.
Let's look at some ways you can be prepared.

LOWS

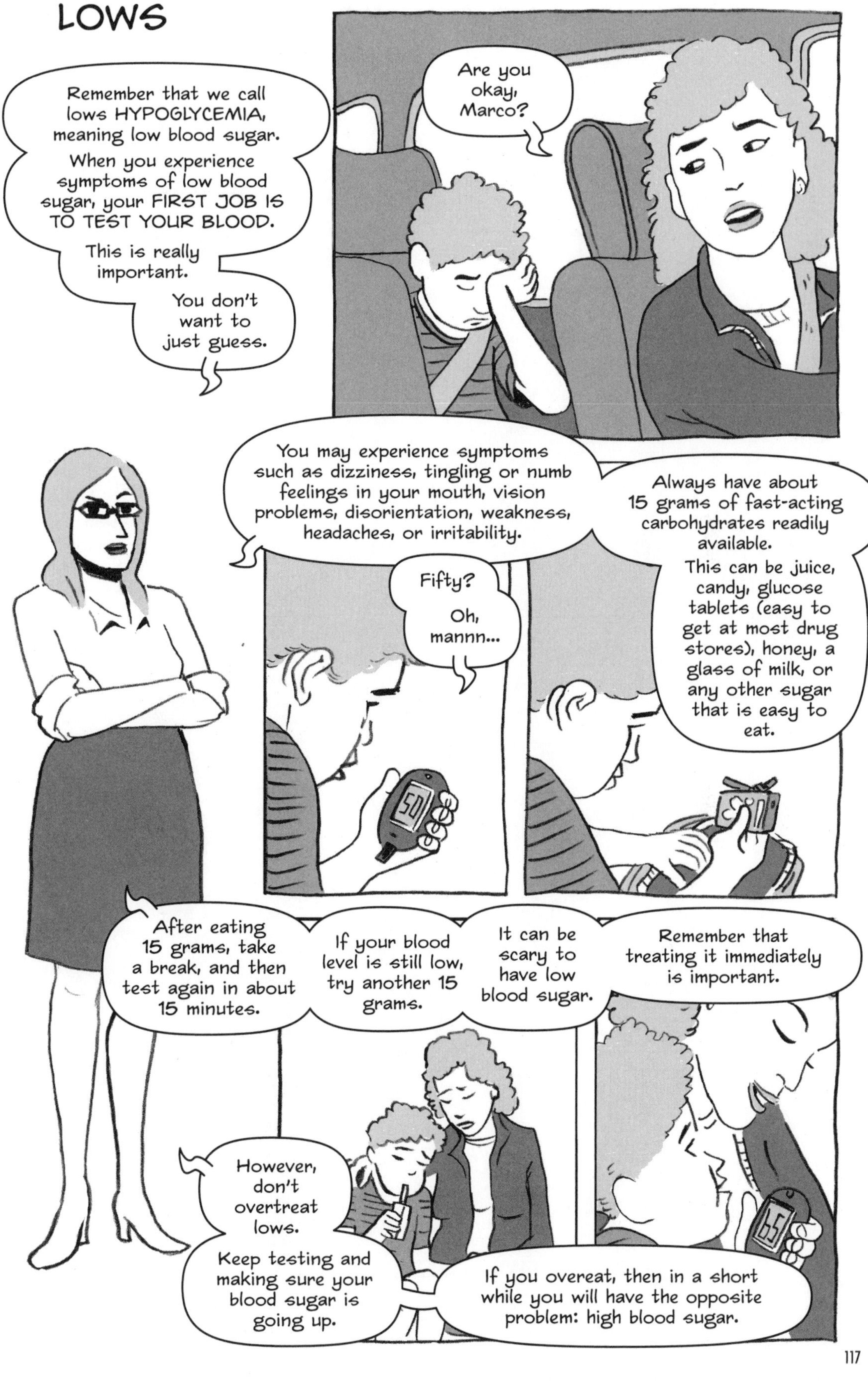
Remember that we call lows HYPOGLYCEMIA, meaning low blood sugar.
When you experience symptoms of low blood sugar, your FIRST JOB IS TO TEST YOUR BLOOD.
This is really important.
You don't want to just guess.
Are you okay, Marco?
You may experience symptoms such as dizziness, tingling or numb feelings in your mouth, vision problems, disorientation, weakness, headaches, or irritability.
Fifty?
Oh, mannn...
Always have about 15 grams of fast-acting carbohydrates readily available.
This can be juice, candy, glucose tablets (easy to get at most drug stores), honey, a glass of milk, or any other sugar that is easy to eat.
After eating 15 grams, take a break, and then test again in about 15 minutes.
If your blood level is still low, try another 15 grams.
It can be scary to have low blood sugar.
Remember that treating it immediately is important.
However, don't overtreat lows.
Keep testing and making sure your blood sugar is going up.
If you overeat, then in a short while you will have the opposite problem: high blood sugar.

SEVERE LOWS

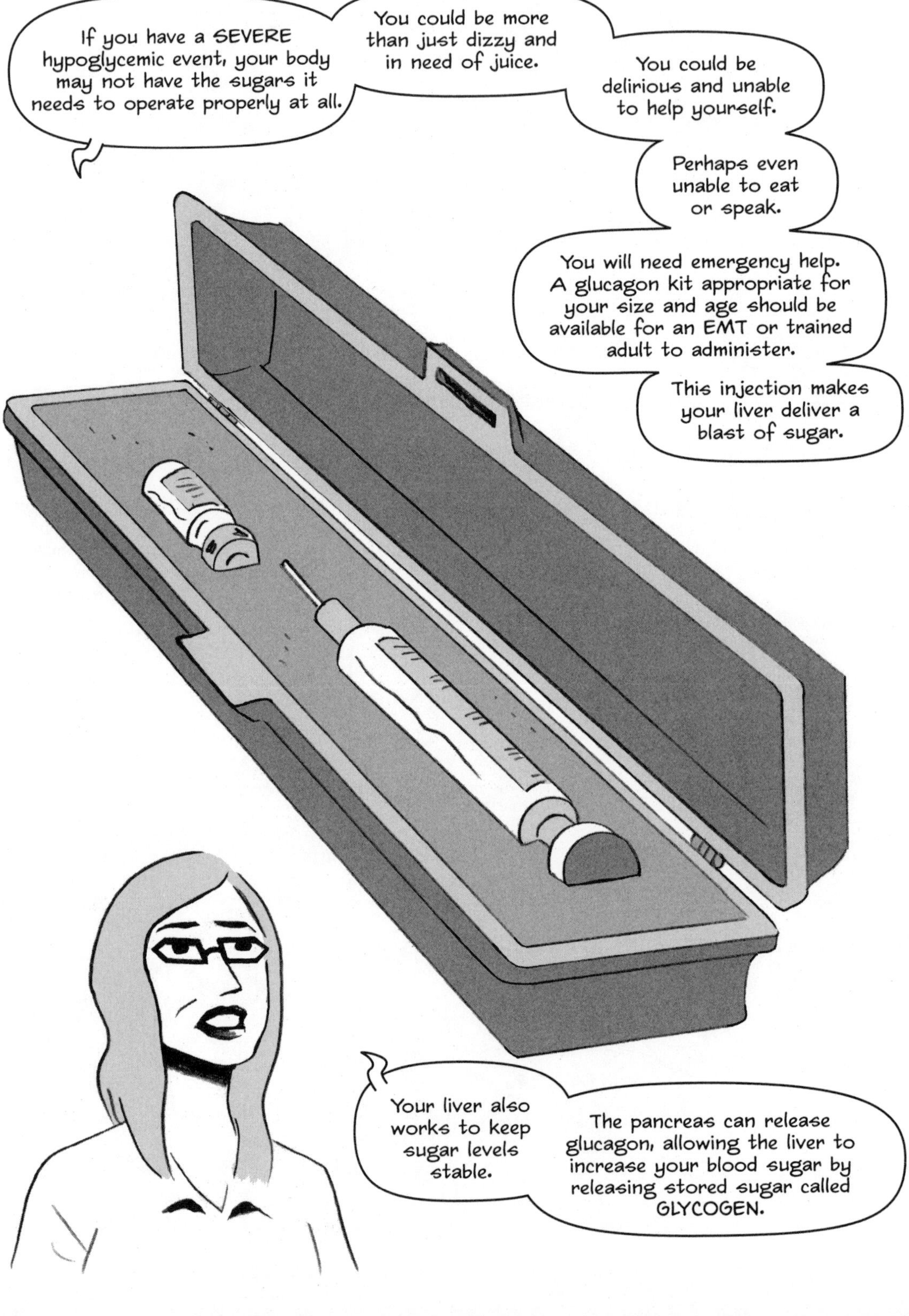

If you have a SEVERE hypoglycemic event, your body may not have the sugars it needs to operate properly at all.
You could be more than just dizzy and in need of juice.
You could be delirious and unable to help yourself.
Perhaps even unable to eat or speak.
You will need emergency help. A glucagon kit appropriate for your size and age should be available for an EMT or trained adult to administer.
This injection makes your liver deliver a blast of sugar.
Your liver also works to keep sugar levels stable.
The pancreas can release glucagon, allowing the liver to increase your blood sugar by releasing stored sugar called GLYCOGEN.

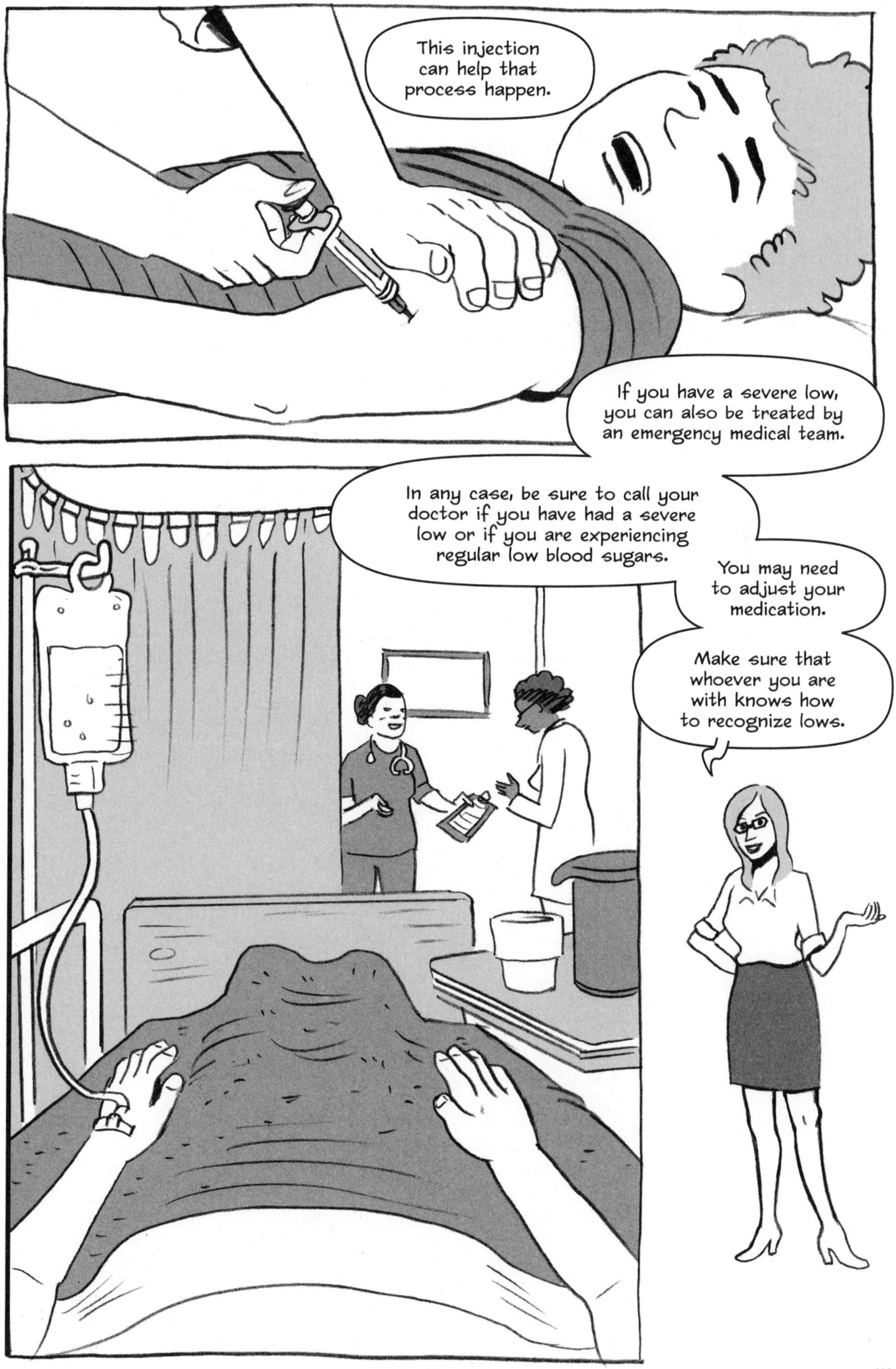
This injection can help that process happen.
If you have a severe low, you can also be treated by an emergency medical team.
In any case, be sure to call your doctor if you have had a severe low or if you are experiencing regular low blood sugars.
You may need to adjust your medication.
Make sure that whoever you are with knows how to recognize lows.

PART FIVE: ON THE FIELD

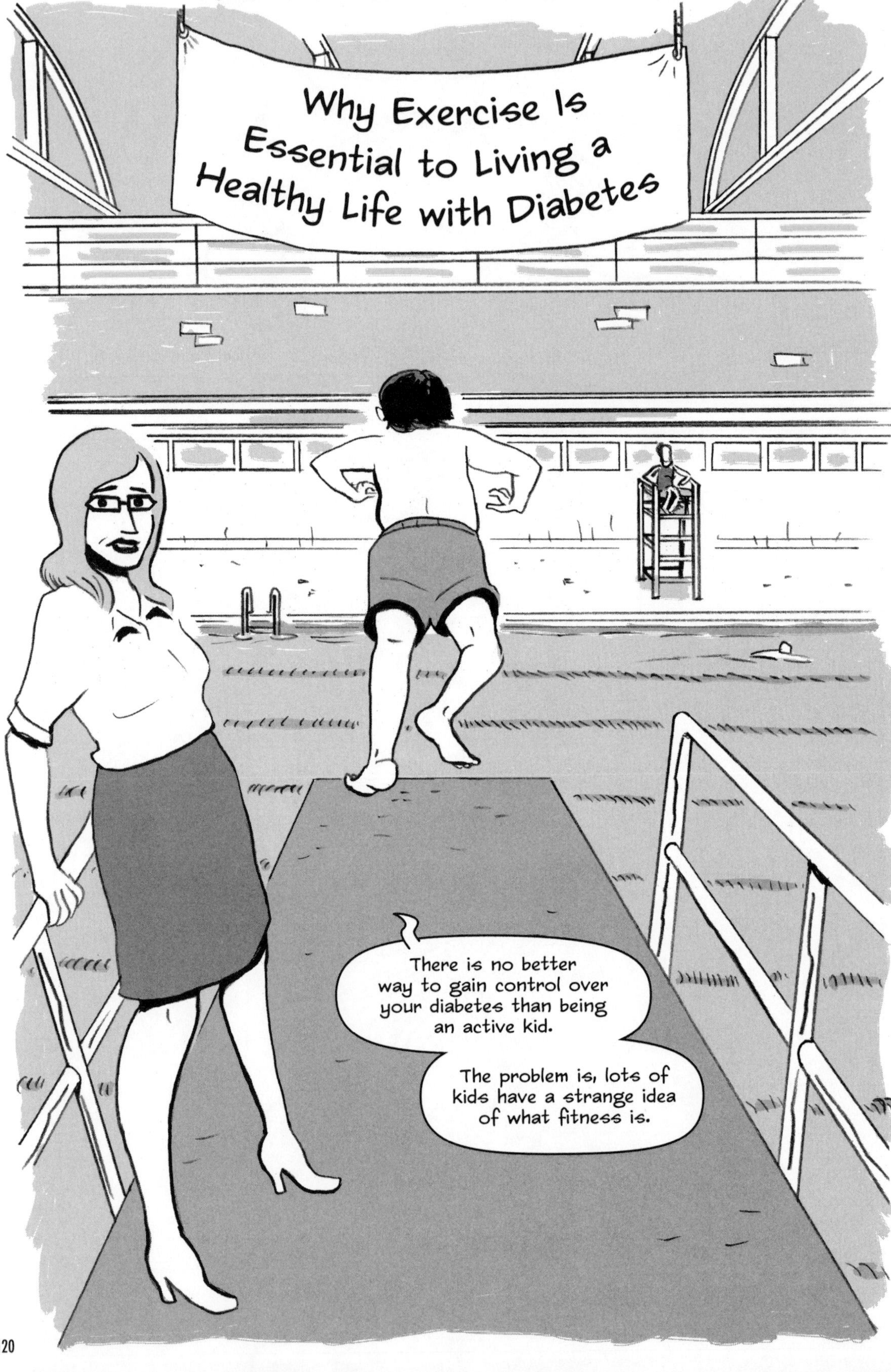
Why Exercise Is Essential to Living a Healthy Life with Diabetes
There is no better way to gain control over your diabetes than being an active kid.
The problem is, lots of kids have a strange idea of what fitness is.

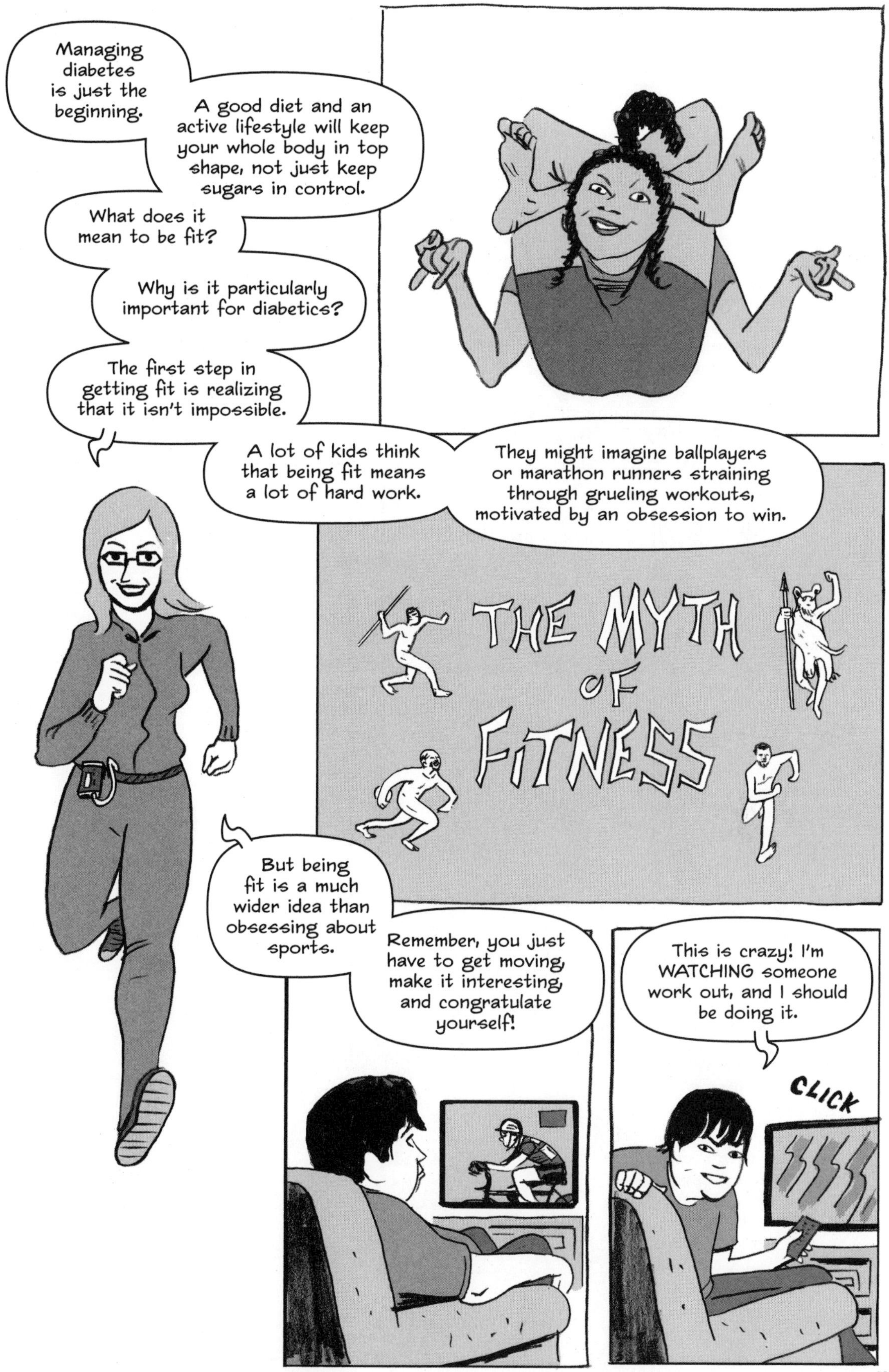
Managing diabetes is just the beginning.
A good diet and an active lifestyle will keep your whole body in top shape, not just keep sugars in control.
What does it mean to be fit?
Why is it particularly important for diabetics?
The first step in getting fit is realizing that it isn't impossible.
A lot of kids think that being fit means a lot of hard work.
They might imagine ballplayers or marathon runners straining through grueling workouts, motivated by an obsession to win.
THE MYTH OF FITNESS
But being fit is a much wider idea than obsessing about sports.
Remember, you just have to get moving, make it interesting, and congratulate yourself!
This is crazy! I'm WATCHING someone work out, and I should be doing it.
CLICK

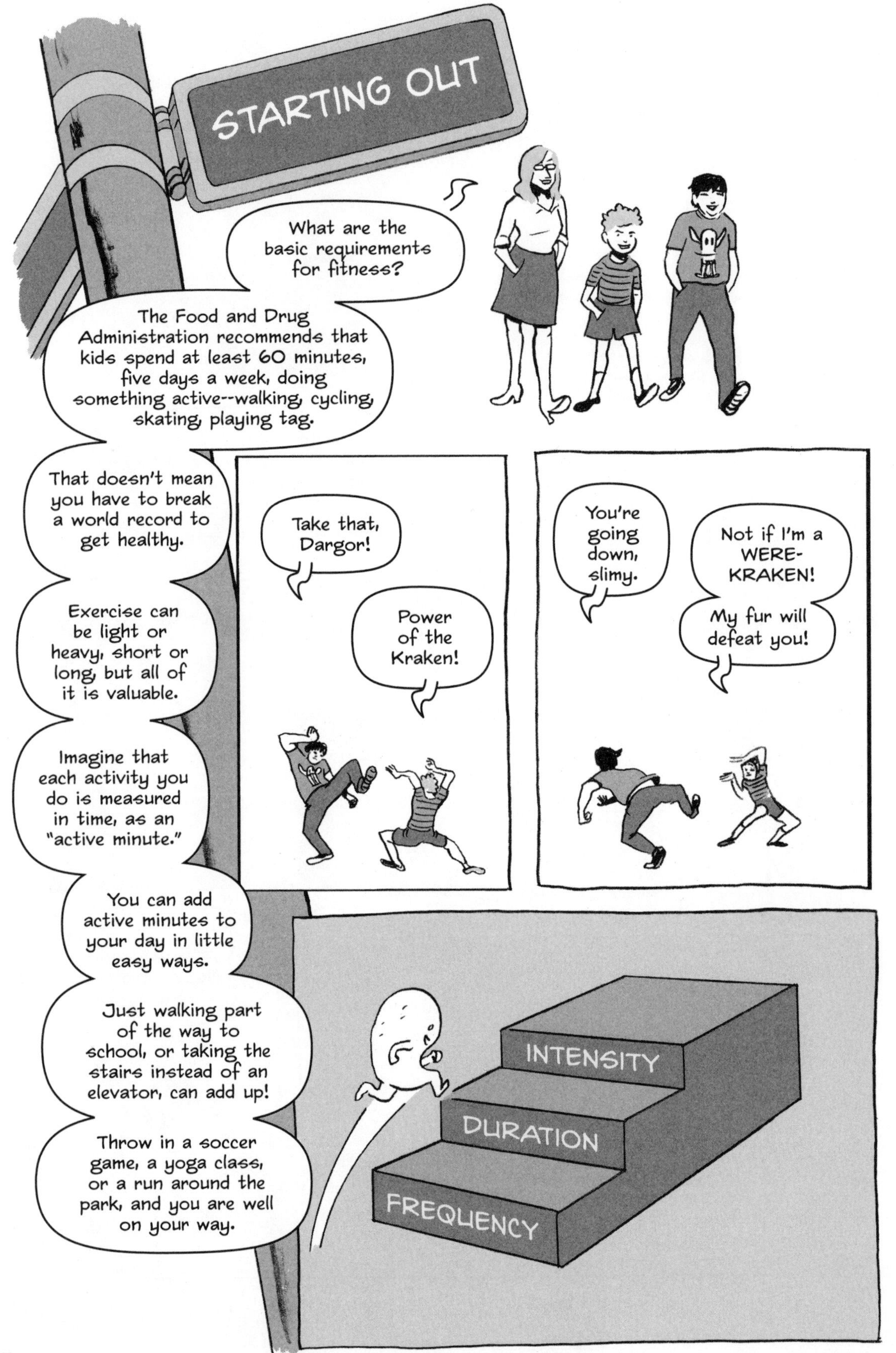
STARTING OUT
What are the basic requirements for fitness?
The Food and Drug Administration recommends that kids spend at least 60 minutes, five days a week, doing something active--walking, cycling, skating, playing tag.
That doesn't mean you have to break a world record to get healthy.
Exercise can be light or heavy, short or long, but all of it is valuable.
Imagine that each activity you do is measured in time, as an "active minute."
Take that, Dargor!
Power of the Kraken!
You're going down, slimy.
Not if I'm a WERE-KRAKEN!
My fur will defeat you!
You can add active minutes to your day in little easy ways.
Just walking part of the way to school, or taking the stairs instead of an elevator, can add up!
Throw in a soccer game, a yoga class, or a run around the park, and you are well on your way.
INTENSITY
DURATION
FREQUENCY

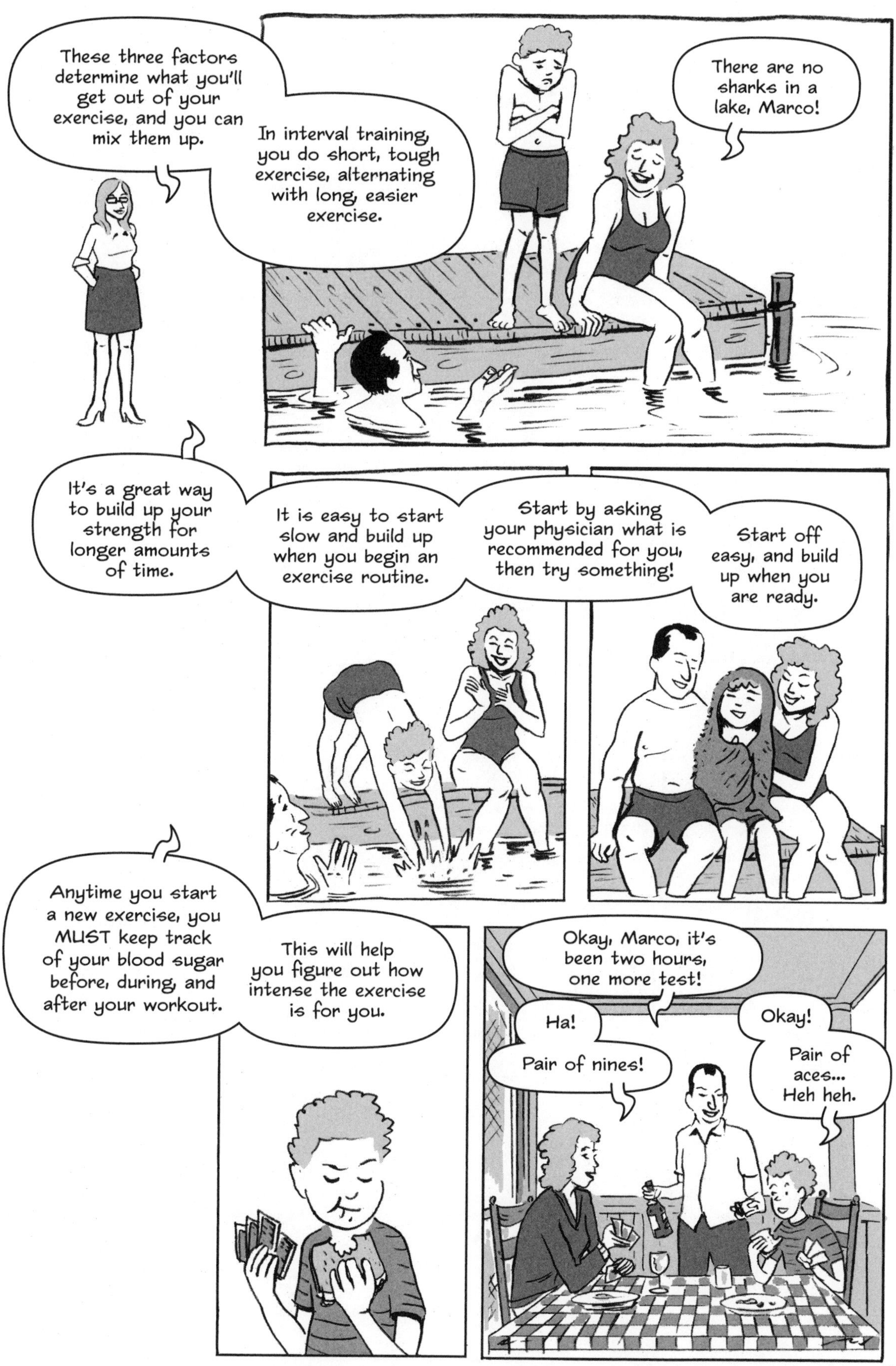
These three factors determine what you'll get out of your exercise, and you can mix them up.
In interval training, you do short, tough exercise, alternating with long, easier exercise.
There are no sharks in a lake, Marco!
It's a great way to build up your strength for longer amounts of time.
It is easy to start slow and build up when you begin an exercise routine.
Start by asking your physician what is recommended for you, then try something!
Start off easy, and build up when you are ready.
Anytime you start a new exercise, you MUST keep track of your blood sugar before, during, and after your workout.
This will help you figure out how intense the exercise is for you.
Okay, Marco, it's been two hours, one more test!
Ha!
Pair of nines!
Okay!
Pair of aces... Heh heh.

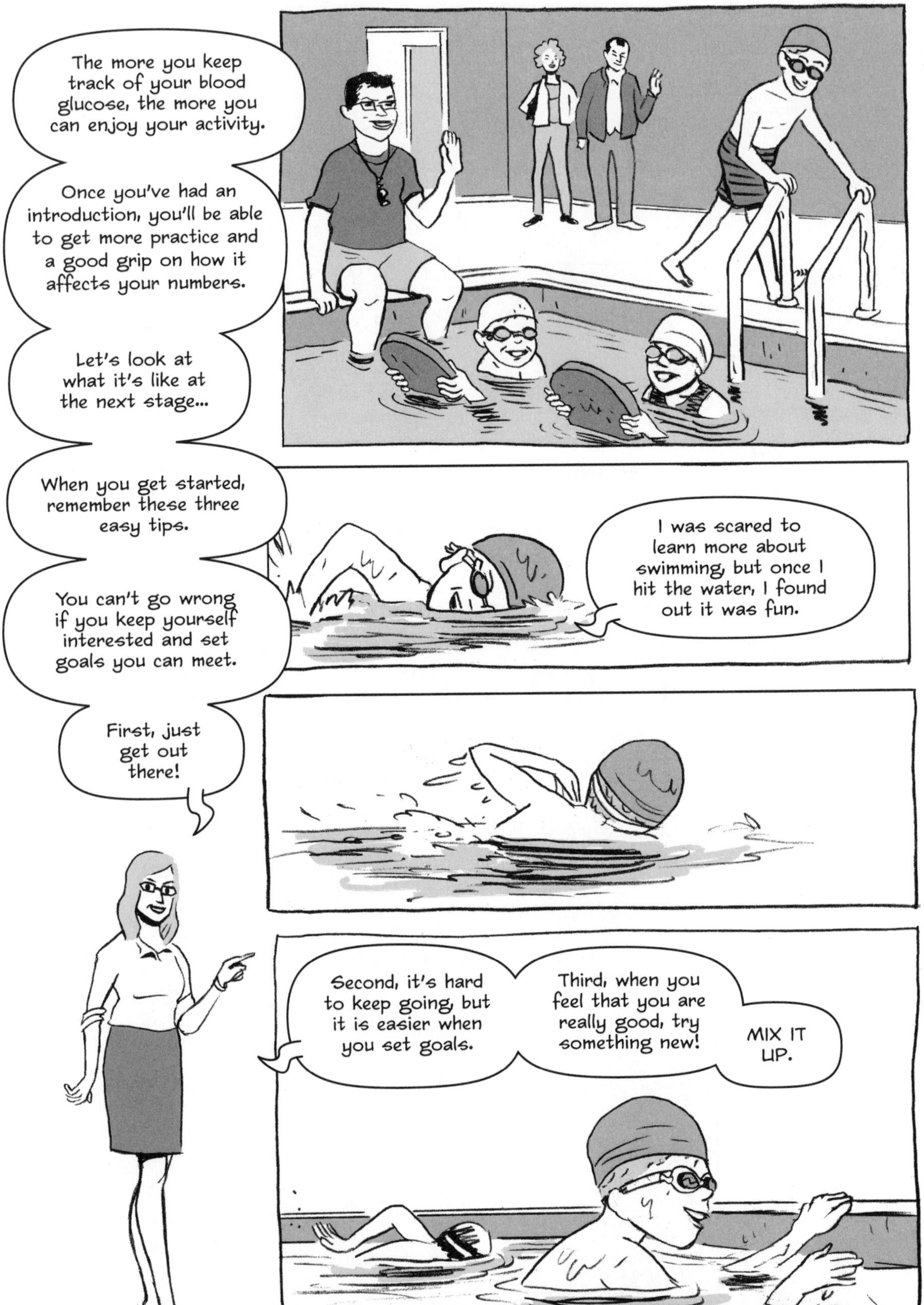
The more you keep track of your blood glucose, the more you can enjoy your activity.
Once you've had an introduction, you'll be able to get more practice and a good grip on how it affects your numbers.
Let's look at what it's like at the next stage...
When you get started, remember these three easy tips.
I was scared to learn more about swimming, but once I hit the water, I found out it was fun.
You can't go wrong if you keep yourself interested and set goals you can meet.
First, just get out there!
Second, it's hard to keep going, but it is easier when you set goals.
Third, when you feel that you are really good, try something new!
MIX IT UP.

TAKING IT TO THE NEXT LEVEL

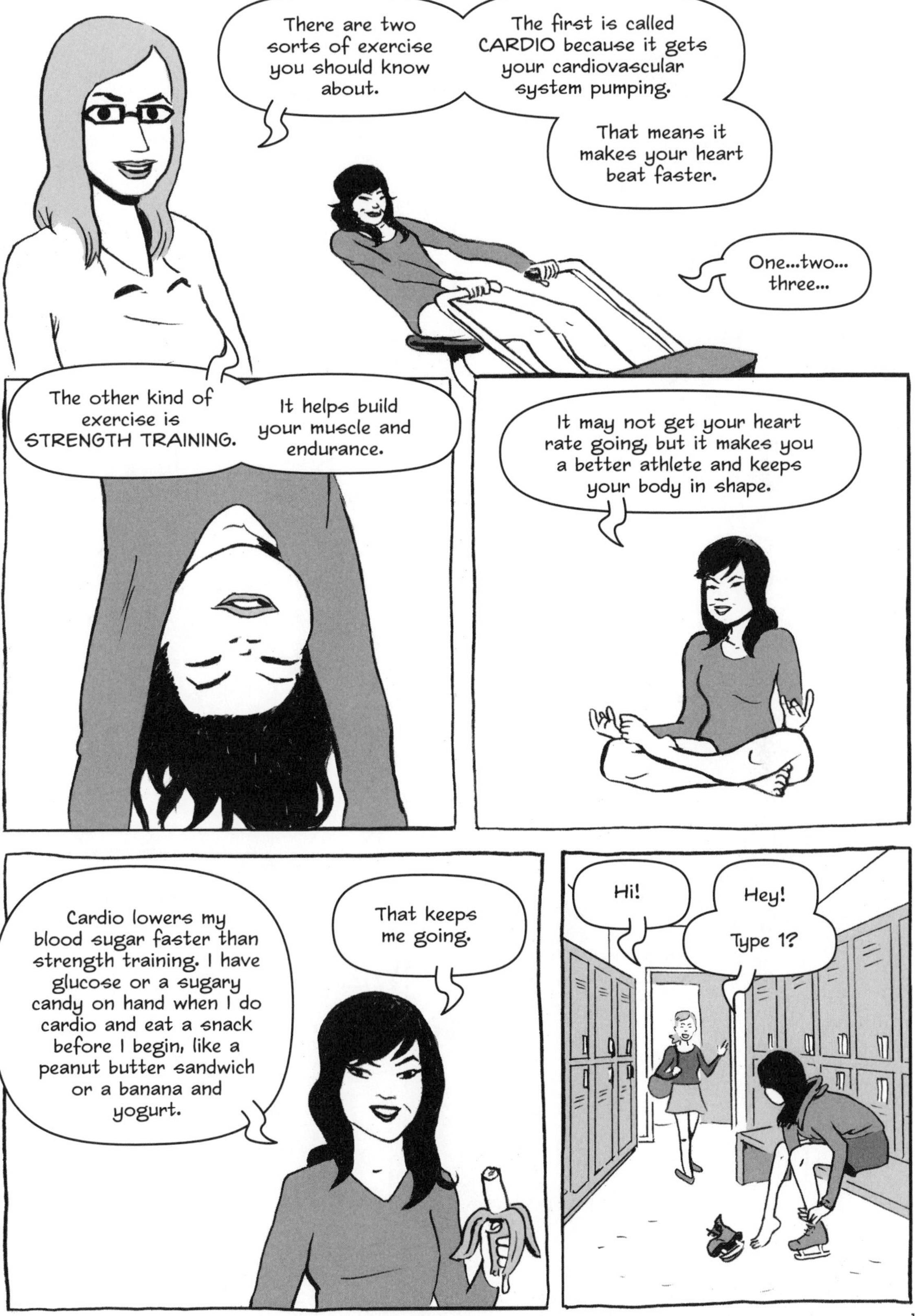

There are two sorts of exercise you should know about.
The first is called CARDIO because it gets your cardiovascular system pumping.
That means it makes your heart beat faster.
One...two... three...
The other kind of exercise is STRENGTH TRAINING.
It helps build your muscle and endurance.
It may not get your heart rate going, but it makes you a better athlete and keeps your body in shape.
Cardio lowers my blood sugar faster than strength training. I have glucose or a sugary candy on hand when I do cardio and eat a snack before I begin, like a peanut butter sandwich or a banana and yogurt.
That keeps me going.
Hi!
Hey!
Type 1?

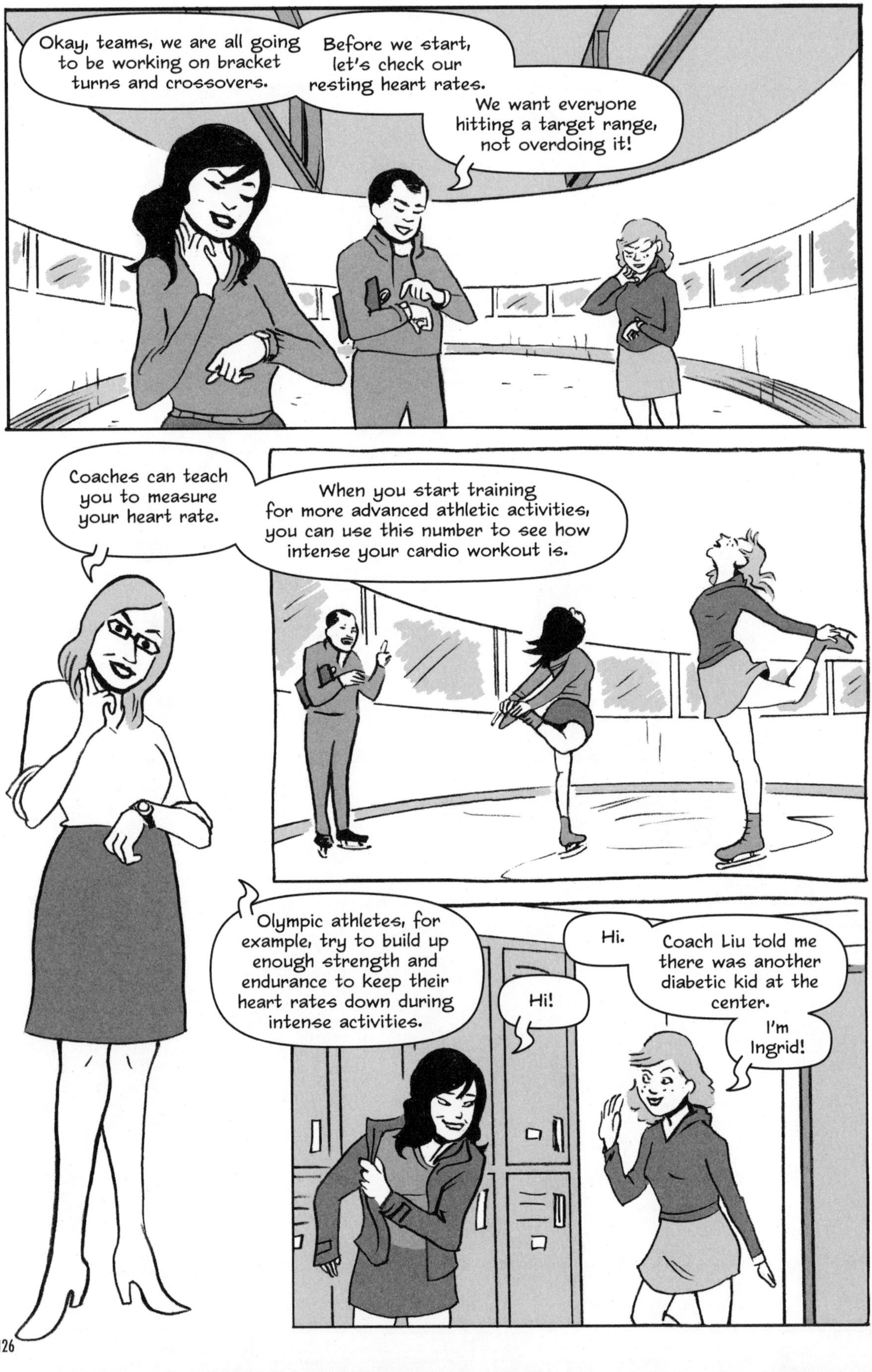
Okay, teams, we are all going to be working on bracket turns and crossovers.
Before we start, let's check our resting heart rates.
We want everyone hitting a target range, not overdoing it!
Coaches can teach you to measure your heart rate.
When you start training for more advanced athletic activities, you can use this number to see how intense your cardio workout is.
Olympic athletes, for example, try to build up enough strength and endurance to keep their heart rates down during intense activities.
Hi.
Hi!
Coach Liu told me there was another diabetic kid at the center.
I'm Ingrid!

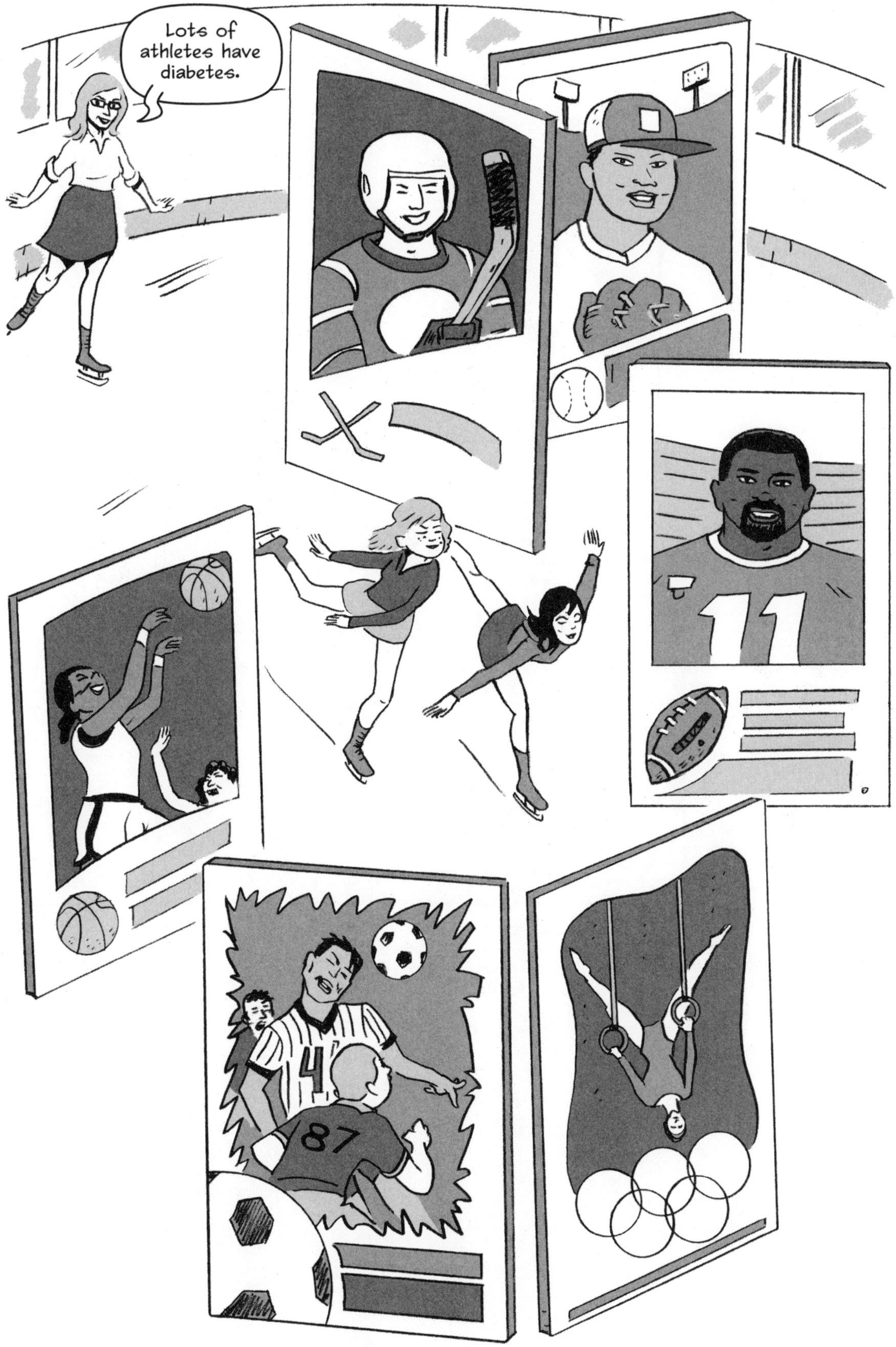
Lots of athletes have diabetes.
11
4
87

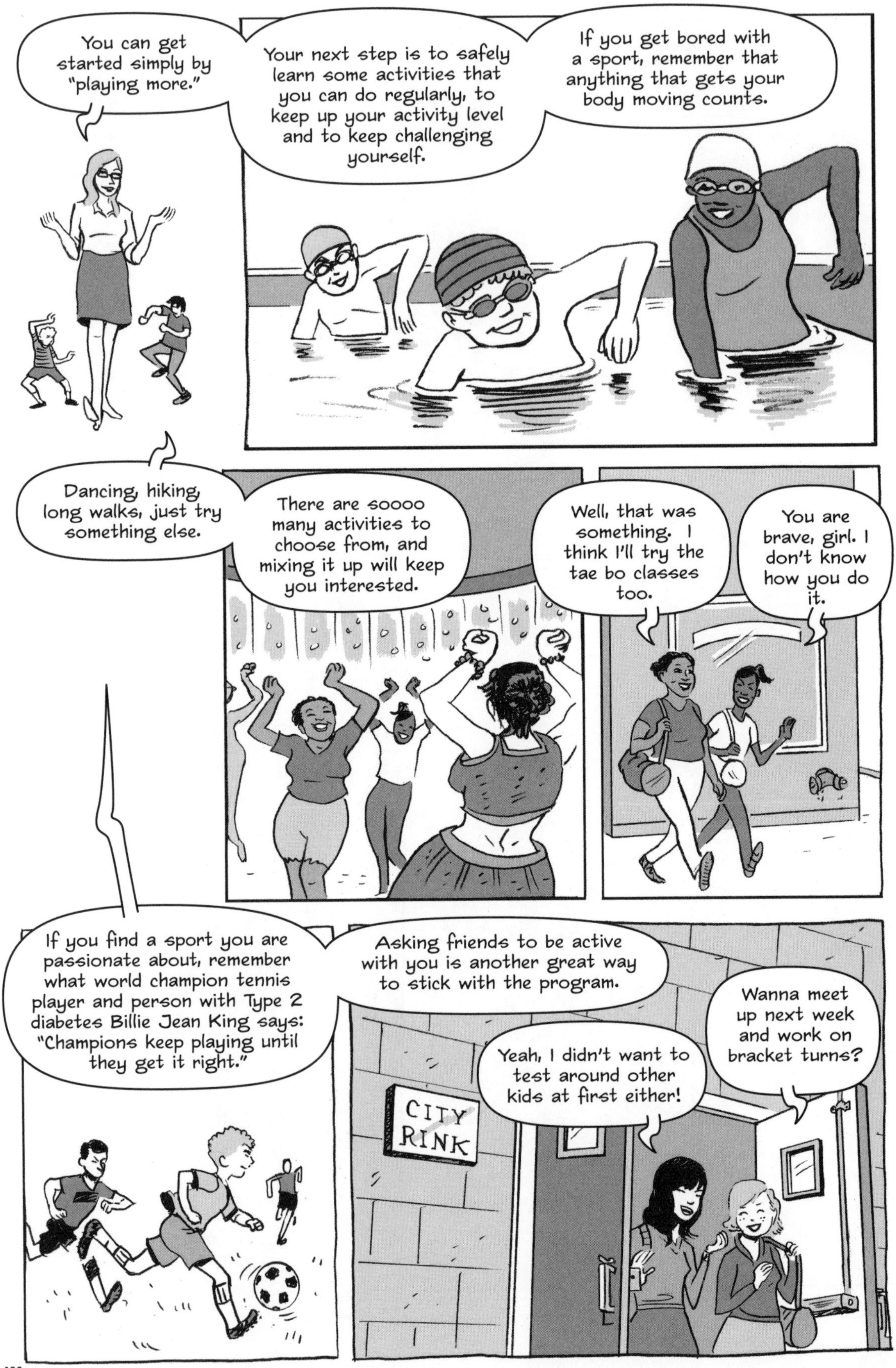
You can get started simply by "playing more."
Your next step is to safely learn some activities that you can do regularly, to keep up your activity level and to keep challenging yourself.
If you get bored with a sport, remember that anything that gets your body moving counts.
Dancing, hiking, long walks, just try something else.
There are soooo many activities to choose from, and mixing it up will keep you interested.
Well, that was something. I think I'll try the tae bo classes too.
You are brave, girl. I don't know how you do it.
If you find a sport you are passionate about, remember what world champion tennis player and person with Type 2 diabetes Billie Jean King says: "Champions keep playing until they get it right."
Asking friends to be active with you is another great way to stick with the program.
Wanna meet up next week and work on bracket turns?
Yeah, I didn't want to test around other kids at first either!
CITY RINK

RUNNING INTERFERENCE

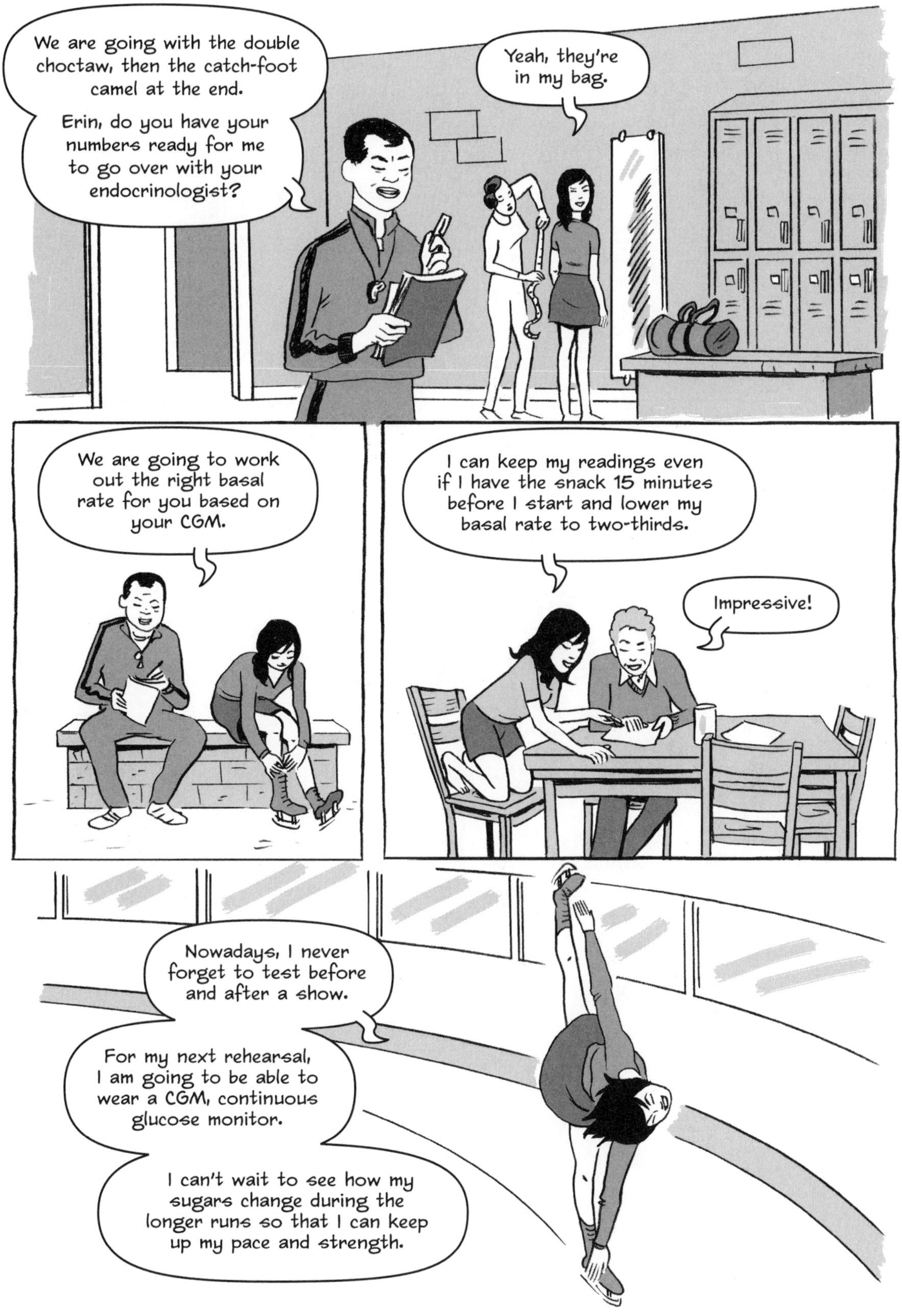
We are going with the double choctaw, then the catch-foot camel at the end.
Erin, do you have your numbers ready for me to go over with your endocrinologist?
Yeah, they're in my bag.
We are going to work out the right basal rate for you based on your CGM.
I can keep my readings even if I have the snack 15 minutes before I start and lower my basal rate to two-thirds.
Impressive!
Nowadays, I never forget to test before and after a show.
For my next rehearsal, I am going to be able to wear a CGM, continuous glucose monitor.
I can't wait to see how my sugars change during the longer runs so that I can keep up my pace and strength.

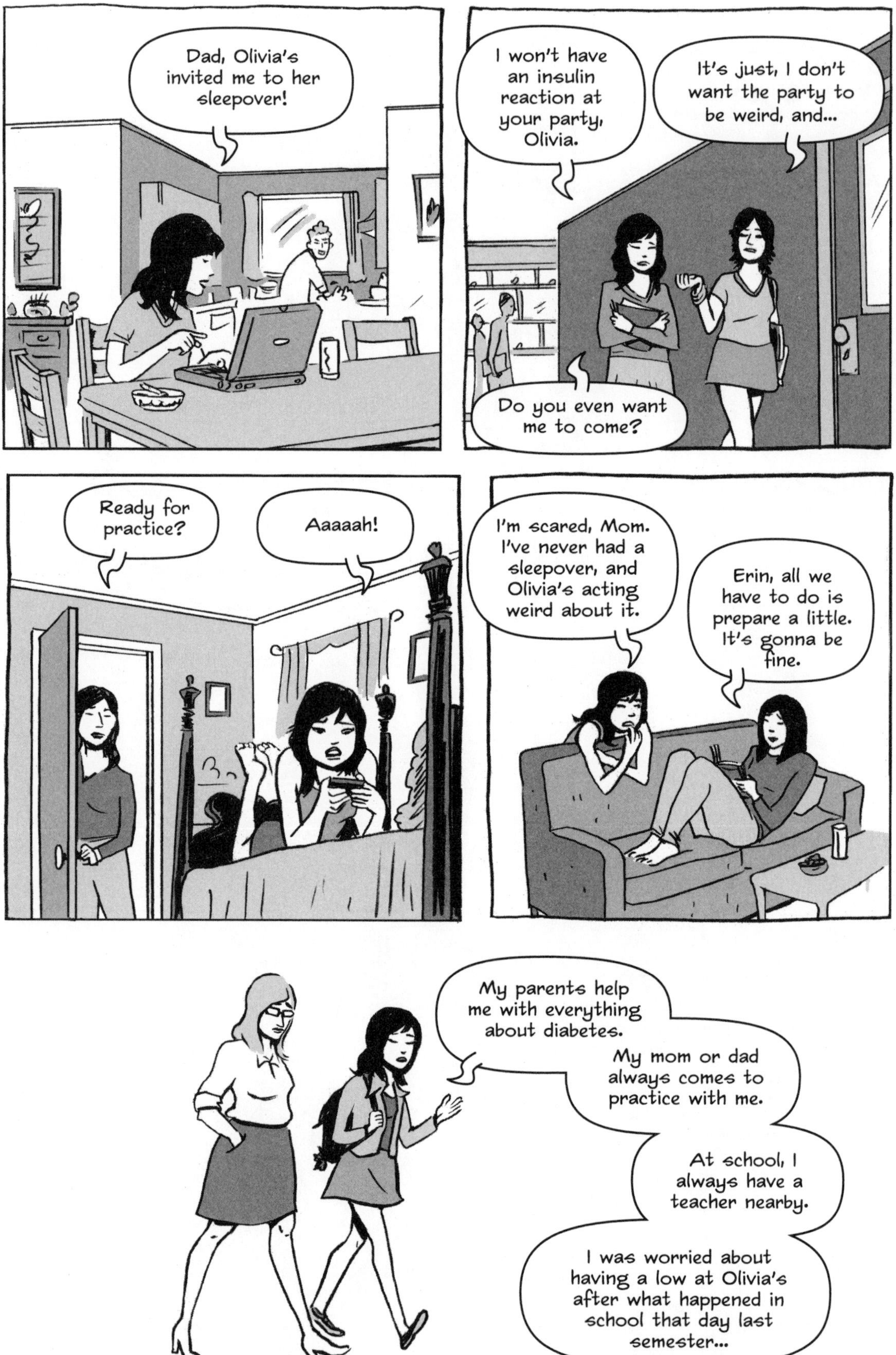
Dad, Olivia's invited me to her sleepover!
I won't have an insulin reaction at your party, Olivia.
It's just, I don't want the party to be weird, and...
Do you even want me to come?
Ready for practice?
Aaaaah!
I'm scared, Mom. I've never had a sleepover, and Olivia's acting weird about it.
Erin, all we have to do is prepare a little. It's gonna be fine.
My parents help me with everything about diabetes.
My mom or dad always comes to practice with me.
At school, I always have a teacher nearby.
I was worried about having a low at Olivia's after what happened in school that day last semester...

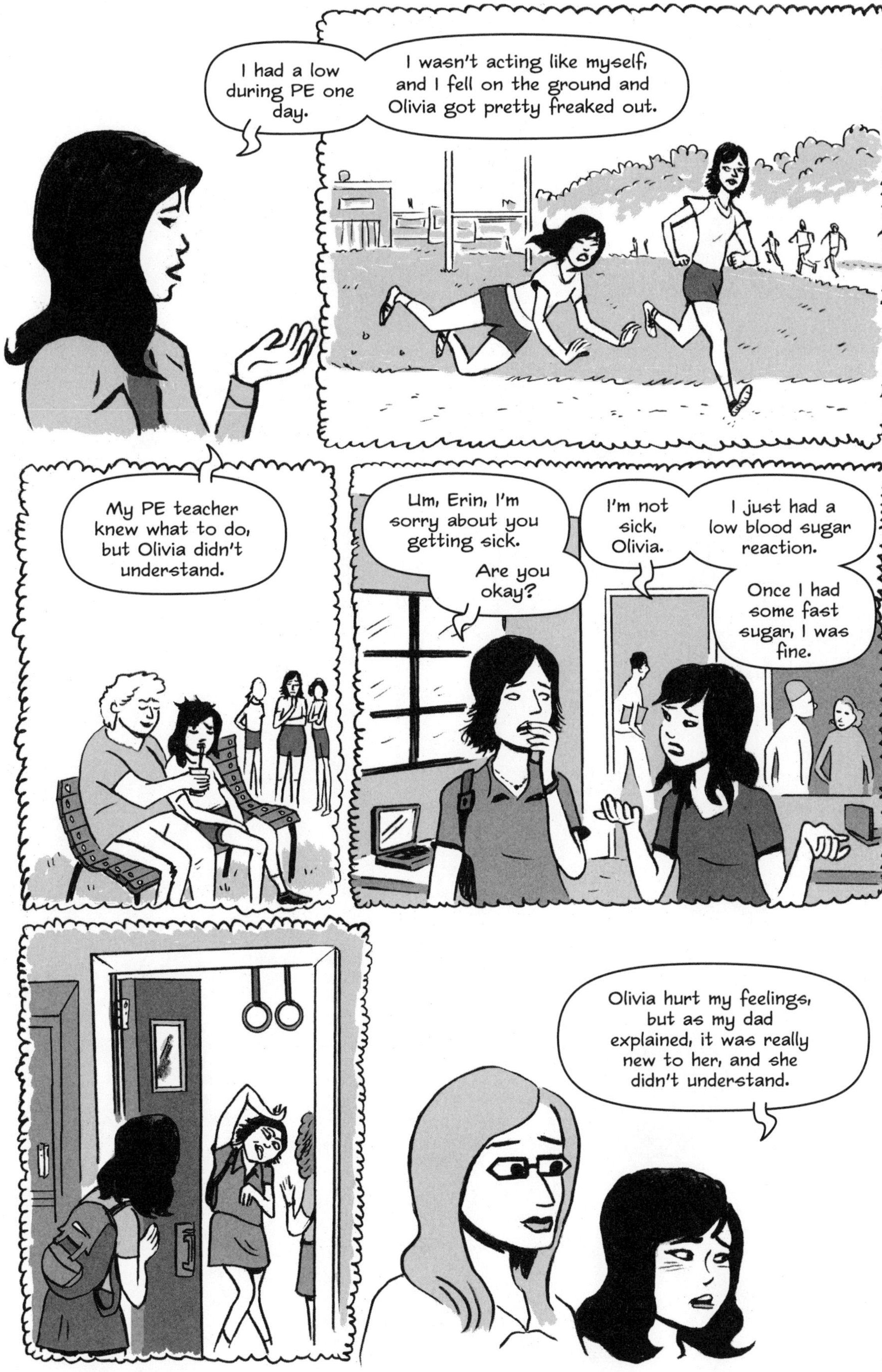
I had a low during PE one day.
I wasn't acting like myself, and I fell on the ground and Olivia got pretty freaked out.
My PE teacher knew what to do, but Olivia didn't understand.
Um, Erin, I'm sorry about you getting sick.
Are you okay?
I'm not sick, Olivia.
I just had a low blood sugar reaction.
Once I had some fast sugar, I was fine.
Olivia hurt my feelings, but as my dad explained, it was really new to her, and she didn't understand.

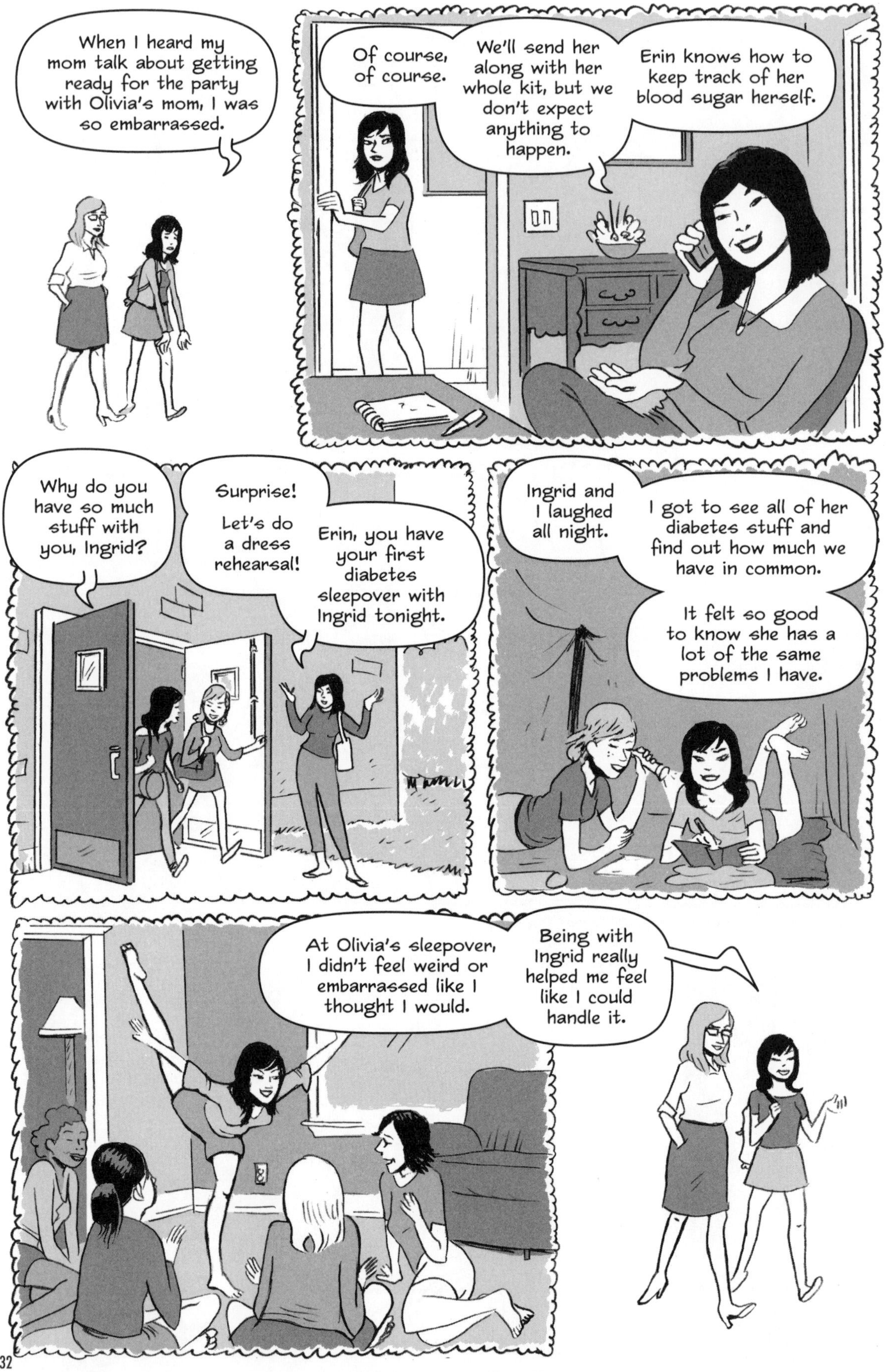
When I heard my mom talk about getting ready for the party with Olivia's mom, I was so embarrassed.
Of course, of course.
We'll send her along with her whole kit, but we don't expect anything to happen.
Erin knows how to keep track of her blood sugar herself.
Why do you have so much stuff with you, Ingrid?
Surprise!
Let's do a dress rehearsal!
Erin, you have your first diabetes sleepover with Ingrid tonight.
Ingrid and I laughed all night.
I got to see all of her diabetes stuff and find out how much we have in common.
It felt so good to know she has a lot of the same problems I have.
At Olivia's sleepover, I didn't feel weird or embarrassed like I thought I would.
Being with Ingrid really helped me feel like I could handle it.

WHAT WILL YOU TRY?

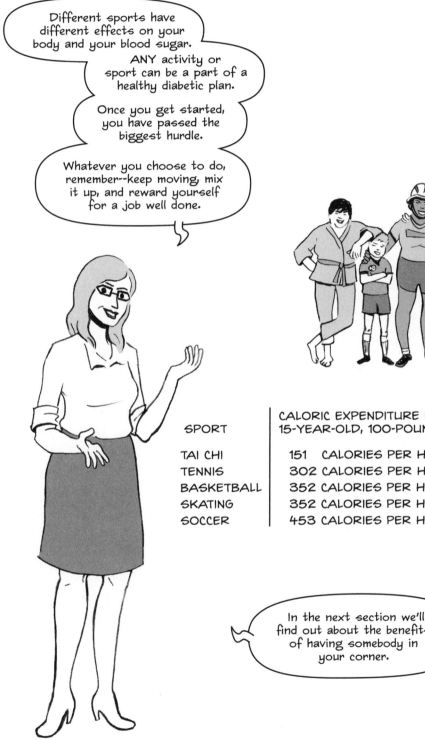

Different sports have different effects on your body and your blood sugar.

ANY activity or sport can be a part of a healthy diabetic plan.

Once you get started, you have passed the biggest hurdle.

Whatever you choose to do, remember--keep moving, mix it up, and reward yourself for a job well done.

SPORT	CALORIC EXPENDITURE IF YOU'RE A 15-YEAR-OLD, 100-POUND, 5-FOOT KID
TAI CHI	151 CALORIES PER HOUR
TENNIS	302 CALORIES PER HOUR
BASKETBALL	352 CALORIES PER HOUR
SKATING	352 CALORIES PER HOUR
SOCCER	453 CALORIES PER HOUR

In the next section we'll find out about the benefits of having somebody in your corner.

PART SIX: HUDDLE! TEAM SUPPORT

FANS

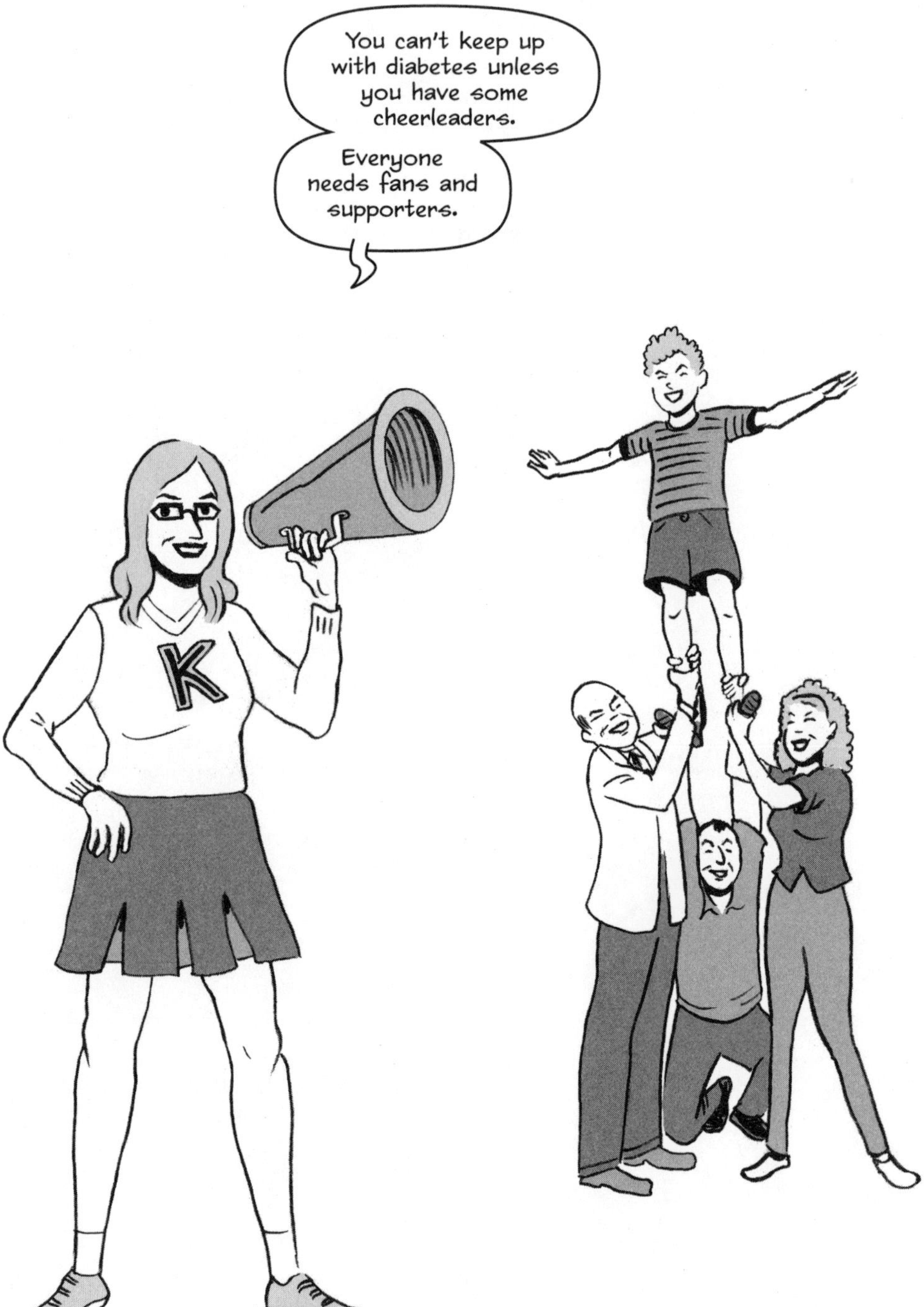
You can't keep up with diabetes unless you have some cheerleaders.
Everyone needs fans and supporters.
K

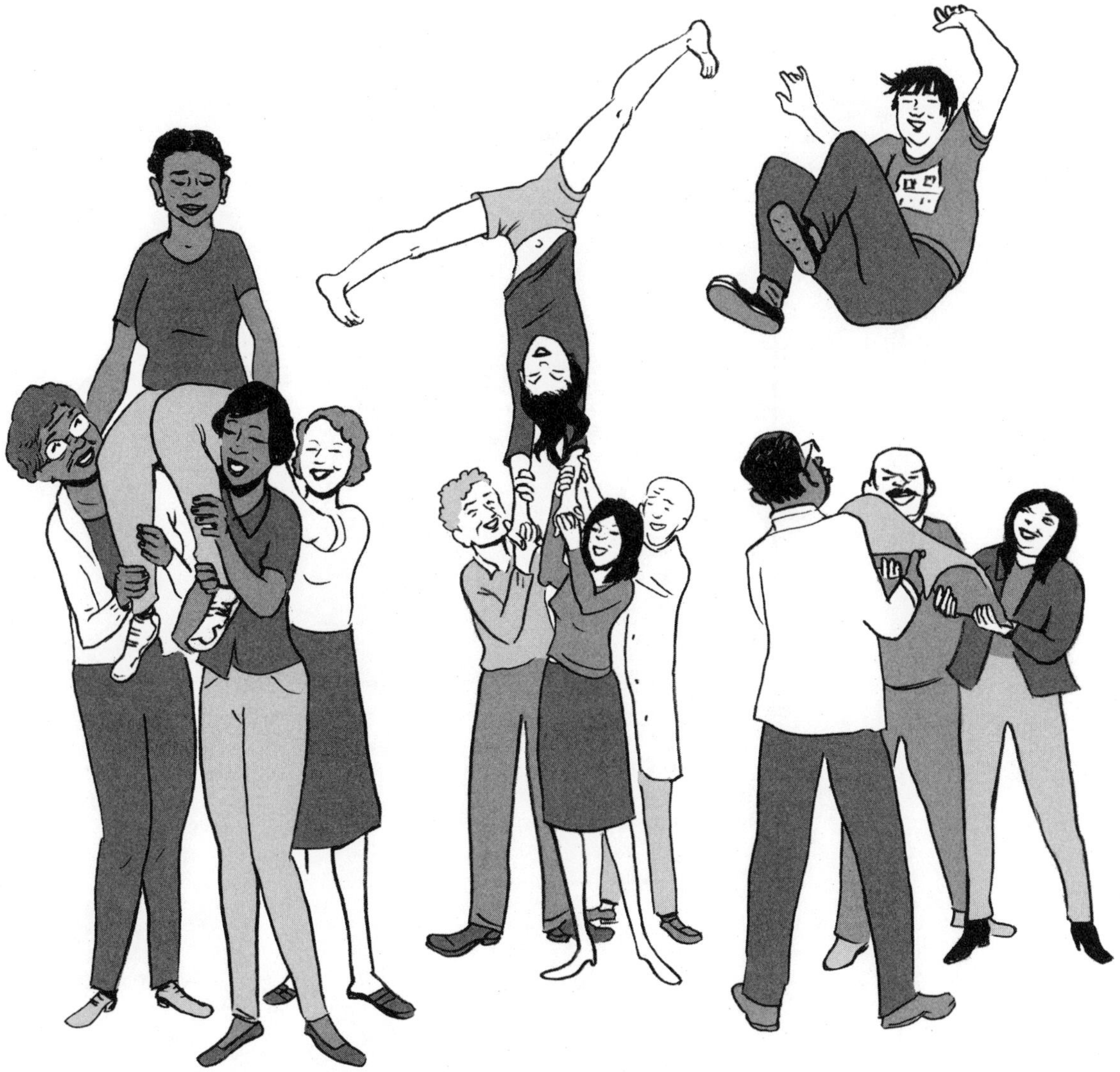

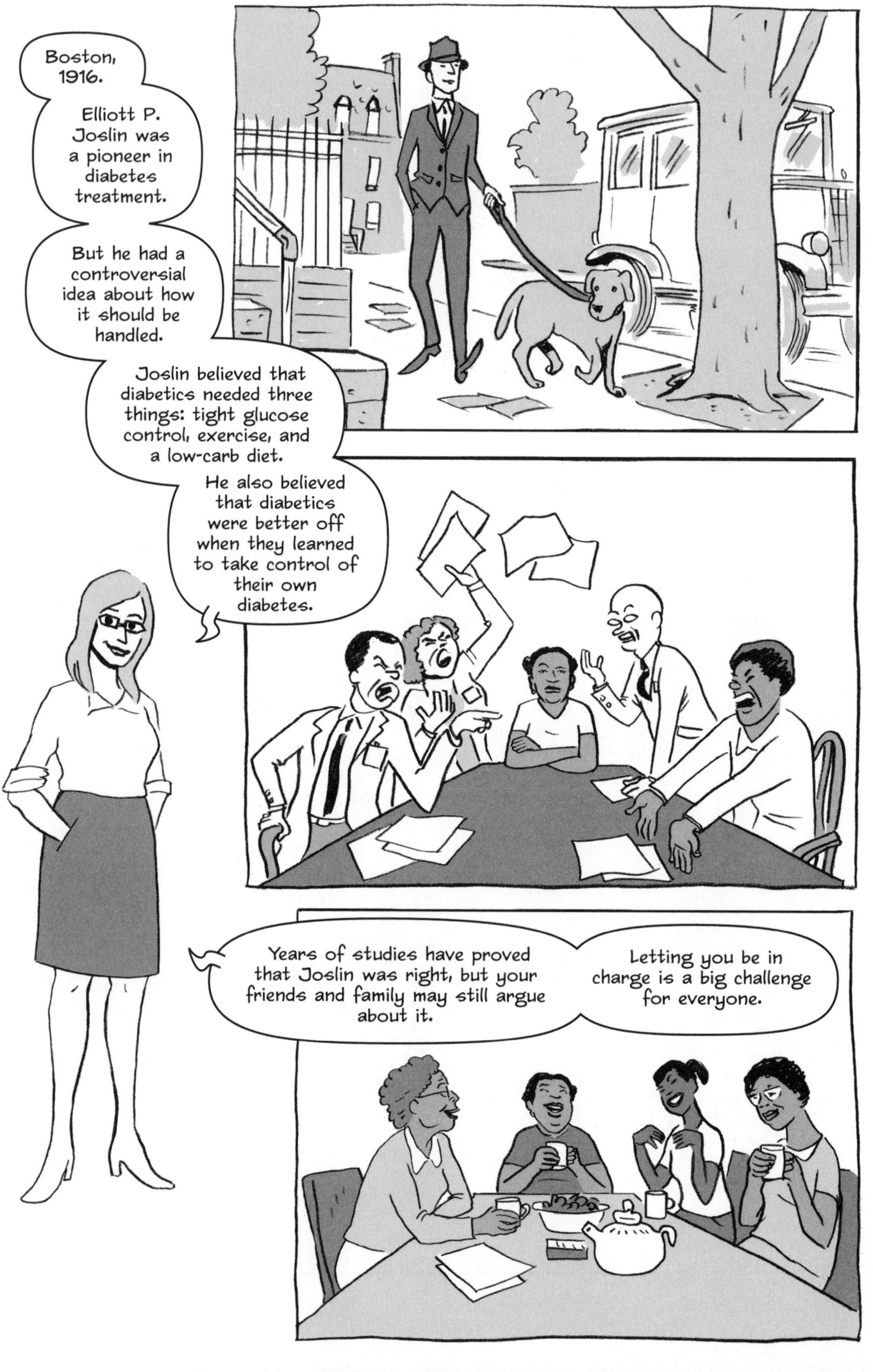
Boston, 1916.
Elliott P. Joslin was a pioneer in diabetes treatment.
But he had a controversial idea about how it should be handled.
Joslin believed that diabetics needed three things: tight glucose control, exercise, and a low-carb diet.
He also believed that diabetics were better off when they learned to take control of their own diabetes.
Years of studies have proved that Joslin was right, but your friends and family may still argue about it.
Letting you be in charge is a big challenge for everyone.

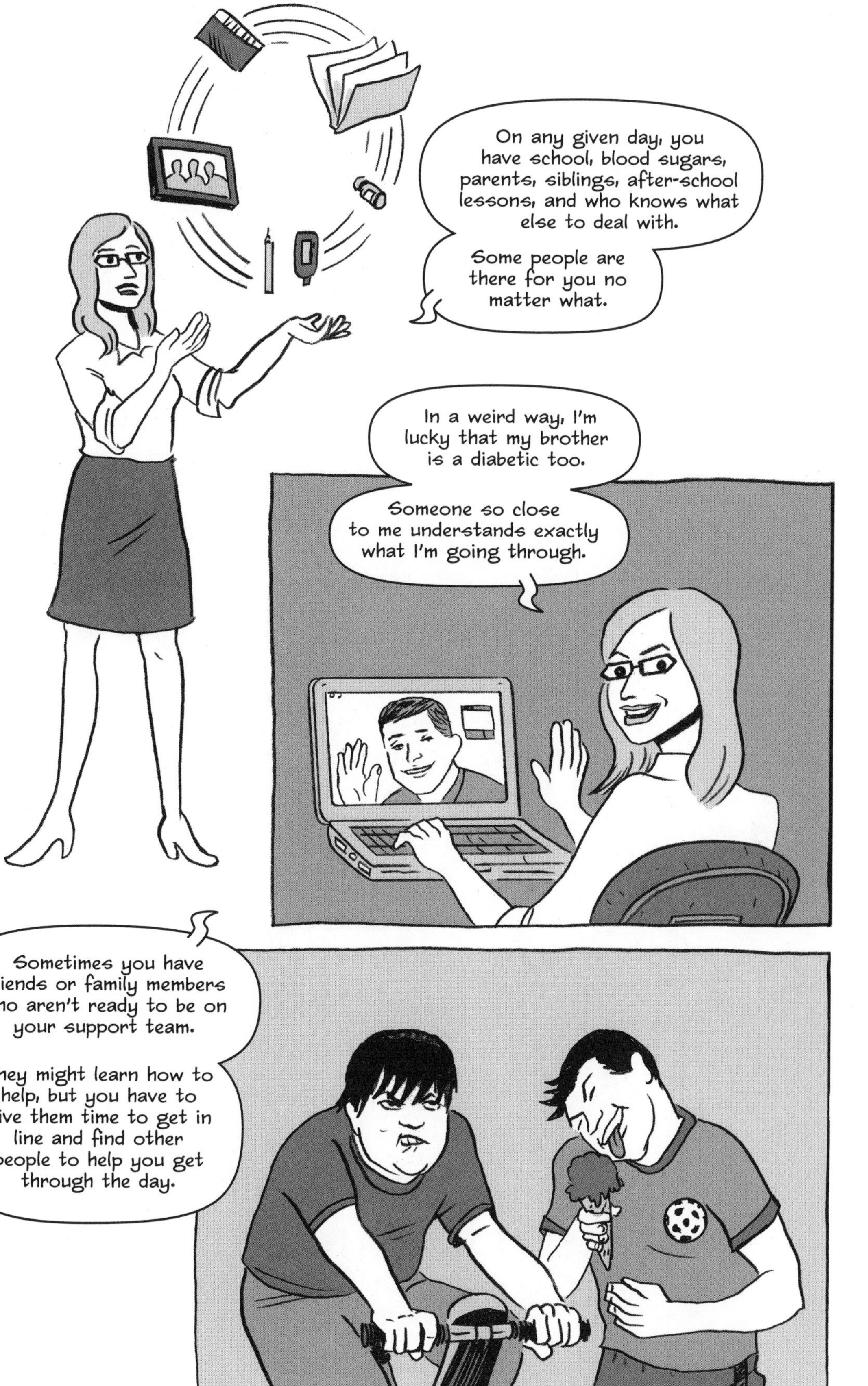
On any given day, you have school, blood sugars, parents, siblings, after-school lessons, and who knows what else to deal with.
Some people are there for you no matter what.
In a weird way, I'm lucky that my brother is a diabetic too.
Someone so close to me understands exactly what I'm going through.
Sometimes you have friends or family members who aren't ready to be on your support team.
They might learn how to help, but you have to give them time to get in line and find other people to help you get through the day.

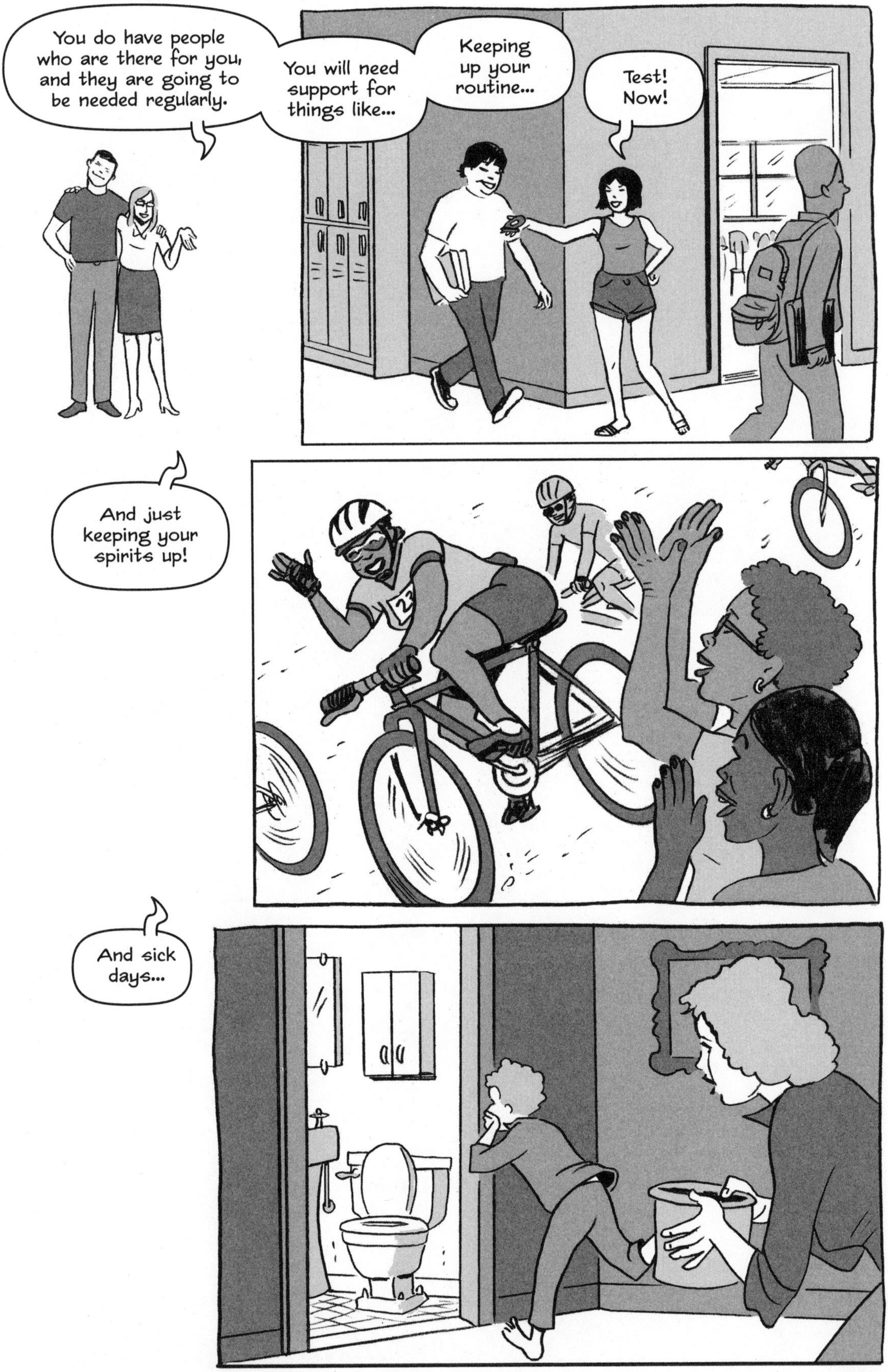
You do have people who are there for you, and they are going to be needed regularly.
You will need support for things like...
Keeping up your routine...
Test! Now!
And just keeping your spirits up!
And sick days...

SICK DAYS

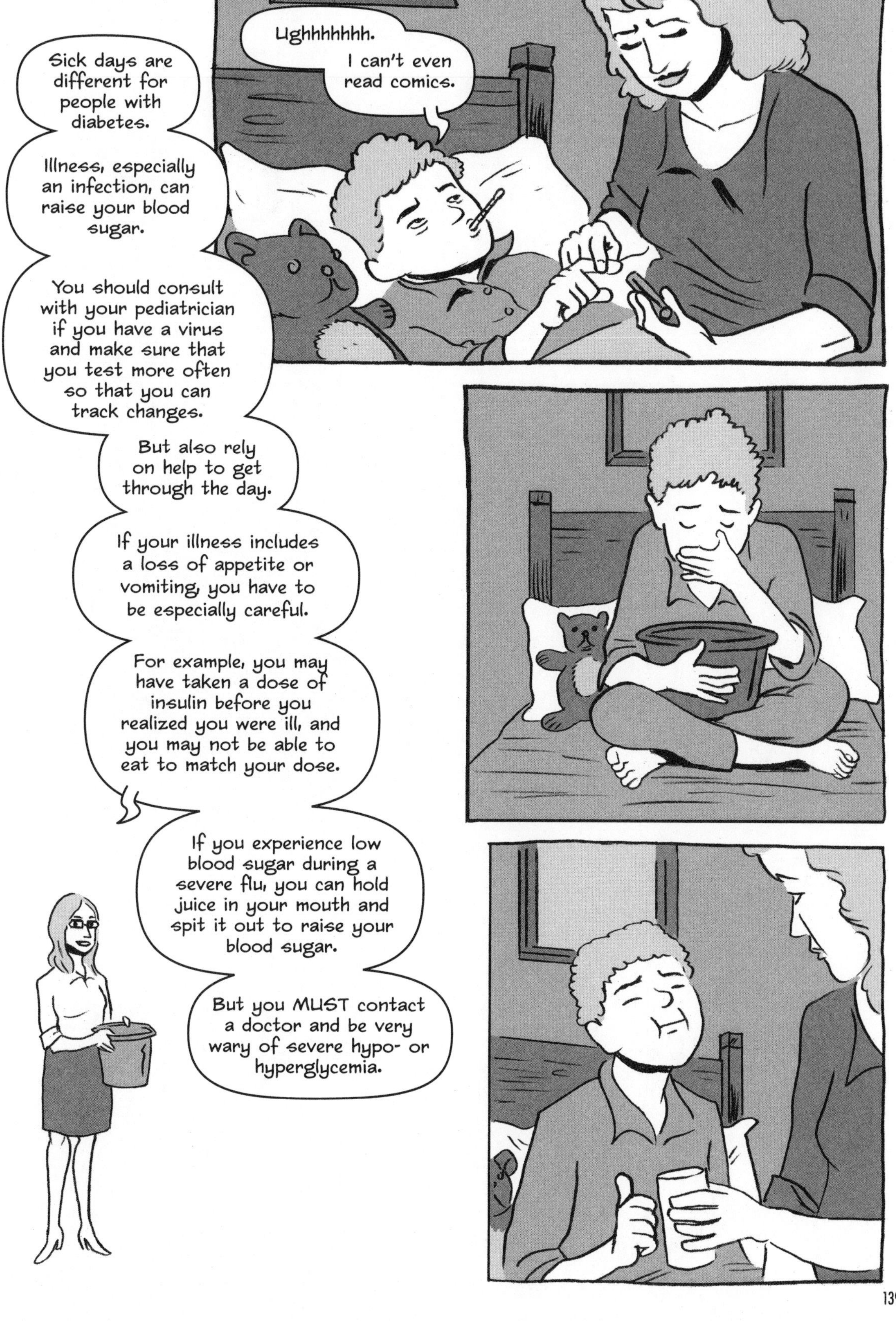

Sick days are different for people with diabetes.
Ughhhhhhh.
I can't even read comics.
Illness, especially an infection, can raise your blood sugar.
You should consult with your pediatrician if you have a virus and make sure that you test more often so that you can track changes.
But also rely on help to get through the day.
If your illness includes a loss of appetite or vomiting, you have to be especially careful.
For example, you may have taken a dose of insulin before you realized you were ill, and you may not be able to eat to match your dose.
If you experience low blood sugar during a severe flu, you can hold juice in your mouth and spit it out to raise your blood sugar.
But you MUST contact a doctor and be very wary of severe hypo- or hyperglycemia.

KEEPING UP YOUR ROUTINE

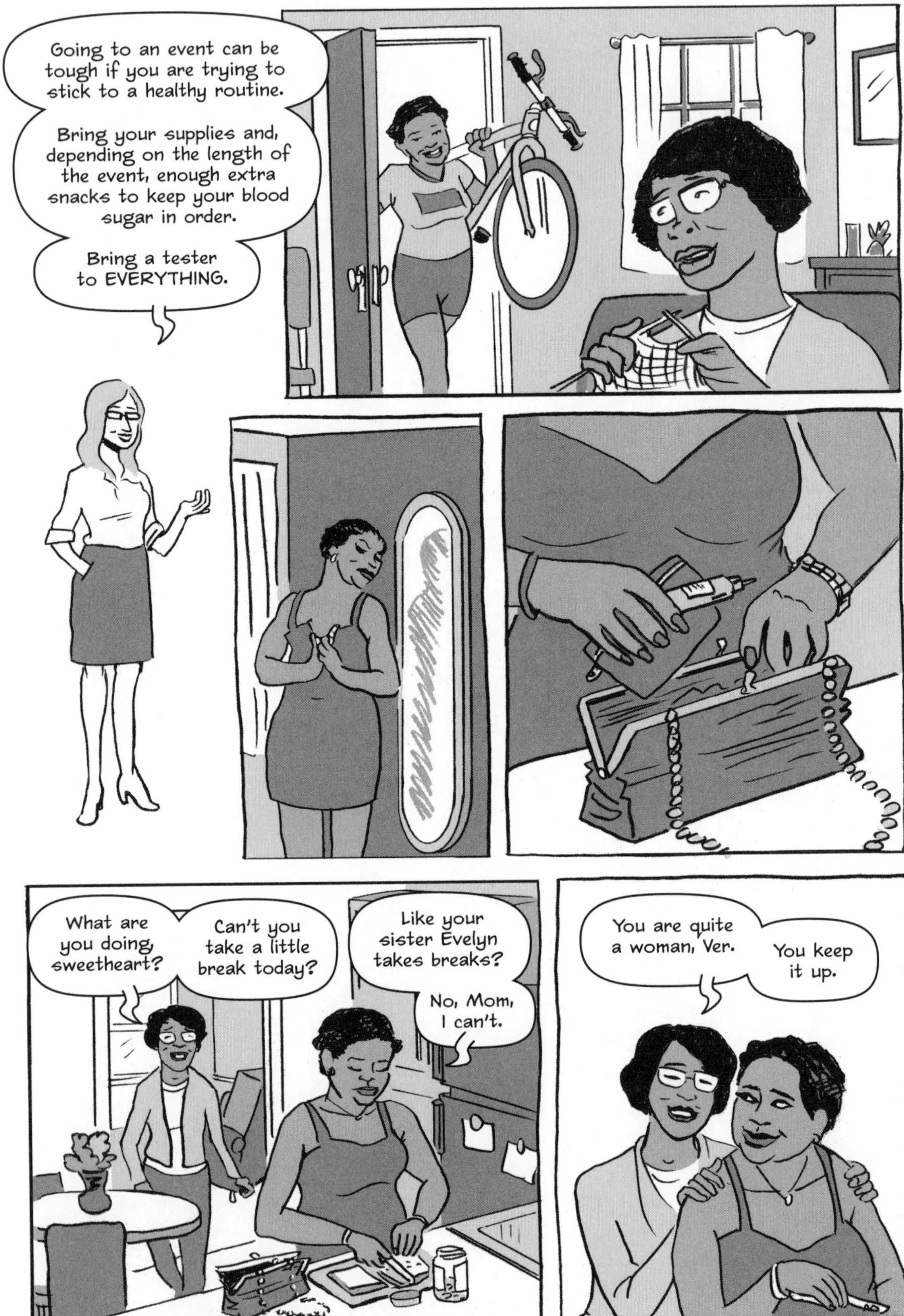
Going to an event can be tough if you are trying to stick to a healthy routine.
Bring your supplies and, depending on the length of the event, enough extra snacks to keep your blood sugar in order.
Bring a tester to EVERYTHING.
What are you doing, sweetheart?
Can't you take a little break today?
Like your sister Evelyn takes breaks?
No, Mom, I can't.
You are quite a woman, Ver.
You keep it up.

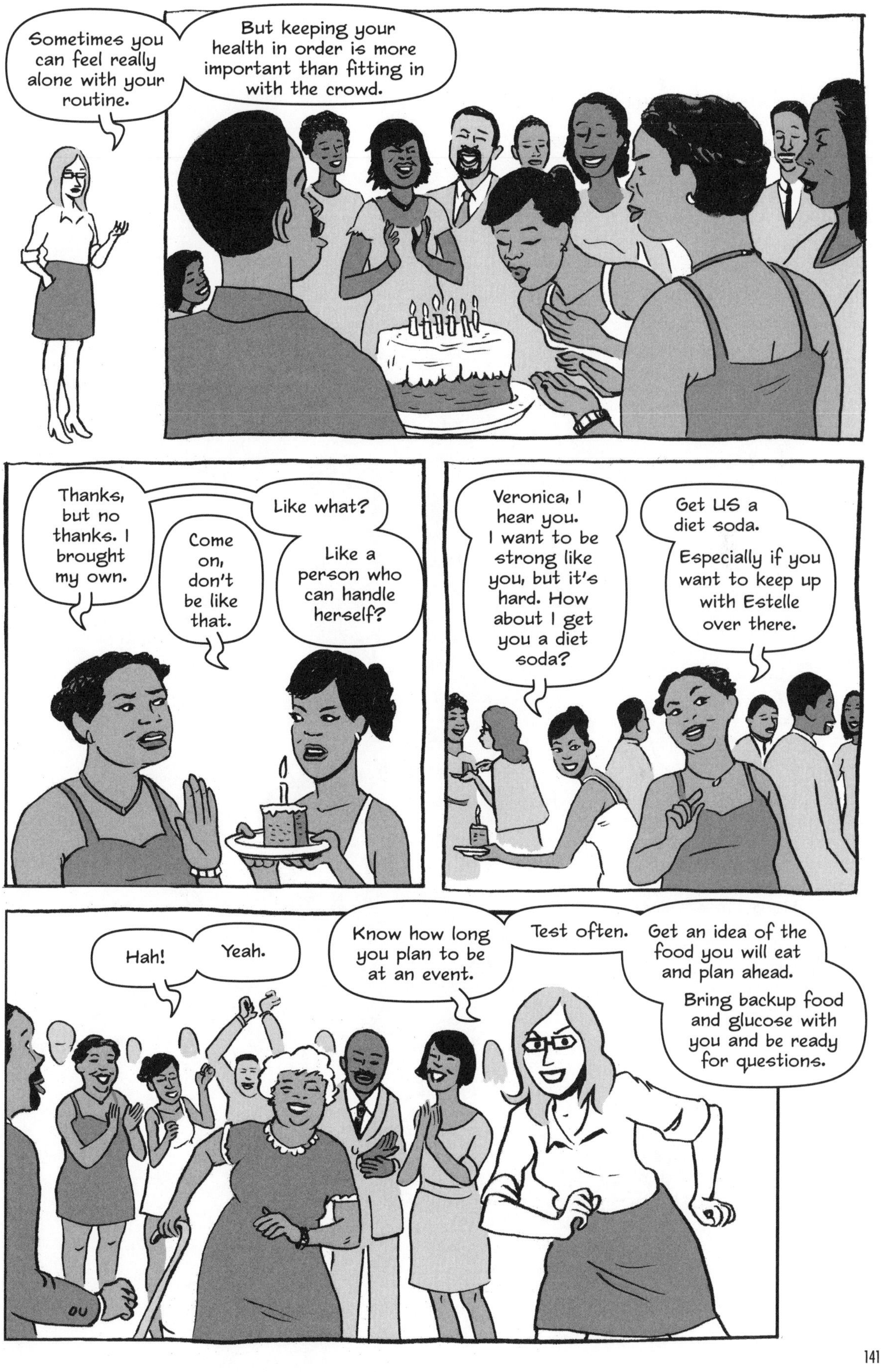

Sometimes you can feel really alone with your routine.
But keeping your health in order is more important than fitting in with the crowd.
Thanks, but no thanks. I brought my own.
Like what?
Come on, don't be like that.
Like a person who can handle herself?
Veronica, I hear you. I want to be strong like you, but it's hard. How about I get you a diet soda?
Get US a diet soda.
Especially if you want to keep up with Estelle over there.
Hah!
Yeah.
Know how long you plan to be at an event.
Test often.
Get an idea of the food you will eat and plan ahead.
Bring backup food and glucose with you and be ready for questions.

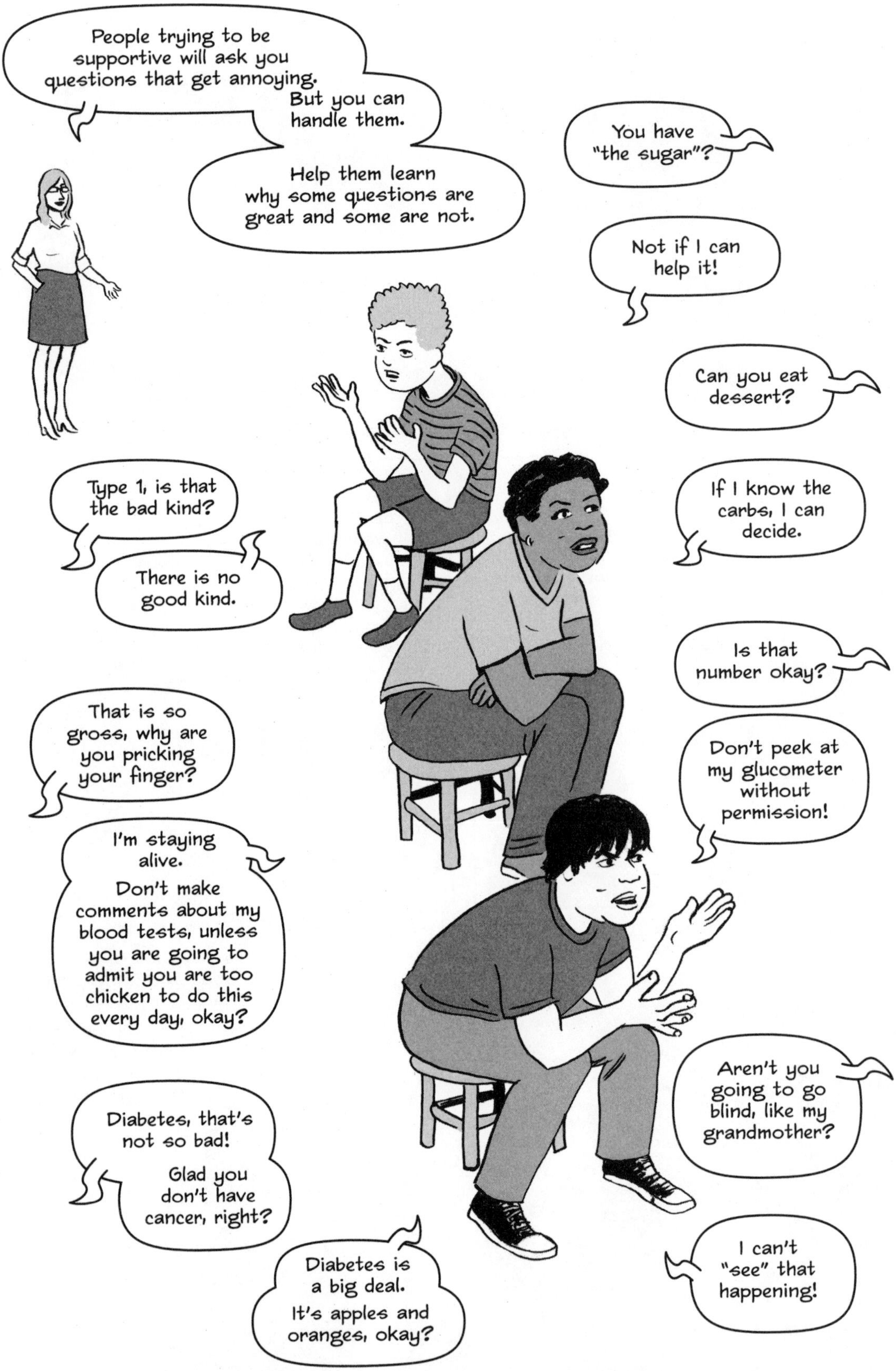
People trying to be supportive will ask you questions that get annoying.
But you can handle them.
Help them learn why some questions are great and some are not.
You have "the sugar"?
Not if I can help it!
Can you eat dessert?
If I know the carbs, I can decide.
Type 1, is that the bad kind?
There is no good kind.
Is that number okay?
Don't peek at my glucometer without permission!
That is so gross, why are you pricking your finger?
I'm staying alive.
Don't make comments about my blood tests, unless you are going to admit you are too chicken to do this every day, okay?
Aren't you going to go blind, like my grandmother?
I can't "see" that happening!
Diabetes, that's not so bad!
Glad you don't have cancer, right?
Diabetes is a big deal.
It's apples and oranges, okay?

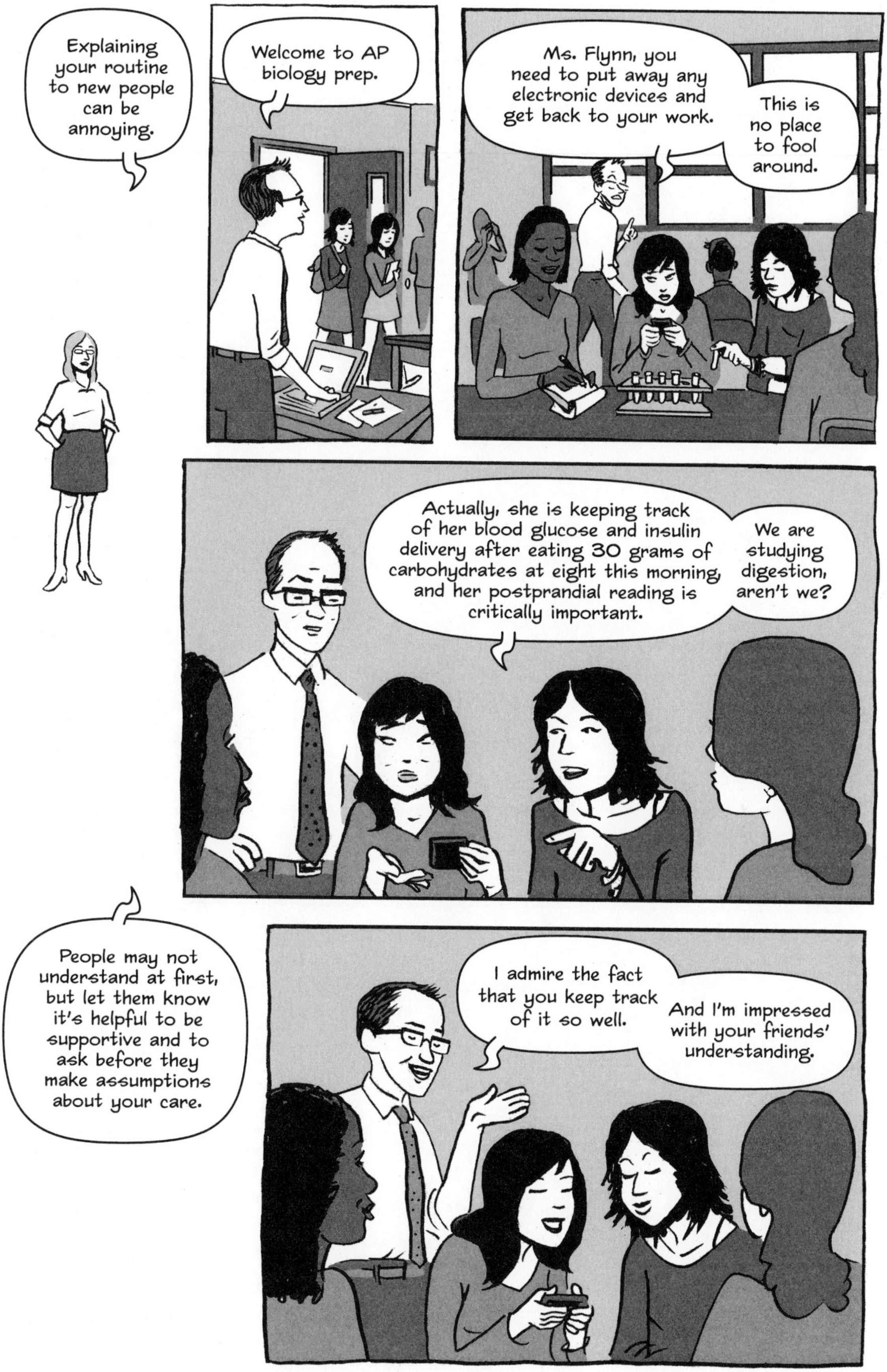
Explaining your routine to new people can be annoying.
Welcome to AP biology prep.
Ms. Flynn, you need to put away any electronic devices and get back to your work.
This is no place to fool around.
Actually, she is keeping track of her blood glucose and insulin delivery after eating 30 grams of carbohydrates at eight this morning, and her postprandial reading is critically important.
We are studying digestion, aren't we?
People may not understand at first, but let them know it's helpful to be supportive and to ask before they make assumptions about your care.
I admire the fact that you keep track of it so well.
And I'm impressed with your friends' understanding.

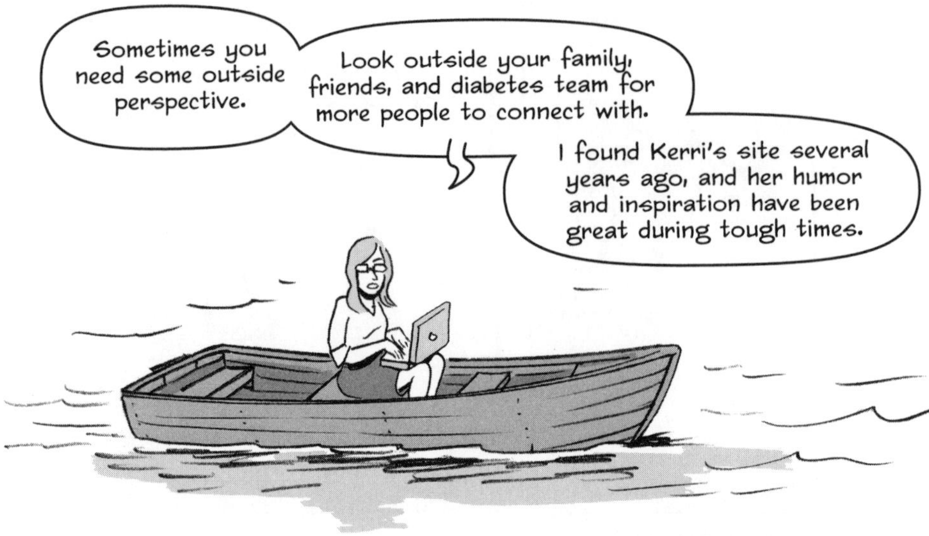
Sometimes you need some outside perspective.
Look outside your family, friends, and diabetes team for more people to connect with.
I found Kerri's site several years ago, and her humor and inspiration have been great during tough times.

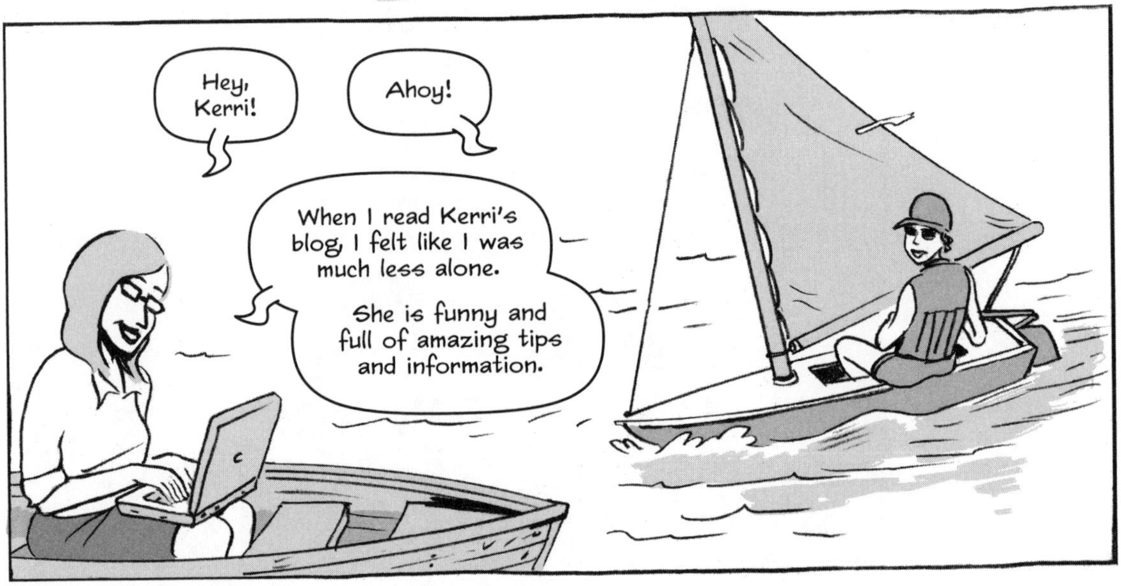
Hey, Kerri!
Ahoy!
When I read Kerri's blog, I felt like I was much less alone.
She is funny and full of amazing tips and information.

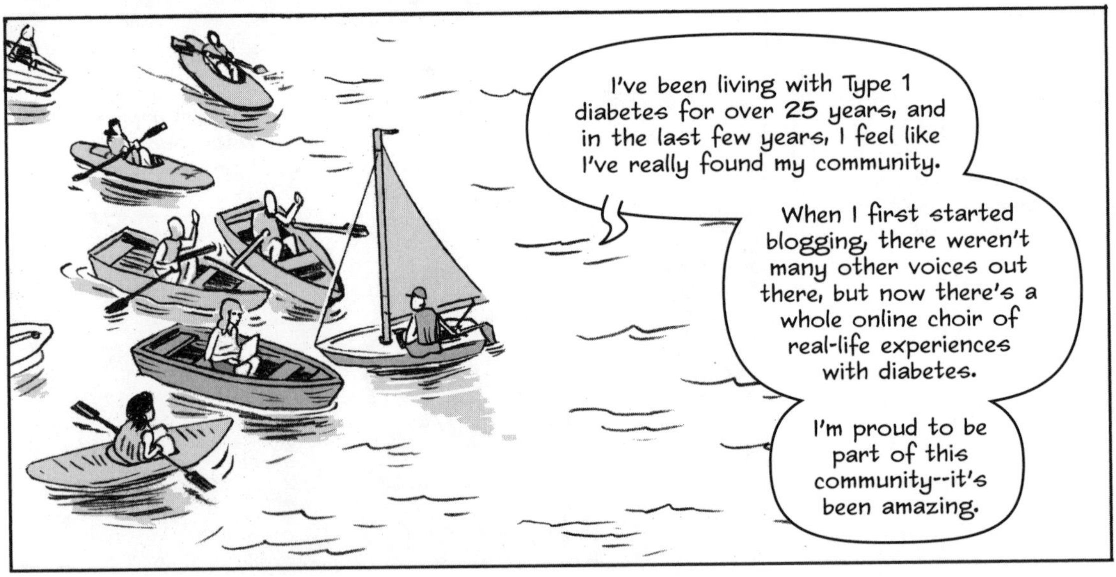
I've been living with Type 1 diabetes for over 25 years, and in the last few years, I feel like I've really found my community.
When I first started blogging, there weren't many other voices out there, but now there's a whole online choir of real-life experiences with diabetes.
I'm proud to be part of this community--it's been amazing.

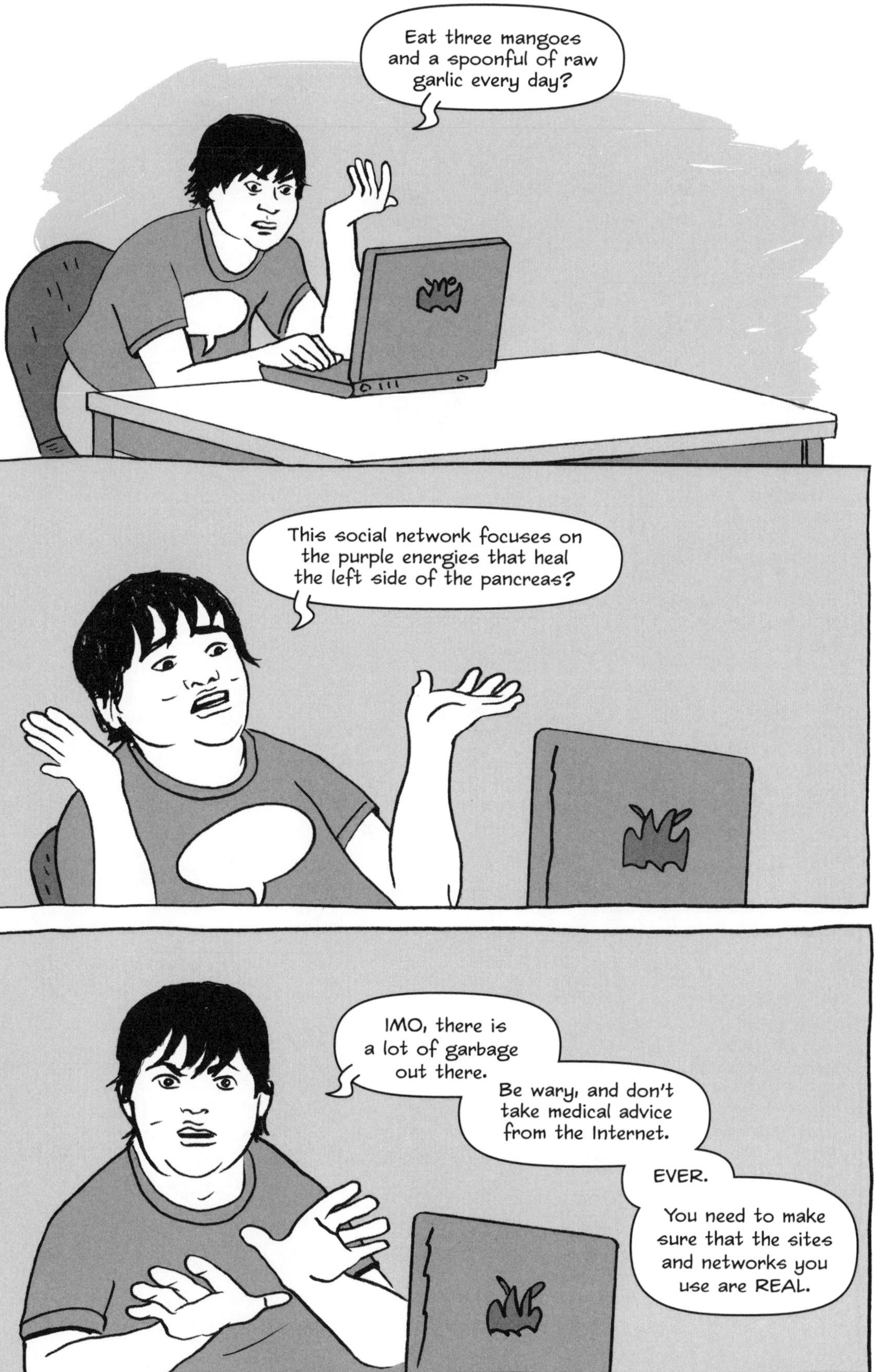
Eat three mangoes and a spoonful of raw garlic every day?
This social network focuses on the purple energies that heal the left side of the pancreas?
IMO, there is a lot of garbage out there.
Be wary, and don't take medical advice from the Internet.
EVER.
You need to make sure that the sites and networks you use are REAL.

MAKING A PUMP ARMBAND/LEG BAND

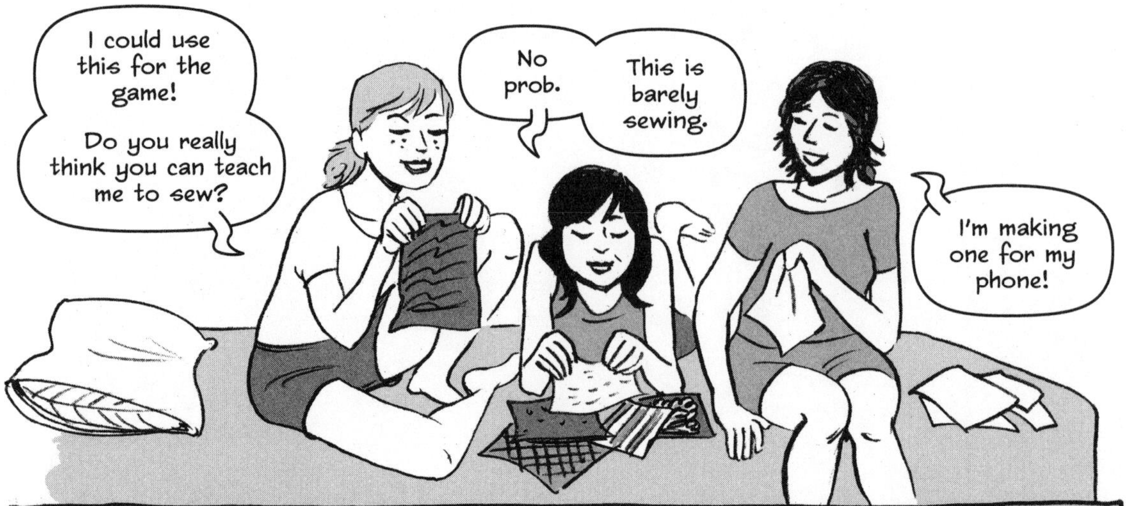
I could use this for the game!
Do you really think you can teach me to sew?
No prob.
This is barely sewing.
I'm making one for my phone!

Materials needed:

- Good scissors
- Needle and thread
- Strong elastic that is at least 2 inches wide and doesn't stretch out easily
- Material for the cover/outside (this works like underwear: subtle colors if you want to hide it, bold colors if you are showing it off)
- Lining material (not entirely necessary but looks nice)
- A fabric pencil
- Your insulin pump or other device

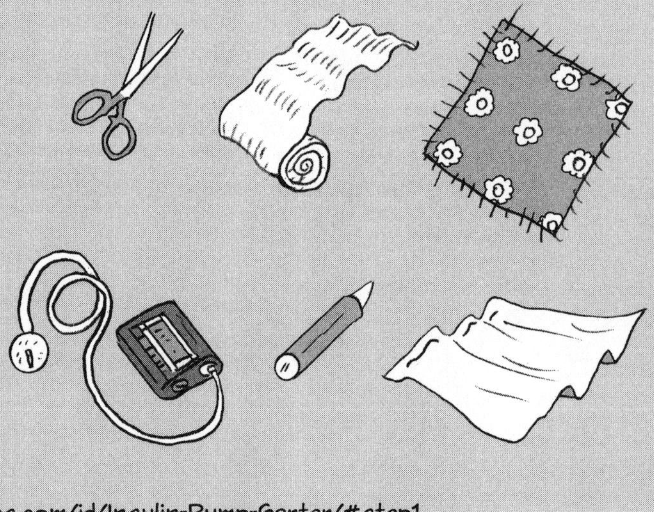

www.instructables.com/id/Insulin-Pump-Garter/#step1

1.

First, measure your pump's dimensions. You will need two pieces of fabric that will wrap around the pump/device as well as create a flap. Don't forget that it's 3-D; add some space horizontally. For my 3½-by-2-inch pump, I measured a rectangle that was 9 inches by 5 inches.

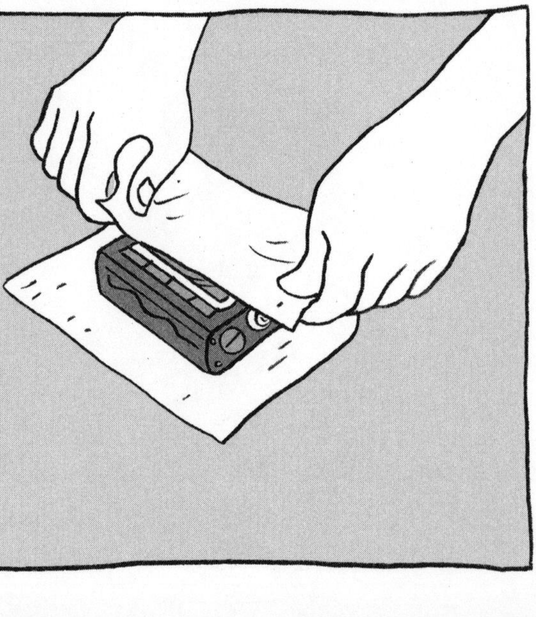

2.

Use this rectangle to cut out two pieces--a lining and a cover.

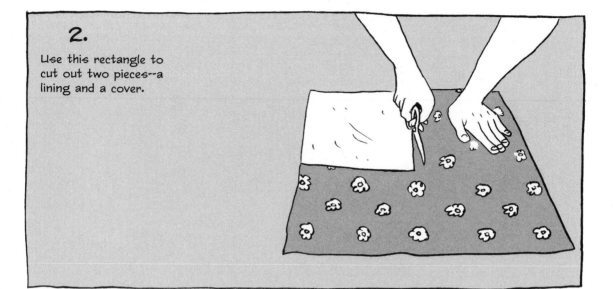

3.

On the top of your two pieces (wrong sides facing), hem along the edge. If your garter is going to be horizontal, hem the short side; vertical, the long side. If you are using lining material, remember that it should just roll over the edge of the cover, and be careful to sew the edges well so that they won't fray.

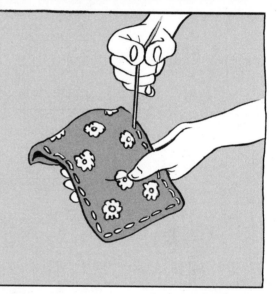

4.

Next, measure a piece of elastic around your chosen appendage. If it is your leg, decide where you want the pump to fall and measure the elastic so that it will be snug (not too tight) and have an extra inch or so on each side to be sewn into the garter. You can always trim the extra edge on the inside later on, but it is not easy to adjust the tightness of the elastic once you've sewn it. Therefore, take some time to feel it out before you cut and sew it.

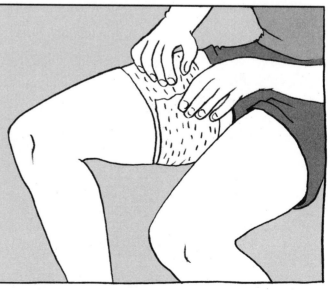

5.

Next, turn the case and lining inside out and fold it up around your actual pump to make sure you have the correct size. Once you've got that lined up, take the pump or device out and put your piece of elastic inside.

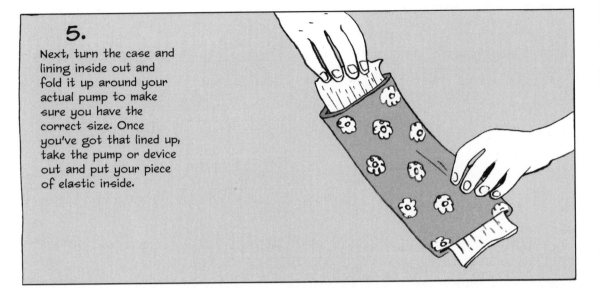

6.

Sew the sides several times so that the binding is strong. If you are hand stitching, use a backstitch. If you are machine stitching, go over it three or four times.

7.

That's it. Really, I'm not kidding--you're done. Check the seams, if you must. Decorate. Enjoy!

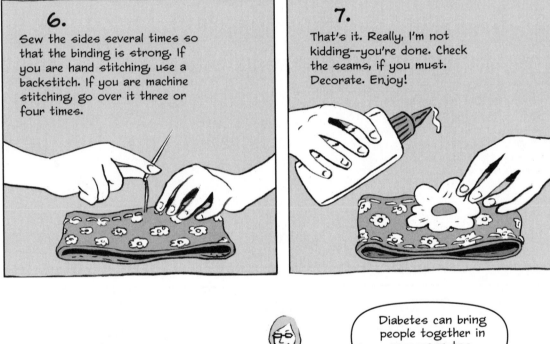

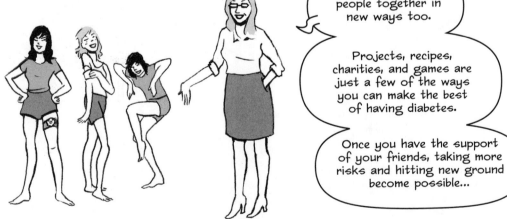

Diabetes can bring people together in new ways too.

Projects, recipes, charities, and games are just a few of the ways you can make the best of having diabetes.

Once you have the support of your friends, taking more risks and hitting new ground become possible...

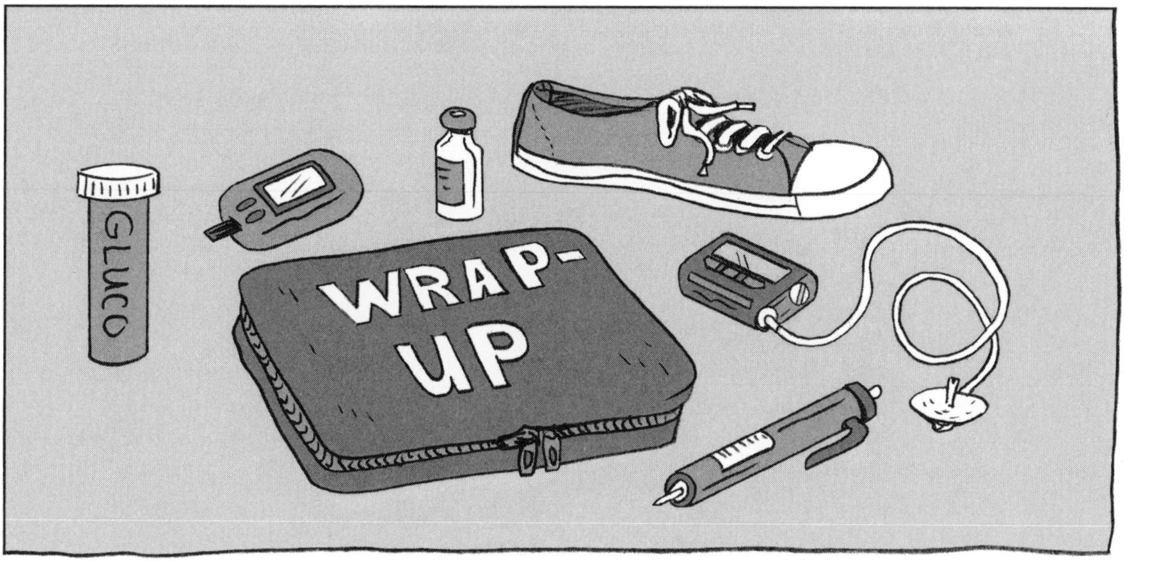
GLUCO
WRAP-UP

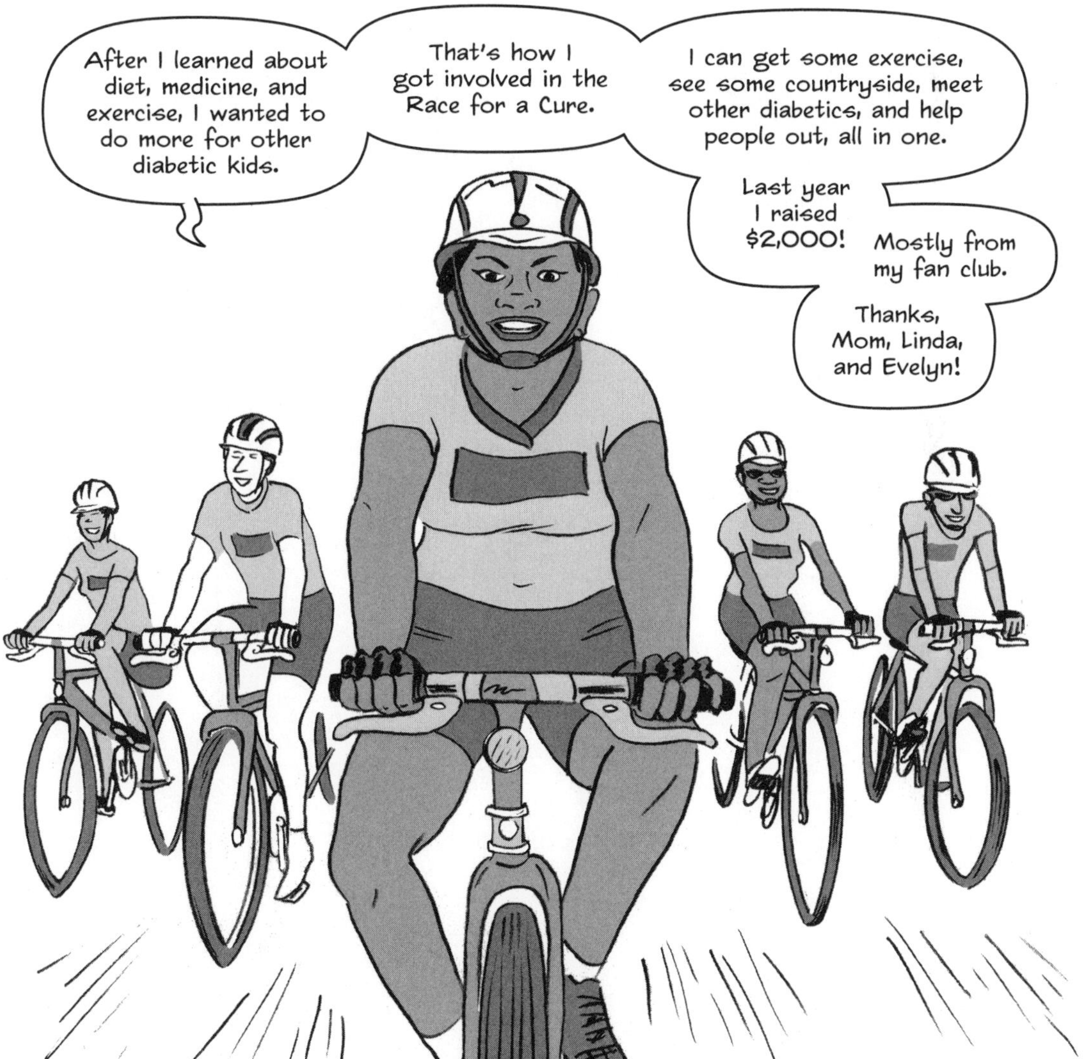
After I learned about diet, medicine, and exercise, I wanted to do more for other diabetic kids.
That's how I got involved in the Race for a Cure.
I can get some exercise, see some countryside, meet other diabetics, and help people out, all in one.
Last year I raised $2,000!
Mostly from my fan club.
Thanks, Mom, Linda, and Evelyn!

Diabetes is not easy, but it is not impossible.

Trust yourself by always testing and learning about diabetes and your body.

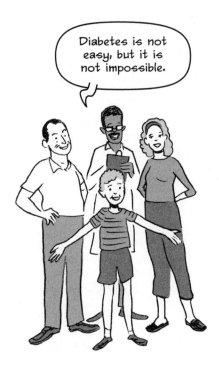

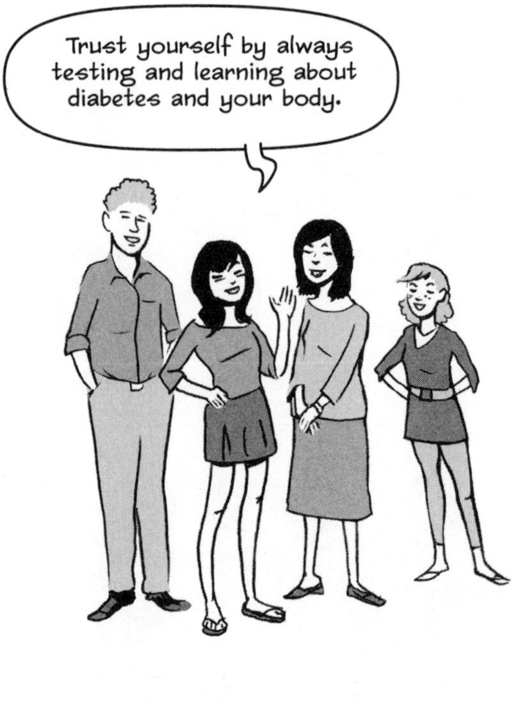

Don't follow old patterns, grow with what you know.

Believe that you can make a difference, that you really can have a healthy future.

You can do this!

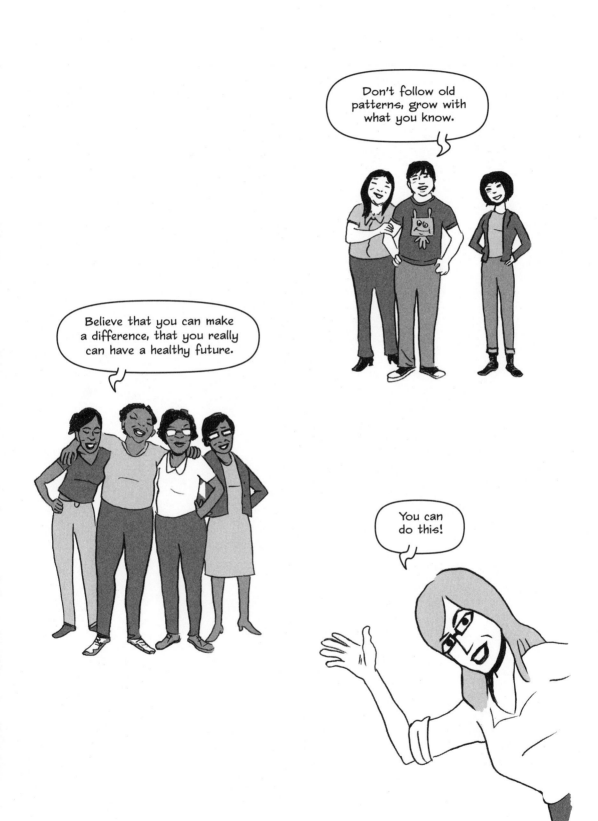

GLOSSARY

Basal rate: This is the amount of insulin you are getting constantly from an insulin pump or from a dose of long-acting insulin.

Bolus rate: This is the amount of insulin you take when you eat a full meal, a snack, or any food that contains carbohydrates. Rates vary for each patient, and a physician will recommend dosage to determine what basal/bolus rates you will use.

Cannula: *Cannula* means "little reed" in Latin. It is a flexible tube that is inserted into the body, right under the skin. Insulin flows through the cannula and is absorbed into your blood.

Carbohydrate: Any of a large group of organic compounds found in foods and living tissues including sugars, starch, and cellulose. Carbohydrates are broken down into smaller sugar molecules, which are critical to all body cells that use sugar as their primary energy source. The main form of this sugar is glucose.

Cardio or cardiovascular exercise: Important to your overall health. It will raise your heart rate and help increase blood circulation and circulatory health. Paired with strength training, it adds to your overall fitness and helps your body maintain healthy blood sugar levels.

Diabetic ketoacidosis: Most common in Type 1 diabetics with untreated high blood sugar. Ketoacidosis is detected when the liver breaks down fat and proteins and forms ketones in the blood. This happens when, due to a lack of insulin, the cells do not have glucose available for energy, and begin breaking down other molecules. The glucose normally available also remains in the bloodstream, rather than entering cells with the help of insulin.

Diabetic retinopathy: The damage to the small blood vessels of the retina caused by prolonged high blood sugars. It can lead to blindness. While this damage was more common in diabetics in the past, yearly checkups and careful attention to blood sugar control can prevent eye damage for most diabetics.

Endocrinologist: A person who studies and works in a branch of biology and medicine that deals with the glands and their secretions, called *hormones*. Endocrine glands are important in metabolism, respiration, excretion, movement, reproduction, and the nervous system. Endocrinologists help patients who have too much or too little function in their endocrine glands to maintain their health. For example, because the pancreas, an endocrine gland, does not release insulin in Type 1 diabetics, the endocrinologist helps the patient with insulin injections and regulating blood glucose.

Glucagon: This is a chemical that is normally released by your pancreas to help your liver add glucose to your bloodstream. During a severe hypoglycemic episode, you can inject glucagon into your body so that you can recover from severe hypoglycemia by causing the liver to initiate the release of glucose more quickly than you could digest glucose by eating it.

Glucometer, or glucose meter: A medical device that determines the concentration of glucose in the blood.

Glucose tablets: Fast-acting carbohydrates, sometimes in gel form, that provide diabetics with a quick increase in blood sugar, relieving them from hypoglycemia, or low blood sugar.

Glucose: A type of simple sugar that is an essential energy source to all living beings. It can be linked together in chains that make other sugars, starches, and carbohydrates.

Glycemic index: A system that ranks foods on a scale from 1 to 100 based on their effect on blood sugar levels. A high glycemic index indicates that a food type will cause blood glucose to rise quickly. A low glycemic index indicates that a food type will cause the blood sugar to rise more slowly, but rise nevertheless. Diabetics are encouraged to be cautious of foods with a high glycemic index.

Hemoglobin A1c (HA1c): This test checks the glucose attached to one form of hemoglobin in your blood, Hemoglobin A. It helps doctors determine your average blood sugar over a long period, roughly three months.

Hyperglycemia (or hyperglycæmia) or high blood sugar: The result of either a lack of insulin or insulin resistance following the consumption of carbohydrates. High blood sugar can damage delicate body tissue, so it should be detected early and treated.

Hypoglycemia: Lower than normal blood glucose. The term literally means "less sugar." Low blood sugar can be dangerous, and should be treated with fast-acting glucose immediately.

Insulin: A hormone that regulates the amount of glucose in the body's cells. It is produced by the pancreas, by the beta cells in the islets of Langerhans. The islets of Langerhans are regions of the pancreas that have endocrine cells including those that produce insulin. A lack of insulin, or insulin resistance, can result in diabetes.

Insulin Pump: This is a medical device that delivers insulin to the body through a subcutaneous tube inserted under the skin. Diabetics can deliver insulin that matches the carbohydrates they eat, as well as receive a "basal rate" (or constant flow) of needed insulin.

Ketones: A chemical compound found in the urine of diabetics with high blood sugar, when prolonged high blood sugars and a lack of insulin have caused the body to start breaking down fats and proteins. When ketones are in the blood, they indicate that treatment, usually with insulin, is necessary. You can test your urine for the presence of ketones.

Metabolism: The sum of chemical and physical reactions that a living being uses to maintain life and keep cell function going.

Neuropathy: The name used to describe damage to nerves of the peripheral nervous system that may be caused either by disease or trauma or as a side effect of illness.

Obesity: A word used to describe people who are overweight. Doctors determine how overweight you are based on your BMI, or body mass index, as well as other indicators of your fitness and health. Your physician determines your BMI using your height, weight, and age. If your BMI is above average, you are considered to be obese. While other factors, such as your activity level, are also used to determine your ideal weight, those who are obese or in danger of becoming obese are at a higher risk for Type 2 diabetes.

Ophthalmologist: A specialist in medical and surgical eye problems. An ophthalmologist performs annual eye exams for diabetic patients that include testing the retina for damage due to high blood sugar.

Oral Medication: Refers to any number of oral medications that can help Type 2 diabetics digest carbohydrates. Each medication is designed to do a different job for Type 2 diabetics. Some oral medications help your pancreas release more insulin, while others help the insulin in your body access cells more effectively.

Pancreas: An endocrine and digestive gland, below the stomach, that releases enzymes and hormones into the small intestine. Inside the tissue of the pancreas are the islets of Langerhans, which create and secrete insulin and glucagon.

Reservoir: This is where the liquid insulin is kept in an insulin "pump" in a small cylindrical tube. The pump itself attaches to the reservoir and delivers measured amounts of insulin through a programmed pump.

LIST OF SOURCES

American Diabetes Association. American Diabetes Association website. Accessed July 2011. www.diabetes.org.

_____. *Complete Guide to Diabetes: The Ultimate Home Reference from the Diabetes Experts.* 5th ed. Alexandria, VA: American Diabetes Association, 2011.

Behavioral Diabetes Institute. Behavioral Diabetes Institute website. Accessed December 2010. www.behavioraldiabetesinstitute.org.

Colberg, Sheri. *The Diabetes Athlete.* Champaign, IL: Human Kinetics, 2001.

Dean, Laura, MD, and Johanna McEntyre, PhD. *The Genetic Landscape of Diabetes.* Bethesda, MD: National Center for Biotechnology Information, 2004. www.ncbi.nlm.nih.gov.

Diabetes Digital Media Ltd. Diabetes.co.uk. Accessed March 6, 2011. www.diabetes.co.uk.

dLife Foundation. dLife website. Accessed March 2011. www.dlife.com.

Greenberg, Riva. *50 Diabetes Myths That Can Ruin Your Life: And the 50 Diabetes Truths That Can Save It.* Philadelphia: Da Capo Press, 2009.

International Diabetes Federation. "Diabetes Atlas." Accessed January 6, 2012. www.idf.org /diabetesatlas.

JDRF. JDRF website. www.jdrf.org.

Joslin Diabetes Center. "Diabetes Information." Accessed January 2011. www.joslin.org/diabetes _information.html.

Naomi Berrie Diabetes Center. The Naomi Berrie Diabetes Center website. Accessed May 2012. www.nbdiabetes.org.

Nobel Media AB. "Dorothy Crowfoot Hodgkin – Biographical." Accessed February 2011. www.nobelprize.org/nobel_prizes/chemistry /laureates/1964/hodgkin-bio.html.

_____. "Frederick G. Banting – Biographical." Accessed February 2011. www.nobelprize.org /nobel_prizes/medicine/laureates/1923/banting -bio.html.

Polonsky, William. *Diabetes Burnout: What to Do When You Can't Take It Anymore.* Alexandria, VA: American Diabetes Association, 1999.

Soltész, Gyula. "Diabetes in Children: Changing Trends in an Emerging Epidemic." *Diabetes Voice* 52 (May 2007): 13–15. Accessed March 13, 2011. www.idf.org/diabetesvoice/files.attachments /article_499_en.pdf.

Vertical Health, LLC. EndocrineWeb. Accessed January 2011. www.endocrineweb.com.

World Diabetes Foundation. World Diabetes Foundation website. Accessed March 19, 2011. www.worlddiabetesfoundation.org.

World Health Organization. "Diabetes." Accessed November 10, 2011. www.who.int/mediacentre /factsheets/fs312/en/index.html.

ACKNOWLEDGMENTS

Many thanks to Amanda Moon, Thomas LeBien, Bob Mecoy, Dean Haspiel, and Daniel Gerstle for their guidance and wise counsel. We are indebted to Dr. Robin Goland of the Naomi Berrie Diabetes Center for providing valuable feedback on the text, and to Dr. Iven Young for providing essential medical advice that has informed my understanding of diabetes. Dr. William Polonsky's writing about the emotional experience of being a diabetic has been a very positive influence, and online writing by Mr. Divabetic, Max Szadek, and Kerri Morrone Sparling of Six Until Me have been a source of motivation and solace.

We would like to thank all the members of our family who have supported Kim in becoming a healthy Type 1 diabetic, and without whom writing this book would not have been possible: Chris Chaloner; Sabina and Ramona Bertozzi; Ted Chaloner; Lydia Walshin; Gretchen, Kurt, and Charlie Haas; and all the Bertozzis—Judith, Edward, Julia, Vanessa, and Allegra. Finally, I would like to thank Dean Kamen, Judith Ambrosini, Jean-Robert Andre, Wendy Small, and Carol Collet for their encouragement and inspiration, and the people at the JDRF for their work in finding a cure.

One of the most empowering things you can do for yourself or your family member is to help support diabetics worldwide by contributing to organizations working toward a cure. We personally recommend the Juvenile Diabetes Research Foundation (www.jdrf.org) and the American Diabetes Association (www.diabetes.org).

A NOTE ABOUT THE AUTHOR

Kim Chaloner is an award-winning middle school science teacher and the dean of community life at an independent private school in Manhattan, where she organizes programs in sustainability, biology, multicultural education, and community service. She was diagnosed with Type 1 diabetes at age sixteen.

A NOTE ABOUT THE ILLUSTRATOR

Nick Bertozzi is an award-winning illustrator and the author of *The Salon* and *Lewis & Clark*. He is the recipient of multiple Harvey Awards and Ignatz Awards, as well as a Xeric Grant. He teaches cartooning at the School of Visual Arts in New York City. He has also taught at the Rhode Island School of Design and the Center for Cartoon Studies in White River Junction, Vermont.

Kim and Nick live with their two daughters in Jackson Heights, New York.